Pain Management

Pain Management

Fact versus Fiction

Myrna Chandler Goldstein and
Mark A. Goldstein, MD

GREENWOOD™

An Imprint of ABC-CLIO, LLC
Santa Barbara, California • Denver, Colorado

This book discusses treatments (including types of medication and mental health therapies), diagnostic tests for various symptoms and mental health disorders, and organizations. The authors have made every effort to present accurate and up-to-date information. However, the information in this book is not intended to recommend or endorse particular treatments or organizations, or substitute for the care or medical advice of a qualified health professional, or be used to alter any medical therapy without a medical doctor's advice. Specific situations may require specific therapeutic approaches not included in this book. For those reasons, we recommend that readers follow the advice of qualified health care professionals directly involved in their care. Readers who suspect they may have specific medical problems should consult a physician about any suggestions made in this book.

Library of Congress Cataloging-in-Publication Data

Names: Goldstein, Myrna Chandler, 1948- author. | Goldstein, Mark A. (Mark Allan), 1947- author.
Title: Pain management : fact versus fiction / Myrna Chandler Goldstein and Mark A. Goldstein, MD.
Description: First edition. | Santa Barbara, California : Greenwood, an Imprint of ABC-CLIO, LLC, [2022] | Includes bibliographical references and index.
Identifiers: LCCN 2022008184 | ISBN 9781440876950 (print ; acid-free paper) | ISBN 9781440876967 (ebook)
Subjects: LCSH: Pain—Treatment. | BISAC: HEALTH & FITNESS / Pain Management | HEALTH & FITNESS / Alternative Therapies
Classification: LCC RB127 .G656 2022 | DDC 616/.0472—dc23/eng/20220315
LC record available at https://lccn.loc.gov/2022008184

ISBN: 978-1-4408-7695-0 (print)
978-1-4408-7696-7 (ebook)

26 25 24 23 22 1 2 3 4 5

This book is also available as an eBook.

Greenwood
An Imprint of ABC-CLIO, LLC

ABC-CLIO, LLC
147 Castilian Drive
Santa Barbara, California 93117
www.abc-clio.com

This book is printed on acid-free paper ∞
Manufactured in the United States of America

We dedicate this book with love to our five grandchildren:

Aidan Zev Goldstein
Payton Maeve Goldstein
Milo Adlai Kamras
Erin Abigail Goldstein
Zoe "Scout" Eames Kamras

Contents

Acknowledgments

Once again, we would like to thank our editor, Maxine Taylor, who has edited several of our more recent books. Over the years that we have worked together, Maxine has repeatedly offered excellent suggestions and advice.

Introduction: A Primer on Pain

WHAT EXACTLY IS PAIN?

Pain is an uncomfortable feeling anywhere in the body; it is a signal to the body that something is wrong and that tissues, such as bones, soft tissues, and organs, have been damaged. Part of the body's defense mechanism, pain allows the body to react and attempt to prevent further tissue damage. Pain is experienced when special nerves, known as nociceptors, detect tissue damage and send signals about the damage along the spinal cord to the brain. Nociceptors detect extremes in temperature and pressure and injury-causing chemicals and convert these stimuli into long-ranging electrical signals that are relayed to higher brain cells. Then, the brain quickly decides what to do.

But sometimes the signal does not need to go all the way to the brain. For example, if a person touches an extremely cold object, the message rapidly travels to the spinal cord, and, even before the message reaches the brain, the person will automatically pull away from the object. Obviously, the same response occurs with a hot object. It is important to note that people experience pain in different ways; whereas some people tolerate intense pain, others have difficulty dealing with even low levels of pain. People may have the same diagnosis but experience the related pain in vastly varying ways. Their bodies modulate pain in different ways; the very structure of the brain differs.

Though they are often treated as the same entity, pain threshold and pain tolerance are different. Pain threshold defines the level at which people experience a stimulus as painful. Pain tolerance is how much pain a person can manage. Because they process pain quickly, people with chronic pain may have a lower pain threshold. But because they are used to living with chronic pain, they have a higher pain tolerance.

Though the brain releases chemicals, such as dopamine, that help counter the unpleasantness of pain, pain appears in many different forms. Depending on the underlying cause, pain may pinch, throb, ache, or stab. Although it may be uncomfortable, most people function with their pain, especially mild pain. However, in many instances, pain may be debilitating and seriously disrupt life.

Frequently, pain occurs with other physical symptoms such as nausea, weakness, fatigue, and dizziness, as well as emotional symptoms such as irritability, depression, anxiety, mood changes, and anger. It is not uncommon for pain and these associated problems to take a toll on relationships with family, friends, and coworkers.

Types of Pain

There are two main types of pain: acute and chronic. Acute pain generally appears suddenly, and it may be quite profound. But, it lasts for a relatively brief period of time. Acute pain tends to be caused by damage to bone, skin, muscle, or organ tissue. Common causes of acute pain include broken bones, surgery, dental work, labor and childbirth, cuts, and burns. Treating the injury helps to resolve the pain. There are three types of acute pain. Somatic pain is superficial pain that is felt on the skin or the soft tissues below the skin; visceral pain is in the internal organs and linings of the cavities of the body; and referred pain is pain at a different location than the original pain. Thus, a person may have a neck injury but feel intense pain down both arms.

Chronic pain, which ranges from mild to severe, continues for an indeterminate period of time, usually between three and six months—long after the initial injury has healed. However, chronic pain may also be the result of gradual tissue degeneration, as with the pain associated with osteoarthritis, or it may be the result of damage to the nociceptors. Chronic pain may occur intermittently, as with migraines; it may be localized, or it may spread throughout the body. Chronic pain is more resistant to medical treatment than acute pain, and although it may be the consequence of damaged tissue, it often is a result of nerve damage. Because they are dealing with ongoing pain, people with chronic pain are at increased risk for psychological problems, such as depression and anxiety. And these psychological concerns may increase the levels of pain. Other symptoms associated with chronic pain include tense muscles, lack of energy, and limited mobility. Millions of adults in the United States deal with chronic pain associated with medical problems, such as low back pain, arthritis, fibromyalgia, and headaches.

The distinction between acute and chronic pain is important. Acute pain serves as an alarm; something is wrong and needs to be addressed immediately. Conversely, chronic pain has no positive function, and it persists far too long, often radiating to different parts of the body, taking a long-term physical and emotional toll.

In addition to describing pain as either acute or chronic, there are a few other pain designations. Neuropathic pain, which is pain that is shooting, burning, tingling or numbing, is frequently chronic. Often, it is caused by nerve damage or a nervous system that is not functioning properly. This may be associated with alcoholism, chemotherapy, diabetes, facial nerve problems, HIV or AIDS infection, multiple myeloma, multiple sclerosis, nerve or spinal cord compression, shingles, spine surgery, syphilis, or thyroid problems. Phantom limb syndrome is an example of neuropathic pain. With this condition, people still feel pain associated with an arm or leg that had been removed because of illness or injury. Even though the arm or leg is gone, the brain continues to receive pain messages from the misfiring nerves. At present, the exact cause of phantom pain in unclear. Still, it appears to come from the spinal cord and brain. Imaging tests have shown that during phantom pain, sections of the brain that were previously connected to the amputated limb show activity. Other factors may contribute to this pain such as mixed signals from the brain, damaged nerve endings, scar tissue, tangled sensory wires, and remapping of the body's sensory circuitry. People who had pain in the limb before amputation are likely to have it after amputation.

With central pain syndrome, another type of pain, there is damage or dysfunction to the central nervous system, which includes the brain, brainstem, and spinal cord. This syndrome may be triggered by several medical problems such as tumors, brain or spinal cord trauma, stroke, multiple sclerosis, epilepsy, or Parkinson's disease. Central pain syndrome may affect nearly the entire body or may be isolated to specific areas. And while the amount of pain varies from person to person, the pain tends to be constant, and it becomes more intense with cold temperatures, touch, movement, and emotional experiences. Burning is the most common type of pain in people with central pain syndrome. Other associated pains include pins and needles, pressing, lacerating, aching pain, and brief bursts of sharp pain. The symptoms tend to be more severe in the extremities.

Pain may also be classified by the type of tissue that is involved or the part of the body that is affected. Examples of these are joint pain, muscular pain, chest pain, or back pain.

Prevalence of Pain

According to an article published in 2018 in the *MMWR Morbidity and Mortality Weekly Report*, chronic pain, which is one of the most common reasons that people seek medical care, has been linked to other medical problems such as restrictions in mobility and daily living, dependence on opioids, anxiety, depression, poor perceived health, and reduced quality of life. Hence, it is important to know the prevalence of chronic pain. Yet, population estimates of adults in the United States have ranged from 11 to 40 percent, and there has been a good deal of variation in population subgroups. As a result, the Centers for Disease Control and Prevention (CDC) decided to analyze the 2016 National Health Interview Survey, a cross-sectional, in-person, household health survey, for incidence of chronic pain and high-impact chronic pain. Chronic pain was defined as pain on most days or every day during the past six months; high-impact chronic pain was defined as chronic pain that limited life or work activities on most days or every day during the past six months. The survey included pain-related questions: "In the past six months, how often have you had pain? Would you say never, some days, most days, or every day?" and "Over the past six months, how often did pain limit your life or work activities? Would you say never, some days, most days, or every day?"

The researchers learned that 20.4 percent of the adults in the United States, or 50 million adults, had chronic pain, and 8 percent of the adults, or 19.6 million adults, had high-impact chronic pain. Women and older adults were more likely to have chronic pain and high-impact chronic pain, as were previously but not currently employed adults, adults with less than a high school education, adults living in poverty, adults with public health insurance, and rural residents. Among adults under the age of 65 years, higher prevalence of chronic pain and high-impact pain was observed among those with public health-care coverage, such as Medicaid, than among those with private insurance or those who were uninsured. Among adults 65 years or older, people with both Medicare and Medicaid had higher rates of chronic pain and high-impact chronic pain than did adults with other types of coverage. The prevalence of chronic pain and high-impact chronic pain was lower among adults with a bachelor's degree or higher education. Non-Hispanic white adults had a significantly higher prevalence of chronic pain compared with all other racial and ethnic subgroups, and veterans had a significantly higher prevalence of chronic pain compared to nonveterans. Why are these statistics so important? The authors commented that "chronic pain contributes to an estimated $560 billion each year in direct medical costs, lost productivity, and disability programs."[1]

Though there are no comparable surveys on the incidence of pain in children, a January 21, 2019, article published in the *New York Times* cites interviews with pediatric pain specialists. According to these specialists, as many as one in five children may experience chronic pain, which is pain that lasts for three months or more. In the United States, about four to eight million children have missed school during previous months because of pain.[2]

Measuring Pain

Probably the most common way to assess pain is the numerical rating scale. This scale measures pain on a scale of 0 to 10; 0 means there is no pain, and 10 is the worst pain imaginable. In medical settings, many health-care providers use this scale to assess the pain levels of their patients. Obviously, this is a subjective rating. People may experience and rate the same levels of pain in different ways. In addition, memories vary. People may easily under- or overrate past pain.

In another type of assessment, known as the Faces Scale, there are a series of faces in various stages, ranging from happy to profoundly distressed. This type of evaluation is primarily useful for children. The Verbal Descriptor Scale consists of a series of descriptive phrases that refer to different levels of pain severity or intensity. This scale is used for assessing pain in older adults with mild or moderate levels of cognitive impairment. (Other indicators of pain in older adults with cognitive issues are restlessness, crying, moaning and groaning, grimacing, resistance to care, reduced social interactions, increased wandering, reduced intake of food, and sleeping problems.) The Brief Pain Inventory is a detailed questionnaire that is used to evaluate the effect of pain on mood, activity, sleep patterns, and how the pain affects interpersonal relationships. In addition, it uses a timeline to detect pain patterns. And, often mentioned in research studies, the McGill Pain Questionnaire, which is also known as the McGill Pain Index, is a self-reporting measure of pain used for people with a number of different medical problems. Evaluating the quality and intensity of subjective pain, this test is composed of 78 adjectives, which respondents select to best describe their pain.

History of Pain Treatment and Management

For as long as people have existed, they have been compelled to deal with pain. Unless someone has a rare genetic disorder in which he or she is unable to feel pain, pain is an unwelcome part of life. Fortunately, for many people, pain is a relatively rare event. A child might fall and scrape his or her knees, and an adult might break a finger. Within a relatively short time, the problem is healed. However, large numbers of people deal with more frequent bouts of pain.

Historically, European physicians used opium to relieve their patients' pain, sometimes mixing it with sherry (laudanum). By the 19th century, in Europe and the United States, opiates were the standard treatment for both acute pain from injuries and recurrent pain, such as periodic headaches. Though it may be hard to believe, opium and alcohol-based products were unregulated and sold in pharmacies in liquids, pills, and "headache powders." People simply walked into pharmacies and purchased these products at will. Without a doubt, at least some of these people developed an addiction. Eventually, physicians became concerned about this misuse of opium.

Meanwhile, in 1846, at Massachusetts General Hospital in Boston, the American dentist William T. G. Morton demonstrated the utility of treating pain with ether anesthesia. And, two years later, in 1848, the British obstetrician James Young Simpson advocated the use of chloroform in childbirth and surgery. Clearly, the use of surgical anesthesia represented a monumental change for medicine. Still, anesthesia was not universally welcomed. Some physicians thought that anesthesia would impair the ability of the body to heal, and certain religious writers considered it a violation of God's law. Nevertheless, the many benefits of anesthesia become abundantly evident, and it prevailed. During the Civil War, anesthesia was used for surgical procedures, and morphine treated the pain suffered by countless numbers of soldiers. But problems arose when soldiers continued to use morphine long after their injuries were healed. This led to restrictions on the use of morphine in the early 1900s and on the use of heroin in the 1920s.

Near the close of the 19th century, the Bayer Company of Germany began selling diacetylated morphine as a remedy for coughing. The trade name was Heroin. It was believed to be less habit-forming than morphine. Yet, by the early 20th century, working-class Americans were crushing this product into powder and inhaling it. In 1899, Bayer chemists introduced acetylated salicylic acid, a plant compound known as aspirin. Although it had the potential to cause gastric upset, it proved to be an extremely useful analgesic (medication that reduces pain) and antipyretic (medication that reduces fever). In 1917, aspirin became an over-the-counter medication in America, and it became the drug of choice for mild to moderate pain. But it was not as useful for severe pain as the opiates, especially in seriously ill and dying people. Physicians were frequently worried that treating their patients in chronic serious pain with opiates would lead to addiction, a problem that continues to plague physicians to this day.

Reid Hunt, a Harvard pharmacologist, emphasized the need to develop a nonaddictive medication that would treat stronger pain. His input triggered the development of the Committee on Drug Addiction, which was formed in 1929 under the National Research Council. In 1938, it moved to the National Institutes of Health. Over the years, this program has tested a number of analgesics including oxycodone, meperidine, methadone, and pentazocine.

During World War II, while treating soldiers with complicated injuries, physicians were able to learn more about the effective treatment of pain. Henry K. Beecher, a Harvard anesthesiologist, observed that his seriously wounded battlefield patients appeared to experience less pain than his civilian patients in the recovery area at Massachusetts General Hospital. According to Beecher, there had to be a cognitive and emotional component to pain. Another anesthesiologist, John Bonica, who practiced during the war at the Madigan Army Hospital in Washington, advocated the founding of multidisciplinary pain clinics that would promote the sharing of clinical and laboratory evidence.

Creation of the Medical Field of Pain Management

In the early 1970s, Dr. Bonica invited 300 researchers and clinicians to a three-day meeting near Seattle, Washington. All of the participants had either worked in pain management or written about the topic. The International Association for the Study of Pain was founded; it would have a journal entitled *Pain*. Dr. Bonica become the group's first president.

During the past two or three decades, researchers have developed alternative or adjuncts to opiates for ongoing intractable pain. These include medications such as tricyclic antidepressants and amitriptyline and imipramine, which increase levels of norepinephrine in the nervous system; in so doing, these medications relieve chronic pain. Another group of pain treatments are the counterstimulation methods; of these, the most successful is the transcutaneous electrical nerve stimulation device (TENS). It appears to stimulate endorphins. Cognitive behavioral therapy programs have been effective in improving mood and function and reducing levels of pain. Today, many providers believe that chronic pain is best treated with a multidisciplinary approach. Medical providers should not consider chronic pain as a solely physical problem; rather, they should reach out to other disciplines and work to provide the best treatments for their patients with chronic pain.

Treating Pain with Medications May Cause Complications and Side Effects

In 1986, the World Health Organization (WHO) created a Pain Relief Ladder, in which pain and treatment are divided into three steps. Step 1 includes treatment with nonopioid analgesics, including nonsteroidal anti-inflammatory drugs (NSAIDs), acetaminophen, and aspirin. If the pain persists or worsens, the medical provider should prescribe "weak" opioids, such as codeine. Patients with moderate to severe pain should take "strong" opioids.

Though these medications may bring relief, they all have numerous negative side effects. Side effects for NSAIDs include stomach pain, heartburn, stomach ulcers, excessive bleeding, headaches and dizziness, ringing in the ears, liver or kidney problems, and high blood pressure. Side effects of acetaminophen include nausea, stomach pain, loss of appetite, itching, rash, headache, dark urine, and clay-colored stools. Allergic reactions to acetaminophen include difficulty breathing or swallowing, swelling of the face, lips, throat, or tongue, hives, and severe itching, peeling, or blistering of the skin. The overuse of acetaminophen may cause liver damage. Symptoms of liver damage include yellowing of the skin or the whites of the eyes, pain in the upper right area of the abdomen, nausea, vomiting, loss of appetite, fatigue, excessive sweating, pale skin, unusual bruising or bleeding, dark or tea-colored urine, and dark, tarry stools. Side effects of aspirin include rash, gastrointestinal ulcerations, abdominal pain, upset stomach, heartburn, drowsiness, headache, and cramping.

Opioids

Opioids are a class of drugs that are naturally found in the opium poppy plant. They work in the brain to block pain signals between the body and the brain. In so doing, they relieve moderate to severe levels of pain. (Opiates are drugs derived from or related to opium.) Some people find that opioids make them feel happy, relaxed, and "high." Opioids available legally by prescription include oxycodone (OxyContin, the most popular opioid medication), hydrocodone (Vicodin), codeine, and morphine. Another opioid is the synthetic medication known as fentanyl, which is 50 to 100 times more potent than morphine, and then there is the illegal drug heroin, which is also known as diamorphine. Heroin, a synthetic derivate of the opium plant, produces intense feelings of euphoria and is far stronger than most common low-dose prescription opioids, such as codeine and Vicodin.

Still, opioids come with a host of concerns. They have side effects such as slowed breathing, constipation, nausea, confusion, and drowsiness. More important, as many are aware, they may be addictive. After the pain has passed, the body may become physically and emotionally dependent on the opioid. And this may occur in a relatively brief period of time. Moreover, the body develops a tolerance of opioids and requires increasing doses. When misused, opioids may lead to fatal overdoses. According to the National Institute on Drug Abuse, every day in the United States, more than 130 people die of opioid overdoses. Between 21 and 29 percent of the people who receive prescriptions for opioids misuse them; between 4 and 6 percent of those who misuse opioids transition to heroin. The statistics are truly daunting. From July 2016 to September 2017, opioid overdoses increased 30 percent in 52 areas in 45 states; during that same time period, the Midwest saw overdoses increase by 70 percent. "The issue has become a public health crisis with devastating consequences."[3]

How did this happen? In the mid-to-late 1990s, the huge opioid-producing pharmaceutical companies reassured the medical community that their products were safe and nonaddictive. Knowing they were effective and believing that they were safe, health-care providers began prescribing increasing amounts of opioids. The opioids did their job; patients received quick relief from their pain. By the time the providers realized that the opioids were highly addictive and not safe, it was too late. In 2010, the number of overdoses began to rise rapidly; an opioid epidemic was raging and escalating. Three years later, in 2013, there were significant increases in overdoses from synthetic opioids, particularly illicitly manufactured fentanyl. In 2017, more than 47,000 Americans died from opioid overdoses; the rates were highest among men under the age of 50 years and among those who also took benzodiazapines, a class of medicines that are primarily used for anxiety. During that same year, about 1.7 million people in the United States suffered from substance abuse disorder related to prescription opioid pain relievers, and 652,000 suffered from heroin use disorder.[4] The overwhelming majority of people who are addicted to heroin started with an opioid prescription to relieve pain. When they are no longer able to take their prescriptive opioid medication, when their medical provider refuses to continue writing prescriptions, or when the cost becomes too high, they may turn to heroin, which is cheaper and readily available from a host of different sources. The overwhelming majority of heroin uses appeared to have begun with prescription opioids. Yet, once people abuse heroin, they are unlikely to return to opioid medications. In addition, whereas prescription opioids are generally swallowed, in the United States, heroin is usually injected, which introduces a whole new set of potential problems, such as risk of serious infections; other diseases, such as HIV infection; and an increased danger of overdose.

And the epidemic affects people in all walks of life and income groups, as well as their relatives, friends, and coworkers. The economic and emotional burdens tend to be overwhelming. While it is heartening to know that the vast majority of people who take prescription opioids stop before they become addicted, in the United States, addiction and related problems have become serious public health issues. That is one of the primary reasons that people need to learn other effective ways to relieve pain, especially chronic pain.

Complementary and Integrative Pain Treatments

Historically, people have probably always used various forms of complementary and integrative medical practices to relieve pain. For example, in ancient Egypt, one can easily imagine a pyramid builder massaging his leg after a long day of work. In fact, until the rise of scientific medicine in the 19th century, medicine included a whole host of eclectic complementary and integrative practices. When scientifically based medicine began to emerge, these practices fell by the wayside and remained there until the 1960s and 1970s, when complementary and integrative medicine reappeared and gained momentum.

For most of those years, there was no U.S. agency in charge of proving or disproving the efficacy of these treatments. In 1998, that situation changed: the National Center for Complementary and Alternative Medicine was created as part of the National Institutes for Health. Now known as the National Center for Complementary and Integrative Medicine, this center sponsors research and attempts to determine the safety and usefulness of the various complementary and alternative modalities. It also has a variety of outreach efforts, such as a website filled with information about the topic, with the goal of integrating proven aspects of complementary and integrative medicine into conventional medicine. Also, there are scores of medical integrative programs, practices, and departments throughout the country. Though the actual offerings may vary, they all attempt to relieve the pain associated with chronic medical problems.

Each year, often with little solid scientific evidence, millions of Americans spend billions of dollars on complementary and integrative ways to relieve their pain. Visits to acupuncturists, chiropractors, massage therapists, and practitioners of meditation and relaxation techniques and others have become commonplace. Fortunately, recent years have witnessed more evidence, and this book will outline the research in the various relevant entries.

NOTES

1. Dahlhamer, James, Jacqueline Lucas, Carla Zelaya, et al. "Prevalence of Chronic Pain and High-Impact Chronic Pain among Adults—United States, 2016." *MMWR Morbidity and Mortality Weekly Report* 67, no. 36 (September 14, 2018): 1001–1006.
2. Klass, Perri. "Helping Children Conquer Chronic Pain." *New York Times* (January 19, 2019): NA.
3. National Institute on Drug Abuse. https://www.drugabuse.gov.
4. National Institute on Drug Abuse.

REFERENCES AND FURTHER READINGS

Dahlhamer, James, Jacqueline Lucas, Carla Zelaya, et al. "Prevalence of Chronic Pain and High-Impact Chronic Pain among Adults—United

States, 2016." *MMWR Morbidity and Mortality Weekly Report* 67, no. 36 (September 14, 2018): 1001–1006.

Klass, Perri. "Helping Children Conquer Chronic Pain." *New York Times* (January 21, 2019): NA.

Meldrum, Marcia L. "A Capsule History of Pain Management." *JAMA* 290, no. 18 (November 12, 2003): 2470–2475.

National Center for Complementary and Integrative Medicine, formerly known as the National Center for Complementary and Alternative Medicine. http://nccim.nih.gov.

National Institute on Drug Abuse. https://drugabuse.gov.

Acetaminophen

INTRODUCTION

Although no one has been able to determine exactly how acetaminophen works, it is both a pain reliever (analgesic) and a fever reducer (antipyretic). It is generally believed that acetaminophen acts on the central nervous system and reduces the production of prostaglandins in the brain. Prostaglandins are chemicals that play a role in the development of pain, fever, inflammation, and swelling. Research has shown that acetaminophen relieves pain by elevating the pain threshold—by requiring more pain to develop before it is felt. Also, it reduces fever by acting on the heat-regulating center of the brain. Moreover, as acetaminophen is not an opioid, it has no mood-altering effects. Metabolized by the liver, acetaminophen is converted into inactive compounds. However, in excess amounts, acetaminophen may be toxic.

Acetaminophen is the most common drug ingredient in the United States. It is found in more than 600 different over-the-counter and prescription medicines. (Actifed and Dayquil are over-the-counter medications with acetaminophen, and Oxycodone, Tylenol with codeine, and Vicodin are prescription medications with acetaminophen.) Each week, approximately 23 percent of U.S. adults—or 52 million consumers—use a medicine containing acetaminophen. Acetaminophen treats mild to moderate pain and reduces fever; it may be combined with an opioid to treat moderate to severe pain. (Outside the United States, acetaminophen is often called paracetamol.)

Acetaminophen was discovered by accident in the late 19th century. A chemical known as acetanilide was mistakenly administered to a patient who had intestinal parasites. Although the medication failed to resolve the parasite issue, the patient's fever was reduced. Subsequently, the chemical became the focus of more research on its painkilling properties. In 1951, the U.S. Food and Drug Administration (FDA) first issued a patent for acetaminophen. Developed by McNeil Laboratories, in 1955, acetaminophen was sold under the brand name of Tylenol.

ADMINISTRATION AND REGULATION

Acetaminophen is sold as tablets, chewable tablets, gelcaps, geltabs, capsules, caplets, liquid, solution/suspension/syrup, oral disintegrating tablets (tablet that quickly dissolves in the mouth), and suppositories. After opening, it is best to store the liquid in a refrigerator, and the suppositories should be stored in a refrigerator or freezer. Acetaminophen may also be used intravenously.

In general, adults should take 500 to 1,000 mg of over-the-counter acetaminophen four times per day. Although that is the maximum anyone should take during a 24-hour period, problems and negative effects may appear with lower doses. For children, the recommended dose depends on the age and weight. Never give children acetaminophen products made for adults. Always follow the instructions on the label. Do not take more medicine than is indicated on the label. At any given time, do not take more than one medicine that contains acetaminophen. Unless directed by a medical provider, acetaminophen should not be used for more than 10 days. Although considered safe for pregnant and nursing women, acetaminophen leaches into breast milk. Therefore, if a nursing mother is taking acetaminophen, she should avoid breastfeeding.

The FDA has found the over-the-counter use of acetaminophen to be safe and effective, when used in accordance with the instructions on the label. The FDA requires a wider margin of safety for prescription forms of acetaminophen. For example, in 2014, the FDA recommended that doctors and other health professionals prescribe acetaminophen at dose of 325 mg or less. Any products containing acetaminophen should have a black box warning to highlight the risk for severe liver damage as well as a warning for potential allergic reactions, such as swelling of the face, mouth, and throat; difficulty breathing; itching; or rash.

BENEFITS AND RISKS

Acetaminophen is used to relieve aches and pain and fevers associated with many medical problems, such as headache, arthritis pain, back and body pain, tooth pain, menstrual cramps, colds, reactions to vaccinations, sore throats, sinus infections, sprains, and strains. However, while acetaminophen relieves pain, it has no effect on inflammation. If pain is not a result of inflammation, acetaminophen is as effective as the NSAID aspirin, and it is considered as effective as ibuprofen in relieving the pain of osteoarthritis of the knee.

Because it has no anti-inflammatory properties, it is less likely than NSAIDs to irritate the stomach lining, harm the kidneys, or alter blood clotting.

When used as directed, acetaminophen tends to have few side effects. The most common side effects are rash, nausea, vomiting, insomnia, and headaches. Other side effects include hypersensitivity reactions, hoarseness, serious skin reactions, mouth or throat swelling, difficulty urinating, lightheadedness, itching, fainting, sweating, weakness, unusual bruising or bleeding, chest tightness, breathing difficulties, a reduced number of platelets in the blood (thrombocytopenia), a reduced number of white blood cells in the blood, swelling under the skin, anemia, and kidney damage. There is an increased risk of gastrointestinal bleeding or liver problems, especially among people who frequently drink alcohol. Acetaminophen may cause the skin or whites of the eyes to yellow, which is a sign of liver damage.

Symptoms of an acetaminophen overdose may occur in as little as 12 hours or take as long as 4 days. Early signs of acetaminophen overdose include stomach cramping, loss of appetite, fatigue, nausea, stomach pain, sweating, flu-like symptoms, and vomiting. Worsening symptoms include pain in the right side of the abdomen, urinating less than normal, and an enlarged liver. Acetaminophen overdose is a relatively common medical emergency. Overdoses have resulted in liver damage, the need for a liver transplant, and death. Acetaminophen is the leading cause of nonalcoholic liver damage in the United States.

Acetaminophen should not be mixed with alcohol and drugs known to cause liver damage. It should not be taken with carbamazepine, rifampin, or isoniazid, which increases liver enzyme activity, decreasing its effectiveness. Cholestyramine decreases the absorption of acetaminophen from the intestine, thus reducing its effectiveness. Warfarin, a blood thinner, may be enhanced by acetaminophen. So people who take warfarin should avoid higher doses of acetaminophen.

RESEARCH FINDINGS

Intravenous Acetaminophen Appears to Be Useful for Postcraniotomy Pain

In a systematic review and meta-analysis published in 2020 in the journal *World Neurosurgery*, researchers from Iran and the United States (Los Angeles, California, Baltimore, Maryland, and Boston, Massachusetts) wanted to determine if intravenous acetaminophen would help with postcraniotomy pain. Five randomized, controlled trials were held with 2,635 patients who met their criteria for inclusion; there were 1,327 in the intervention groups and 1,308 in the control groups. The trials were published between 2002 and 2018. The researchers learned that the use of intravenous acetaminophen was significantly associated with a number of pain-relieving factors, such as reduced rescue doses, need for fewer total doses of rescue medication, reduced length of stay in intensive care units, and lower visual analog scale scores. The overall comfort of the patients was improved. The researchers commented that "intravenous paracetamol is a safe and efficient agent for controlling postoperative pain in those undergoing elective craniotomy."[1]

Acetaminophen Seems to Be a Good Treatment for Pain Associated with Acute Musculoskeletal Injuries

In a systematic review and meta-analysis published in 2021 in the journal *Emergency Medicine Australasia*, researchers from New Zealand and Australia evaluated the use of oral acetaminophen and combination oral acetaminophen analgesics for acute musculoskeletal injuries. The researchers located six randomized, controlled trials with 1,254 subjects who met their criteria. In all instances, the subjects presented at an emergency department, an urgent care facility, or a primary care provider with an acute musculoskeletal injury. The primary outcome studied was the difference in pain scores at rest. Pain scores were analyzed at baseline and up to 2 hours later, at 24 hours, and at 72 hours. The researchers learned that there was high-quality evidence that there was no significant difference between acetaminophen monotherapy and acetaminophen combination therapy in terms of the reductions in pain score. In addition, there was moderate-quality evidence that there was no difference between the groups in adverse events and the need for more analgesia. The researchers concluded that there was "no difference in analgesic efficacy between oral paracetamol and oral paracetamol used in combination with other oral analgesic agents in the management of acute musculoskeletal injuries."[2]

Acetaminophen with Caffeine Seems to Help Acute Dental Pain

In a systematic review published in 2019 in the *Saudi Dental Journal*, researchers from New Hope, Minnesota (USA), Italy, and Saudi Arabia examined the efficacy and safety of acetaminophen and caffeine for acute dental pain. The researchers located three randomized, controlled trials that met their criteria. One trial evaluated the efficacy of 500 mg acetaminophen and 65 mg caffeine compared to acetaminophen alone or placebo. Though this trial initially had 200 subjects, only 173 were used for statistical calculations. The trial found that the mean response for the combination therapy was better than the mean response for acetaminophen alone. A second trial compared the efficacy of 500 mg acetaminophen and 30 mg caffeine to 400 mg ibuprofen for the management of postoperative pain in 15 dental patients. During the first and second hours after surgery, the mean pain scores were lower in the acetaminophen and caffeine group, but 6, 7, and 8 hours after surgery, the mean pain scores were lower in the ibuprofen group. On the day after surgery, there were no differences between the groups. A third trial compared the efficacy of 300 mg acetaminophen and 20 mg caffeine to 300 mg acetaminophen and 30 mg codeine for postsurgical dental pain in 76 patients. Each subject received one dose of medication 30 minutes before surgery. They rated their pain before surgery and at several intervals after surgery. At 3, 6, and 12 hours after surgery, the pain was lower in the acetaminophen and codeine group; at other times, there were no differences in pain levels. The researchers noted that acetaminophen and caffeine seemed to work well together to relieve dental pain. They may be considered "an efficacious alternative to NSAIDs and opioids, with minimal contraindications and side effects in the therapeutic dosage."[3]

Acetaminophen Does Not Work as Well as Ibuprofen in Treating Short-Term Pain and Fever in Children Younger Than Two Years

In a systematic review and meta-analysis published in 2020 in the journal *JAMA Network Open*, researchers from New Zealand compared the use of acetaminophen and ibuprofen for the treatment of pain and fever in children younger than two years. The researchers included 11 randomized and 8 nonrandomized studies with a total of 241,138 subjects. The studies were conducted in the United States, the United Kingdom, France, the Netherlands, Israel, Turkey, and Iran. They took place in various settings, including pediatric and mixed emergency departments, pediatric wards, hospital-based clinics, and community clinics. Though no data were available for pain reduction during the first four hours, moderate-quality evidence found that ibuprofen was associated with more pain relief than acetaminophen from 4 to 24 hours after treatment. There was low-quality evidence that children treated with acetaminophen and ibuprofen had similar pain levels at one to three days. The researchers concluded that there is a need for more research on the use of these medications in young children. "Large, randomized trials are needed to address these knowledge gaps."[4]

Patients with Liver Disease Appear to Have Limited Knowledge about Acetaminophen

In an observational, cross-sectional study published in 2016 in the *Journal of Clinical and Translational Hepatology*, researchers from Los Angeles and Pasadena, California (USA), noted that unintentional acetaminophen intake is the leading cause of acute liver failure in the United States. People with underlying liver disease are at a higher risk of poor outcomes from acetaminophen overdoses. The researchers wanted to learn if patients with liver disease were aware of the problems associated with the use of acetaminophen. The cohort consisted of 401 patients with liver disease who were treated at the Pfleger Liver Institute at the University of California in Los Angeles during a 15-month period of time. The patients completed a demographic questionnaire and an acetaminophen knowledge survey. The majority of the patients were male (53.4%), and their median age was 60. Most of the patients were non-Hispanic white and had at least a college education. Hepatitis C, hepatitis B, and nonalcoholic fatty liver disease were the most common diagnoses; the mean length of time since the patients' liver disease diagnosis was seven years. About two out of every three patients had underlying cirrhosis. The majority of patients (59.6%) had taken pain medication during the previous six months. Only 30 patients could identify the maximum daily dose of acetaminophen for a person without liver disease. A few patients knew that the maximum daily dose of acetaminophen for a person with cirrhosis was less than 3 g per day. Most did not know that commonly prescribed pain medications often had acetaminophen. Two hundred thirty of the patients believed that people with liver disease could not safety take any acetaminophen. The researchers commented that the patients appeared to have "limited" knowledge about acetaminophen. Interestingly, females were more likely than males to know that Vicodin and Percocet contained acetaminophen. According to the researchers, this "may explain why unintentional acetaminophen overdose makes up such a large portion of cases of acute liver failure." Furthermore, it may result in the underutilization of pain medication and inadequate pain management. The researchers concluded that patients with liver disease had very low levels of knowledge about acetaminophen. This placed them at increased risk for both acetaminophen overdose and the "under-medication and inadequate management of chronic pain."[5]

Acetaminophen May Not Be Useful for Spinal Pain and May Have Only a Limited Usefulness for People with Osteoarthritis of the Hip or Knee

In a systematic review and meta-analysis published in 2015 in the journal *BMJ*, researchers from Australia wanted to learn if acetaminophen would be useful for spinal pain or the pain associated with osteoarthritis of the hip or knee. The researchers located 13 randomized, controlled trials that met their criteria; one of these could not be included in the meta-analysis. All of the trials compared the use of acetaminophen to a placebo. Trials with mixed populations of patients with spinal pain and osteoarthritis were excluded. Three trials with a total of 1,825 patients investigated the efficacy of acetaminophen in people with low back pain, and 10 trials with 3,541 patients investigated the efficacy of acetaminophen in people with hip or knee osteoarthritis. In all but one of the trials, acetaminophen was administered orally. Doses and dose regimens varied. The researchers learned that while acetaminophen did not offer relief to people with low back pain, it had a significant but small short-term effect in people with hip or knee osteoarthritis. Unfortunately, there was strong evidence that acetaminophen increased the risk of having an abnormal result on liver function tests by nearly fourfold. The researchers observed that acetaminophen alone "might not be sufficient to treat hip or knee osteoarthritis and might need to be accompanied by other management strategies, such as exercise and advice/education."[6]

Intravenous Acetaminophen May Lower the Blood Pressure of Hospitalized Patients, Especially Those Who Are Critically Ill

In a study published in 2019 in the journal *Annals of Pharmacotherapy*, researchers from Jacksonville, Florida (USA), investigated the belief that intravenous acetaminophen lowered blood pressure levels of hospitalized patients, especially those who are critically ill. Why is this important? When blood pressure drops too low, therapeutic interventions may be needed. The researchers identified five randomized, controlled trials (n = 205), six prospective open-label trials (n = 279), and eight retrospective reviews (n = 2,986) that met their criteria. Fourteen of these studies were conducted with critically ill patients in an emergency department or an intensive care unit. The researchers determined that among the included studies, 10 to 60 percent of the patients experienced a reduction in blood pressure. Of these, between 10 and 30 percent required an intervention. These reactions were usually seen shortly after the acetaminophen infusion. The researchers noted that "Intravenous acetaminophen use in the critically ill may contribute to clinically relevant hypotension, and these risks should be considered when treating this population."[7]

Other Medications Seem to Work Better Than Acetaminophen for Knee or Hip Osteoarthritis

In a systematic review and meta-analysis published in 2018 in the journal *Clinical and Experimental Rheumatology*, researchers from China compared the usefulness of acetaminophen, glucosamine, chondroitin, glucosamine and chondroitin, placebo, and celecoxib for the pain associated with knee or hip osteoarthritis. The researchers identified 61 randomized, controlled trials that met their criteria. Forty-seven trials had participants with only knee osteoarthritis; 2 trials had participants with only hip osteoarthritis; and 12 trials had subjects with knee and hip osteoarthritis. None of the trials had poor methodological quality, and all were believed to have a low risk of bias. The researchers found that the celecoxib, a prescription NSAID, was the most effective pain relief alternative. However, it also had the most adverse side effects. The combination of glucosamine and chondroitin was the next most effective. Other than the placebos, acetaminophen was the least efficacious option. The researchers concluded that their findings should help clinicians make treatment recommendations.[8]

Ibuprofen Seems to Relieve Pain Better Than Acetaminophen

In an overview of systematic reviews and meta-analyses published in 2015 in the *European Journal of Pain*, researchers from the United Kingdom and Canada compared the degree of pain relief obtained from acetaminophen and ibuprofen, a NSAID. The researchers identified 16 systematic reviews and four individual patient data meta-analyses that met their criteria. The typical single oral doses of acetaminophen were between 500 and 1,000 mg; the typical single doses of ibuprofen were between 200 and 400 mg. The researchers learned that ibuprofen was consistently better than acetaminophen for reducing pain over a range of different conditions, such as acute pain, migraine, and osteoarthritis. In almost all circumstances, single doses of ibuprofen offered good pain relief in more people than single doses of acetaminophen. For dysmenorrhea, pediatric pain, cancer pain, back pain, and rheumatoid arthritis, there were limited data. When data were available, the favored medication was ibuprofen. The researchers noted that their findings "call into question the widespread practice of routinely using paracetamol as a first line analgesic in preference to ibuprofen or other analgesics."[9]

Acetaminophen May or May Not Be Useful for Pain in Newborns

In a review published in 2020 in the *Cochrane Database of Systematic Reviews*, researchers from Toronto, Canada, evaluated the efficacy and safety of the use of acetaminophen for the prevention and treatment of pain in newborns. Although even healthy newborns will have routine tests, newborns who have more difficult births or who are hospitalized may experience a good deal of pain. The researchers located nine trials with 728 infants who met their criteria; all of the trials had a low risk of bias. The painful procedures that were addressed in these trials included heel lancing, assisted vaginal births, eye examination for retinopathy of prematurity assessment, and postoperative care. The results of the studies varied. For example, in one study, which measured premature infant pain profile (PIPP) scores, the pain levels were higher in the acetaminophen group than in the oral glucose group. In another study, which used the Bernese Pain Scale, infants treated with acetaminophen for a heel lancing had higher pain scores and spent more time crying than the infants in the placebo group. In still another study, during eye examinations, the PIPP scores were significantly lower in the acetaminophen group than in the water group. And during postoperative care after major surgery, the total amount of morphine administered over 48 hours was significantly less in the infants in the acetaminophen group than in the infants in the morphine group. No adverse events were observed in any of the studies. Still the researchers felt that the quality of the evidence was low. The researchers concluded that "the paucity and low quality of existing data do not provide sufficient evidence to establish the role of paracetamol in reducing the effects of painful procedures in neonates." On the other hand, acetaminophen may reduce the amount of morphine needed by infants undergoing major surgery.[10]

Many People Who Take Products Containing Acetaminophen Know Little about the Proper Administration of Their Medication(s)

In a study published in 2018 in the *Journal of the American Pharmacists Association*, researchers from Boston and Arlington, Massachusetts, Pittsburgh, Pennsylvania, and Titusville, New Jersey (USA), investigated the level of acetaminophen knowledge among users of acetaminophen over-the-counter and prescription products. (This research was funded by Johnson & Johnson, which markets the Tylenol-brand acetaminophen medications.) The nationwide study had an internet one-week diary design; 9,629 participants provided information on acetaminophen knowledge, attitudes, and self-dosing practices. The median age of the subjects was 44 years; 61 percent were female, and 26 percent were nonwhite. Eighty percent had more than a high school education. The subjects were asked specific questions about their use of medication that contained acetaminophen. In their diaries, the subjects listed what medications they took, how much they took and at what time(s) of the day, and what symptoms the medications treated. They also provided other information, such as label reading behavior. The subjects were asked to identify, without consulting their medication labels, the main ingredient or ingredients in each medication they had taken from the following products: acetaminophen, ibuprofen, naproxen, and aspirin. For over-the-counter medications, the subjects were asked how much to take per dose and the minimum interval between doses. Respondents were considered knowledgeable only if they correctly identified acetaminophen as an ingredient in all of the medications they took and were aware of correct dosing and intervals. The subjects were asked if it was acceptable to take a medicine containing acetaminophen with a second medicine containing acetaminophen, ibuprofen, naproxen, or aspirin. The researchers learned that recent users of acetaminophen products had a low-level knowledge about products containing acetaminophen and how they should be used. Only one-third were aware that two acetaminophen products should not be taken at the same time, and only 15 percent of the subjects taking two or more medicines had ingredient knowledge and were aware of the dangers of concomitant use. Most users of over-the-counter acetaminophen medicines did not know redosing intervals. Most of the problems were associated with combination products, especially over-the-counter medications that treat respiratory illnesses. Why are these shortfalls important? The lack of correct information is associated with the intake of medicine contrary to directions on the label, which may result in improper use. The researchers concluded that "there is clearly a great deal of room for improvement in users' knowledge about Rx [prescription] and OTC [over-the-counter] medications that contain acetaminophen."[11]

NOTES

1. Ghaffarpasand, Fariborz, Ehsan Dadgostar, Ghazal Ilami, et al. "Intravenous Acetaminophen (Paracetamol) for Postcraniotomy Pin: Systematic Review and Meta-Analysis of Randomized Controlled Trials." *World Neurosurgery* 134 (February 2020): 569–576.

2. Scott, Gemma, Jiayi Gong, Carl Kirkpatrick, and Peter Jones. "Systematic Review and Meta-Analysis of Oral Paracetamol *versus* Combination Oral Analgesics for Acute Musculoskeletal Injuries." *Emergency Medicine Australasia* 33, no. 1 (February 2021): 107–113.

3. Abou-Atme, Youssef S., Marcello Melis, and Khalid H. Zawawi. "Efficacy and Safety of Acetaminophen and Caffeine for the Management of Acute Dental Pain: A Systematic Review." *Saudi Dental Journal* 31 (2019): 417–423.

4. Tan, Eunicia, Irene Braithwaite, Christopher J. D. McKinlay, and Stuart R. Dalziel. "Comparison of Acetaminophen (Paracetamol) with Ibuprofen for Treatment of Fever or Pain in Children Younger Than 2 Years: A Systematic Review and Meta-Analysis." *JAMA Network Open* 3, no. 10 (October 1, 2020): e2022398.

5. Saab, Sammy, Peter G. Konyn, Matthew R. Viramontes, et al. "Limited Knowledge of Acetaminophen I Patients with Liver Disease." *Journal of Clinical and Translational Hepatology* 4 (2016): 281–287.

6. Machado, Gustavo C., Chris G. Maher, Paulo H. Ferreira, et al. "Efficacy and Safety of Paracetamol for Spinal Pain and Osteoarthritis: Systematic Review and Meta-Analysis of Randomised Placebo Controlled Trials." *BMJ* 350 (March 31, 2015): h1225.

7. Maxwell, Erin N., Brittany Johnson, Joseph Cammilleri, and Jason A. Ferreira. "Intravenous Acetaminophen-Induced Hypotension: A Review of

Current Literature." *Annals of Pharmacotherapy* 53, no. 10 (October 2019): 1033–1041.

8. Zhu, X., Wu, L. Sang, et al. "Comparative Effectiveness of Glucosamine, Chondroitin, Acetaminophen or Celecoxib for the Treatment of Knee and/or Hip Osteoarthritis: A Network Meta-Analysis." *Clinical and Experimental Rheumatology* 36 (2018): 595–602.

9. Moore, R. A., S. Derry, P. J. Wiffen, et al. "Overview Review: Comparative Efficacy of Oral Ibuprofen and Paracetamol (Acetaminophen) across Acute and Chronic Pain Conditions." *European Journal of Pain* 19, no. 9 (October 2015): 1213–1223.

10. Ohlsson, Arne, and Prakeshkumar S. Shah. "Paracetamol (Acetaminophen) for Prevention or Treatment of Pain in Newborns." *Cochrane Database of Systematic Reviews* 1, no. 1 (January 2020): CD011219.

11. Kelly, Judith P., Deena R. Battista, Saul Shiffman, et al. "Knowledge of Dosing Directions among Current Users of Acetaminophen-Containing Medications." *Journal of the American Pharmacists Association* 58, no. 5 (September–October 2018): 492–498.

REFERENCES AND FURTHER READINGS

Abou-Atme, Youssef S., Marcello Melis, and Khalid H. Zawawi. "Efficacy and Safety of Acetaminophen and Caffeine for the Management of Acute Dental Pain: A Systematic Review." *Saudi Dental Journal* 31 (2019): 417–423.

Ghaffarpasand, Fariborz, Ehsan Dadgostar, Ghazal Ilami, et al. "Intravenous Acetaminophen (Paracetamol) for Postcraniotomy Pain: Systematic Review and Meta-Analysis of Randomized Controlled Trials." *World Neurosurgery* 34 (February 2020): 569–576.

Kelly, Judith P., Deena R. Battista, Saul Shiffman, et al. "Knowledge of Dosing Directions among Current Users of Acetaminophen-Containing Medications." *Journal of the American Pharmacists Association* 58, no. 5 (September–October 2018): 492–498.

Machado, Gustavo C., Chris G. Maher, Paulo H. Ferreira, et al. "Efficacy and Safety of Paracetamol for Spinal Pain and Osteoarthritis: Systematic Review and Meta-Analysis of Randomised Placebo Controlled Trials." *BMJ* 350 (March 31, 2015): h1225.

Maxwell, Erin N., Brittany Johnson, Joseph Cammilleri, and Jason A. Ferreira. "Intravenous Acetaminophen-Induced Hypotension: A

Review of the Current Literature." *Annals of Pharmacotherapy* 53, no. 10 (October 2019): 1033–1041.

Moore, R. A., S. Derry, P. J. Wiffen, et al. "Overview Review: Comparative Efficacy of Oral Ibuprofen and Paracetamol (Acetaminophen) across Acute and Chronic Pain Conditions." *European Journal of Pain* 19, no. 9 (October 2015): 1213–1223.

Ohlsson, Arne, and Prakeshkumar S. Shah. "Paracetamol (Acetaminophen) for Prevention or Treatment of Pain in Newborns." *Cochrane Database of Systematic Reviews* 1, no. 1 (January 2020): CD011219.

Saab, Sammy, Peter G. Konyn, Matthew R. Viramontes, et al. "Limited Knowledge of Acetaminophen in Patients with Liver Disease." *Journal of Clinical and Translational Hepatology* 4 (2016): 281–287.

Scott, Gemma, Jiayi Gong, Carl Kirkpatrick, and Peter Jones. "Systematic Review and Meta-Analysis of Oral Paracetamol *versus* Combination Oral Analgesics for Acute Musculoskeletal Injuries." *Emergency Medicine Australasia* 33, no. 1 (February 2021): 107–113.

Tan, Eunicia, Irene Braithwaite, Christopher J. D. McKinlay, and Stuart R. Dalziel. "Comparison of Acetaminophen (Paracetamol) with Ibuprofen for Treatment of Fever or Pain in Children Younger Than 2 Years: A Systematic Review and Meta-Analysis." *JAMA Network Open* 3, no. 10 (October 1, 2020): e2022398.

Zhu, X., D. Wu, L. Sang, et al. "Comparative Effectiveness of Glucosamine, Chondroitin, Acetaminophen or *Celecoxib* for the Treatment of Knee and/or Hip Osteoarthritis: A Network Meta-Analysis." *Clinical and Experimental Rheumatology* 36 (2018): 595–602.

Acupressure

INTRODUCTION

An ancient art of healing, developed in China about 5,000 years ago, acupressure involves the use of fingers, fingernails, knuckles, palms, and sometimes elbows, toes, or specialized tools to press key points on the surface of the skin to stimulate the body's natural ability to heal. According to acupressure theory, the body has 14 primary meridians or energy channels. (The points are the same as those used in acupuncture.) Pressing on these points, termed acupoints, relieves muscle tension, which promotes the circulation of blood and qi. Stimulating these points releases endorphins—chemicals produced by the body that reduce pain—and the flow of blood and oxygen to the affected area is increased.

It should be parenthetically noted that qi, which is pronounced as "chee," is a key element in traditional Chinese medicine, which has its roots in ancient Chinese practices. Qi literally means the vital energy that circulates throughout the body. Practitioners of Western medicine generally believe that there is no scientific proof for qi or qi deficiency.

There are different types of acupressure. Shiatsu (Japanese for finger pressure), the best-known type of acupressure, tends to be vigorous, with firm pressure applied to each point for three to five seconds. Another kind of acupressure holds each point gently for a minute or more. Still another type places pressure with intermittent fast beats. Alternatively, pressure may be increased for about 30 seconds, held for 30 seconds to two minutes, and then gradually decreased for 30 seconds. This may be repeated three to five times.

ADMINISTRATION AND REGULATION

A first session with an acupressure therapist begins with a brief evaluation in which the client identifies painful areas. The client will then lie fully clothed on a massage table, and the acupressure therapy will begin. Normally, a session will last between 30 and 60 minutes.

Acupressure may be used in conjunction with massage therapy, acupuncture, reiki, and tai chi. The combination has the potential to achieve better results.

Licensing laws for acupressure therapy are administered at the state level. In some states, the requirements are fairly easy—as little as 500 to 600 hours of training. But other states require more. In many cases, a longer program may offer more opportunity for a broader education and additional training. Moreover, even after their formal training has ended, acupressure providers tend to enroll in continuing education courses, such as those approved by the National Certification Board of Therapeutic Massage and Bodywork. Often, acupuncturists and massage therapists are also licensed as acupressure therapists. In addition, nurses may train in acupressure. Acupressure training programs are a good source of more information on regulations. Although there do not appear to be any national statistics on the use and cost of acupressure, many people simply teach themselves this technique or purchase devices, such as acupressure wrist bands, to self-administer acu pressure.

People who practice acupressure may work in a wide variety of settings. These include clinics, spas, sports clubs and gyms, massage therapy offices, physical therapy practices, acupuncture settings, and integrative medical practices.

BENEFITS AND RISKS

Acupressure therapy may bring relief from pain, at least in the short term. As acupressure should never be painful, people who experience pain should tell their therapist. After a session, people may feel sore at the acupressure sites. In some instances, people may feel lightheaded.

There are no known risks associated with acupressure. However, because a few points have been identified with increasing the risk of labor, women who are pregnant (unless they are ready to deliver) should use acupressure treatment with extreme caution. And people with certain medical problems, such as heart disease, osteoporosis, cancer, a bleeding disorder, uncontrolled high blood pressure, and diabetes, may wish to discuss acupressure with a health provider before having a session. People who take anticoagulant or antiplatelet medications, such as warfarin, may also want to discuss acupressure with a health provider.

RESEARCH FINDINGS

Acupressure Seems to Be Helpful for Athletes with Acute Musculoskeletal Sports Injuries

In a prospective, three-arm, randomized, placebo-controlled trial published in 2017 in the *Clinical Journal of Sport Medicine*, researchers from New Zealand wanted to learn if acupressure would be useful for athletes with acute musculoskeletal injuries. During 2012, 79 male and female athletes who presented with acute musculoskeletal sports injuries at a sports injury clinic were placed in one of three groups: acupressure (n = 29), sham acupressure (n = 27), or no acupressure (n = 23). The most common musculoskeletal injuries included sprains, strains, and fractures; the most injured body parts were ankles, shoulders, hands, and knees. The mean time from injury to acceptance into the study was 60 minutes. Pain and anxiety measurements were taken before and after the intervention. The researchers determined that the athletes in the acupressure group, which was only administered for three minutes, had significant reductions in pain, and they had less pain than the members of the sham acupressure group and the members of the control group. (There was no difference in anxiety levels between the groups.) "Considering the simplicity and high acceptance of this procedure and lack of adverse effects, it presents as a viable pain management intervention in a sports medicine setting."[1]

Acupressure Seems Useful for Chronic Low Back Pain

In a single-blinded, randomized clinical trial published in 2017 in the *Iranian Journal of Nursing and Midwifery Research*, researchers from Iran wanted to determine if acupressure would help people with chronic low back pain, a very common medical problem among nurses. The cohort consisted of 50 female nurses between the ages of 25 and 55 years. All of the subjects had physician-diagnosed chronic back pain. The subjects were assigned to a treatment or sham group, with 25 nurses in each group. The nurses in the acupressure group received therapy three times per week for three weeks; the nurses in the sham group received placebo interventions. Pain data were collected and analyzed. The researchers found no difference in the preintervention scores between the groups. However, significant differences were seen after interventions. The intervention group had significantly lower pain severity scores than the sham group. And, the researchers advised the use of acupressure for nurses with chronic low back pain. "Acupressure can be used as nonmedicament, inexpensive, and without side effects treatment in reducing pain."[2]

In a systematic review and meta-analysis published in 2017 in the journal *Evidence-Based Complementary and Alternative Medicine*, researchers from China examined the use of auricular or ear acupressure for chronic low back pain. Seven randomized controlled trials met the criteria of the researchers. Of these, four had a low risk of bias. They were conducted in the United States, Hong Kong, and mainland China; six were in English, and one was in Chinese. In four of the trials, the subjects were middle aged or elderly. Trials ranged in size from 19 to 74 subjects, with a total of 369 adults with low back pain, and their duration ranged from two weeks to three months. The researchers learned that auricular acupressure had a large effect in reducing pain within 12 weeks and at a four-week follow-up. "The encouraging evidence of this study indicates that it is recommended to provide auricular acupressure to patients with chronic low back pain."[3]

In a randomized pilot trial published in 2019 in the journal *Pain Medicine*, researchers from Michigan (USA) evaluated the ability of self-administered acupressure to help people with chronic low back pain. The initial cohort consisted of 67 people who had chronic low back pain for at least three months; they were mostly female and middle-aged. The mean body mass index was overweight, and 28 percent were nonwhite. The subjects, who lived in and around southeastern Michigan, were placed in one of three groups. For six weeks, the subjects self-administered relaxing acupressure, stimulating acupressure, or their usual care. Fatigue, pain, sleep, and reported disability measurements were taken. Twelve subjects did not complete the trial. There were four mild adverse events related to the acupressure; all involved applying too much pressure. The researchers learned that both relaxing and stimulating acupressure treatments had a modest positive effect on pain that was higher than what is considered clinically significant. The researchers concluded that "the acupressure interventions had positive preliminary effects on symptoms, and the protocol was feasible and well tolerated by the sample."[4]

Hand Acupressure May Be Useful for Women Who Have Had a Caesarean Delivery with Spinal Anesthesia

In a trial published in 2017 in the journal *Complementary Therapies in Clinical Practice*, researchers from South Korea examined the effect of hand acupressure on opioid-related nausea and vomiting as well as pain after caesarean delivery in a women's hospital. The cohort consisted of 50 women who were randomly assigned to receive hand acupressure or to a control group. The women in both groups had similar demographic, obstetric, and clinical characteristics. The Korean hand acupressure was administered by an obstetric nurse specialist with several years of experience and was certified by a Korean hand acupressure training course. When compared to the control group, the women who received hand acupressure had significantly lower levels of pain and significantly lower requirements for pain medication. "Nevertheless," according to the researchers, "further well-designed research is needed to identify the effect size, optimal duration, and timing of Korean hand acupressure to minimize patient discomfort."[5]

Acupressure May Be Effective for Leukemia-Related Pain

In a controlled trial published in 2017 in the *International Journal of Nursing Practice*, researchers from Iran and Malaysia wanted to learn if hospitalized leukemia patients would benefit from acupressure. The initial cohort consisted of 100 patients who were randomly divided into two groups. The patients in the intervention group received 12 eight-minute acupressure treatments (three sessions per week for four weeks) in addition to standard care; the patients in the other group received only the standard care. Data were collected between February and June 2015. The mean age for the subjects was in the mid-40s, and they had similar sociodemographic backgrounds. The researchers learned that when compared to the control subjects, the subjects in the intervention group experienced a significant reduction in levels of pain after every therapy session. The researchers concluded "that acupressure methods applied to recommended points along with other medical treatments can have pain relieving effects without any side effects."[6]

Stimulation of Specific Acupressure Points May Be Useful during Labor

In a randomized, controlled trial published in 2016 in *Complementary Therapies in Medicine*, researchers from Iran wanted to learn if stimulation of the acupressure points L14 and BL32 might facilitate labor and delivery. (L14 is located on the web between the thumb and index finger; BL32 is midway between the lower spine and the dimple of the buttocks.)

The cohort consisted of 105 women who were pregnant for the first time and in the active phase of the first stage of labor. Thirty-five were assigned to receive acupressure at L14, and 35 were assigned to receive acupressure at BL32. Thirty-five women received no acupressure; they served as controls. Acupressure was applied at cervical dilations of 4–5 cm, 6–7 cm, and 8–10 cm. Each time, the acupressure was applied during six contractions. The women in the control group received the same clinical care, but without any acupressure. The researchers learned that the women who had acupressure therapy experienced significant reductions in pain that continued until the last stage of labor, 8–10 cm. Interestingly, acupressure on BL32 was slightly more effective in relieving labor pain than acupressure on L14. Acupressure application had no effect on uterus contractions, delivery type, or neonatal Apgar scores (newborn evaluation test). As no adverse effects were observed, the researchers concluded that "acupressure could be a safe adjunct for labor pain control."[7]

When Combined with Massage Therapy, Acupressure Is More Effective in Relieving Labor Pain, Reducing Labor Time, and Increasing Delivery Satisfaction

In a randomized controlled trial published in 2020 in *The Journal of Nursing Research*, researchers from Turkey compared the effects of acupressure to massage therapy on labor-related pain management, duration, and satisfaction with delivery. The cohort consisted of 120 women, with a mean age of 23.4 years, who were having their first baby and were not yet dilated to 4 cm. They were placed in one of four groups: acupressure only, massage therapy only, both acupressure and massage, or neither intervention (control). The treatments were administered during the latent, active, and transition phases of labor; acupressure was administered to the Sanyinjiao points (SP6), which are on the inside of the leg just above the ankle. The results were truly notable. Almost all of those in the acupressure group and the massage group were satisfied with their interventions, and 100 percent of those in the combination group expressed such satisfaction. Nearly everyone commented that they would recommend these interventions to other pregnant women. In the acupressure only group, 82.5 percent reported decreased pain, 25 percent reported accelerated delivery, and 17.9 percent reported experiencing relaxation and positive feelings. When combined with massage, those numbers were even higher. Yet, the researchers also found that acupressure therapy applied during the latent phase of delivery had no significant labor pain–reduction effect. "The acupressure intervention significantly reduced the perceived labor pain during the active and transition phases of labor only."[8]

Self-Administered Acupressure Seems to Be Useful for Menstrual Pain

In a two-armed, randomized, "pragmatic" trial published in 2018 in the *American Journal of Obstetrics & Gynecology*, researchers based in Berlin (Germany) noted that menstrual pain is very common among women of reproductive age. That is why they wanted to determine if application-based self-acupressure would be useful for these women. Their cohort consisted of 221 women between the ages of 18 and 34 years (mean age of 24 years) who reported cramping pain of 6 or more on a numeric rating scale. For six consecutive menstrual cycles, 111 women performed app-based self-acupressure and 110 followed their usual care. The app-based intervention provided visual descriptions on how to administer self-acupressure before and during the menstrual cycle. The app also collected study data. Both groups had a reduction in pain at the third and sixth menstrual cycles. However, pain relief was better in the acupressure group. After three months, 37 percent of the women in the acupressure group reported a 50 percent reduction in pain intensity. After six months, that number was up to 58 percent. At the three- and six-month marks, only 25 percent of the control women had such reductions. The researchers concluded that "self-acupressure supported and evaluated by a smartphone app was able to achieve a sustainable reduction in pain and medication in comparison to usual care."[9]

Auricular Acupressure May Help with Postsurgical Pain

In a systematic review and meta-analysis published in 2019 in the *Chinese Journal of Integrative Medicine*, researchers from China investigated the effectiveness of auricular acupressure for acute postoperative pain. They included 26 randomized controlled trials with a total of 1,682 adult patients. The patients in 14 of the trials were middle-aged or elderly; sample sizes ranged from 23 to 301 patients. The researchers found that auricular acupressure was more effective than conventional therapy alone, and pain relief in the auricular acupressure group was most significant at 72 hours after surgery. Yet, there was no statistical significance in patients undergoing ears, nose, and throat surgery. The researchers commented that auricular acupressure has "promising effects in relieving postoperative pain." It is a "relatively safe strategy for pain management."[10]

Shiatsu Acupressure Combined with Amitriptyline May Provide Relief for Refractory Primary Headaches

In a five-month, single-blind, randomized, controlled pilot trial published in 2017 in the journal *Neurological Sciences*, researchers from Italy tested the efficacy and safety of combining shiatsu acupressure with amitriptyline, a tricyclic antidepressant, for treating refractory primary headaches, or incapacitating headaches that are resistant to medical treatment. The cohort consisted of subjects with a diagnosis of primary headache that had not responded to at least two different prophylactic drugs. Initially, 37 women and men, with a mean age of 39.8 years, were treated with shiatsu and amitriptyline; 13 were treated only with shiatsu, 13 were treated only with amitriptyline, and 11 were treated with shiatsu and amitriptyline. The shiatsu treatment consisted of one 45-minute session per week for a total of 12 sessions; oral amitriptyline was started at 5 mg per day and increased to 10 mg per day after one week. At the end of the trial, the researchers found that 55 percent of the subjects on the combination treatment had a more than 50 percent reduction in days with headaches per month. Sixty-nine percent of those on shiatsu and 62 percent of those on amitriptyline alone had similar reductions. About one month after the trial ended, many people still had a more than 50 percent reductions in monthly headaches. Forty-five percent of those on the combination treatment had such reductions, as did 54 percent of those on shiatsu alone and 46 percent of those on amitriptyline alone. The researchers noted that the subjects who had shiatsu alone or in combination "experienced a significant benefit on headache frequency and severity." There were no negative side effects from the shiatsu treatments. Yet, the researchers added, "these findings are only preliminary and should be interpreted cautiously due to the small sample size."[11]

NOTES

1. Mącznik, A. K., A. G. Schneiders, J. Athens, and S. J. Sullivan. "Does Acupressure Hit the Mark? A Three-Arm Randomized Placebo-Controlled Trial of Acupressure for Pain and Anxiety Relief in Athletes with Acute Musculoskeletal Sports Injuries." *Clinical Journal of Sport Medicine* 27, no. 4 (July 2017): 338–343.

2. Movahedi, Maryam, Somayeh, Fateme Nazari, and Mahboubeh Valiani. "The Effects of Acupressure on Pain Severity in Female Nurses with Chronic Low Back Pain." *Iranian Journal of Nursing and Midwifery Research* 22, no. 5 (September–October 2017): 339–342.

3. Yang, Li-Hue, Pei-Bei Duan, Qing-Mei Hou, et al. "Efficacy of Auricular Acupressure for Chronic Low Back Pain: A Systematic Review and Meta-Analysis of Randomized Clinical Trials." *Evidence-Based Complementary and Alternative Medicine* 2017 (2017): Article ID 6383649.

4. Murphy, S. L., R. E. Harris, N. R. Keshavarzi, and S. M. Zick. "Self-Administered Acupressure for Chronic Low Back Pain: A Randomized Controlled Pilot Trial." *Pain Medicine* 20, no. 12 (December 2019): 2588–2597.

5. Ahn, N. Y., and H. J. Park. "Effects of Korean Hand Acupressure on Opioid-Related Nausea and Vomiting, and Pain after Caesarean Delivery Using Spinal Anaesthesia." *Complementary Therapies in Clinical Practice* 28 (August 2017): 101–107.

6. Sharif Nia, H., S. Pahlevan Sharif, A. Yaghoobzadeh, et al. "Effect of Acupressure on Pain in Iranian Leukemia Patients: A Randomized Controlled Trial Study." *International Journal of Nursing Practice* 23, no. 2 (April 2017): e12513.

7. Ozgoli, G., S. Sedigh Mobarakabadi, R. Heshmat, et al. "Effect of L14 and BL32 Acupressure on Labor Pain and Delivery Outcome in the First Stage of Labor in Primiparous Women: A Randomized Controlled Trial." *Complementary Therapies in Medicine* 29 (December 2016): 175–180.

8. Gönenç, I. M., and F. Terzioğlu. "Effects of Massage and Acupressure on Relieving Labor Pain, Reducing Labor Time, and Increasing Delivery Satisfaction." *The Journal of Nursing Research* 28, no. 1 (February 2020): e68.

9. Blödt, S., D. Pach, S. V. Eisenhart-Rothe, et al. "Effectiveness of App-Based Self-Acupressure for Women with Menstrual Pain Compared to Usual Care: A randomized Pragmatic Trial." *American Journal of Obstetrics & Gynecology* 218, no. 2 (February 2018): 227 e 1–9.

10. Zhong, Q., D. Wang, Y. M. Bai, et al. "Effectiveness of Auricular Acupressure for Acute Postoperative Pain after Surgery: A Systematic Review and Meta-Analysis." *Chinese Journal of Integrative Medicine* 25, no. 3 (March 2019): 225–232.

11. Villani, V., L. Prosperini, F. Palombini, et al. "Single-Blind, Randomized, Pilot Study Combining Shiatsu and Amitriptyline in Refractory

Primary Headaches." *Neurological Sciences* 38, no. 6 (June 2017): 999–1007.

REFERENCES AND FURTHER READINGS

Ahn, N. Y., and H. J. Park. "Effects of Korean Hand Acupressure on Opioid-Related Nausea and Vomiting, and Pain after Caesarean Delivery Using Spinal Anaesthesia." *Complementary Therapies in Clinical Practice* 28 (August 2017): 101–107.

Blödt, S., D. Pach, S. V. Eisenhart-Rothe, et al. "Effectiveness of App-Based Self-Acupressure for Women with Menstrual Pain Compared to Usual Care: A Randomized Pragmatic Trial." *American Journal of Obstetrics and Gynecology* 218, no. 2 (February 2018): 227 e 1–9.

Gönenç, I. M. and F. Terzioğlu. "Effects of Massage and Acupressure on Relieving Labor Pain, Reducing Labor Time, and Increasing Delivery Satisfaction." *The Journal of Nursing Research* 28, no. 1 (February 2020): e68.

Mącznik, A. K., A. G. Schneiders, J. Athens, and S. J. Sullivan. "Does Acupressure Hit the Mark? A Three-Arm Randomized Placebo-Controlled trial of Acupressure for Pain and Anxiety Relief in Athletes with Acute Musculoskeletal Sports Injuries." *Clinical Journal of Sport Medicine* 27, no. 4 (July 2017): 338–343.

Movahedi, Maryam, Somayeh Ghafari, Fateme Nazari, and Mahboubeh Valiani. "The Effects of Acupressure on Pain Severity in Female Nurses with Chronic Low Back Pain." *Iranian Journal of Nursing and Midwifery Research* 22, no. 5 (September–October 2017): 339–342.

Murphy, S. L., R. E. Harris, N. R. Keshavarzi, and S. M. Zick. "Self-Administered Acupressure for Chronic Low Back Pain: A Randomized Controlled Pilot Trial." *Pain Medicine* 20, no. 12 (December 2019): 2588–2597.

Ozgoli, G., S. Sedigh Mobarakabadi, R. Hashmat, et al. "Effect of L14 and BL32 Acupressure on Labor Pain and Delivery Outcome in the First State of Labor in Primiparous Women: A Randomized Controlled Trial." *Complementary Therapies in Medicine* 29 (December 2016): 175–180.

Sharif Nia, H., S. Pahlevan Sharif, A. Yaghoobzadeh, et al. "Effect of Acupressure on Pain in Iranian Leukemia Patients: A Randomized

Controlled Trial Study." *International Journal of Nursing Practice* 23, no. 2 (April 2017): e12513.

Villani, V., L. Prosperini, F. Palombini, et al. "Single-Blind, Randomized, Pilot Study Combining Shiatsu and Amitriptyline in Refractory Primary Headaches." *Neurological Sciences* 38, no. 6 (June 2017): 999–1007.

Yang, Li-Hua, Pei-Bei Duan, Qing-Mei Hou, et al. "Efficacy of Auricular Acupressure for Chronic Low Back Pain: A Systematic Review and Meta-Analysis of Randomized Controlled Trials." *Evidence-Based Complementary and Alternative Medicine* 2017 (2017): Article ID 6383649.

Zhong, Q., D. Wang, Y. M. Bai, et al. "Effectiveness of Auricular Acupressure for Acute Postoperative Pain after Surgery: A Systematic Review and Meta-Analysis." *Chinese Journal of Integrative Medicine* 25, no. 3 (March 2019): 225–232.

Acupuncture

INTRODUCTION

A type of traditional Chinese medicine, acupuncture is a technique in which practitioners stimulate specific points on the body, most often by inserting very thin needles into strategic points in the skin. While it is most often used to treat pain, acupuncture may also be part of a wellness and stress reduction program.

Originating thousands of years ago in China, acupuncture is linked to the belief that medical problems and illnesses are caused by a disruption in the flow of energy throughout the body. The insertion of the needles into very specific points stimulates qi (pronounced "chee") or the flow of energy throughout the body. The qi then travels through channels, called meridians. The meridians correspond to the major internal organs of the body. Acupuncture points are located throughout the body; sometimes they are far from the area(s) with pain. While there is no scientific proof that acupuncture points and meridians exist, it is clear that acupuncture works for some people and some conditions.

To explain acupuncture, Westerners may look to neuroscience. Acupuncture points are areas where nerves, muscles, and connective tissues are stimulated. This stimulation increases blood flow while triggering the activity of the body's natural painkillers.

ADMINISTRATION AND REGULATION

Acupuncturists and other health-care professionals who have received training in acupuncture tend to practice in office settings. An initial visit, which may take up to one to two hours, begins with a general health assessment and a review of past medical problems and treatments, patient and family history, diet, digestion, sleeping patterns, and emotional health.

The practitioner will take the pulse of both wrists and will view the tongue for color and coating. Based on these findings, the practitioner will select specific points and insert extremely thin needles into the skin. Only single-use disposable needles are used. After the needles are inserted, the practitioner may gently move or twirl them or apply heat or mild electrical pulses to the needles. Treatment is normally completed on a padded table. Most people feel very relaxed; some fall asleep. During the first three or four weeks of visiting the acupuncturist, four to eight treatments will be scheduled. These will last for up to an hour. If positive results are obtained, additional periodic treatments will be arranged.

Although acupuncture may be covered, at least in part, by health insurance, when it is not covered, fees per session tend to range around $75. Because it is longer, the charge for the first session will probably be higher. In most states, no medical referral is required to see an acupuncturist.

Training to become an acupuncturist requires the completion of three or four years of education in a master's degree–level acupuncture program accredited by the Accreditation Commission for Acupuncture and Oriental Medicine or the completion of an equivalent international education program. In addition, a Diplomate of Acupuncture must pass certain examinations and meet other requirements that vary from state to state. This stands in contrast to other medical providers who only need 100 to 300 hours of abbreviated acupuncture training. However, they must pass an examination conducted by National Certification Commission for Acupuncture and Oriental Medicine. In the United States, there are approximately 18,000 acupuncturists. Of these, about 12,000 are actively practicing. More than half of these practitioners practice in California or New York.

BENEFITS AND RISKS

Studies have found that acupuncture is an effective tool in easing different types of pain, such as low back pain, neck pain, and osteoarthritis knee pain. It may reduce the frequency of tension headaches and prevent migraine headaches. Other conditions that may benefit from acupuncture include dental pain, menstrual cramps, chemotherapy-induced and post-operative nausea and vomiting, infertility, post-traumatic stress disorder, addiction, depression, anxiety, gastrointestinal issues, sleep disturbances, asthma, and respiratory disorders.

When treatment is provided by a certified acupuncture practitioner who uses sterile needles, there is almost no risk from acupuncture. Still, in some instances, there may be soreness, bleeding, or bruising at the site of a needle insertion. Some people have an increased risk of problems from acupuncture. These include people who have a bleeding disorder or are taking blood-thinning medications. As acupuncture may interfere with a pacemaker, people with pacemakers should not have acupuncture. And women who are pregnant should only have acupuncture with the approval of their medical providers.

RESEARCH FINDINGS

Acupuncture Appears to Be Useful for Certain Types of Chronic Pain

In a meta-analysis published in 2018 in *The Journal of Pain*, researchers from multiple locations in the United States and abroad, but based in New York City, evaluated data on the use of acupuncture for nonspecific musculoskeletal pain, osteoarthritis, chronic headache, and shoulder pain. The researchers included data from 39 trials with 20,827 subjects; the randomly controlled trials were published between December 2008 and December 2015. All of the trials had at least one group that received acupuncture and at least one group that received either sham acupuncture or no acupuncture. The researchers found that for all four of the pain problems, acupuncture was superior to either sham acupuncture or no acupuncture. Furthermore, the positive effects of acupuncture persisted over at least a 12-month time period. Moreover, the researchers did not find any obvious differences between the results of trials with varying characteristics, such as the style of acupuncture, the duration of treatment sessions, or the training of the acupuncturists. They also found that acupuncture has a higher than average effect on upper body musculoskeletal pain. The researchers concluded that "acupuncture has a clinically relevant, persistent effect on chronic pain that is not completely explained by placebo effects." As a result, "referral for a course of acupuncture treatment is therefore a reasonable option for a patient with chronic pain."[1]

Acupuncture May Be Helpful for Some People with Low Back Pain

In a systematic review published in 2015 in the journal *Evidence-Based Complementary and Alternative Medicine*, researchers from New Zealand and the United Kingdom wanted to learn if acupuncture would be useful for chronic low back pain, a very common problem. The cohort consisted of 16 randomized controlled trials published between 1998 and 2013; 12 were in English, 3 were in Chinese, and 1 was in Japanese. The trials included various types of low back pain, such as acute, subacute, and chronic low back pain. The researchers found "inconsistent evidence" that acupuncture was better at relieving pain than sham acupuncture, but there is "consistent evidence" that both acupuncture and sham acupuncture improve function. However, for chronic low back pain, acupuncture provides "short-term clinically relevant benefits" and functional improvements. The researchers concluded that acupuncture, either used alone or in conjunction with other therapy, offers short-term improvements in pain and function for chronic low back pain. Still, they underscored the need "to improve both internal and external validity of systematic reviews" of randomized controlled trials.[2]

In a trial published in 2017 in the *Journal of Manipulative and Physiological Therapeutics*, researchers from Whittier, California, and Honolulu, Hawaii (USA) compared the use of acupuncture and spinal manipulative therapy and the combination of both to treat low back pain. A total of 101 subjects were recruited between March 2011 and March 2014 from communities around the Southern California University of Health Sciences. During a 60-day period of time, the subjects were treated with acupuncture ($n = 34$), spinal manipulative therapy ($n = 36$) or both ($n = 31$). Treatments were provided by acupuncturists and licensed doctors of chiropractic. The acupuncture treatments consisted of the needling of acupoints combined with electrotherapy, moxibustion, cupping, and Tui NA (a type of massage). Spinal manipulative therapy used specific contact points on vertebral processes, along with soft tissue therapy and physiotherapy. Follow-ups were held at 14 days, 30 days, and 60 days. Another follow-up was held at 120 days. The final analyses included 32 subjects in the acupuncture group, 36 subjects in the spinal manipulation group, and 30 subjects in the combination group. The researchers determined that the subjects in all three groups improved on the disability scale and pain intensity between baseline and 60 days. However, there were no statistically significant or clinically meaningful differences between the groups. In all three treatments, most of the improvements occurred within the first 60 days. In addition, there were "negligible differences" between the groups in pain frequency, disability days, medication use, patient satisfaction, and overall health status. The researcher commented that both acupuncture and spinal manipulative therapy, either separately or in combination, are effective treatments for low back pain. The participants in all three groups "reported high satisfaction with their care and decreased use of pain pills and missed days of work."[3]

In a clinical trial published in 2018 in the journal *Scientific Reports*, researchers from Egypt, several locations in Korea as well as in New Haven, Connecticut, and Boston, Massachusetts (USA), compared the use of acupuncture to the use of phantom acupuncture on people with low back pain. In this parallel-group trial, 56 people received either real acupuncture ($n = 33$) or phantom acupuncture ($n = 23$). During the procedures, the subjects were supine inside the fMRI machine, and they all believed that they were receiving real acupuncture treatments. Twenty-eight subjects in the real acupuncture group and 19 in the phantom group were included in the analyses. There were no significant differences between the groups in baseline data. Though both groups reported significant acupuncture sensations, the subjects in the real acupuncture group had significantly greater sensations. Interestingly, the subjects who received phantom acupuncture also had reductions in pain. Hence, there was definitely a placebo effect. The researchers concluded that "expectation and belief in acupuncture effectiveness could induce expectation-related placebo analgesic effects, leading to a reduction of subjective pain intensity."[4]

Acupuncture May or May Not Be Helpful for Dysmenorrhea

In a parallel-group, randomized, controlled trial published in 2018 in the *Journal of Acupuncture and Meridian Studies*, researchers from India investigated the use of acupuncture for dysmenorrhea, the pain and discomfort that is sometimes associated with menstruation. The cohort consisted of 60 females between the ages of 17 and 23 years with dysmenorrhea; they were randomly assigned to either the intervention group or the control group. There were no significant differences between the 30 subjects in each group. During a 90-day period, the subjects in the acupuncture group received 45 20-minute treatments. Each 30-day period had 15 sessions. Acupuncture was started on the sixth day of the menstrual cycle and was not performed during the menstrual cycle. Assessments were conducted at baseline, day 30, day 60, and day 90. The primary goal was to determine pain intensity levels. After that, the researchers evaluated muscle cramping and other factors, such as headache and dizziness. Except for headache, the researchers learned that acupuncture triggered a significant reduction in all of the variables studied, at both 30 days and 60 days. With headaches, no reduction was experienced until after the intervention was over. The researchers concluded that "acupuncture could be considered an effective treatment modality for the management of primary dysmenorrhea."[5]

On the other hand, in an analysis published in 2016 in the *Cochrane Database of Systematic Reviews*, researchers from Australia examined the use of acupuncture for dysmenorrhea. Their cohort consisted of 42 randomized controlled trials with a total of 4,640 women of reproductive age; it included published and unpublished trials comparing acupuncture, electroacupuncture, and acupressure with sham acupuncture or placebo. All of the women had moderate to severe symptoms. The researchers found a host of different problems with the studies. For example, some of the trials had inconsistent or inconclusive findings. One study, which was at low risk for bias, found no evidence of a difference between the groups at 3, 6, or 12 months, and the overall quality of the evidence was low. When acupuncture was compared to no treatment, the subjects in the acupuncture groups had lower levels of pain. Yet, in many instances, no data were available on adverse events. There were limitations from risk of bias, poor reporting, and inconsistency. The researchers concluded that "there is insufficient evidence to demonstrate whether or not acupuncture or acupressure are effective in treating primary dysmenorrhoea."[6]

Abdominal Acupuncture Seems to Be Useful for Neck Pain

In a randomized, patient and assessor–blind, sham-controlled trial published in 2017 in the online journal *PLoS ONE*, researchers from Hong Kong (China) investigated the use of abdominal acupuncture for neck pain. The cohort consisted of 154 subjects with neck pain; all of the subjects were between the ages of 18 and 65 years. Seventy-seven subjects received abdominal acupuncture and 77 received nonpenetrating sham abdominal acupuncture. At baseline, there were no significant "sociodemographic characteristics and neck pain-related data" between the two groups. Each participant received six treatments: 30-minute standardized treatments three times per week for two weeks. During their treatments, the subjects wore a black eye mask and lay down with their abdomens exposed. Interestingly, the subjects in both groups experienced improvements in their neck pain and neck pain disability, although the improvement was far better in the acupuncture group. The researchers concluded that in adults with neck pain, abdominal acupuncture results in significantly greater improvements in functional performance, neck pain intensity, and disability than sham abdominal acupuncture. "These findings suggest that abdominal acupuncture is an effective treatment alternative for patients with neck pain."[7]

When Acupuncture Is Combined with a Hyaluronic Acid Injection, There Is More Pain Relief from Knee Osteoarthritis

In a meta-analysis published in 2020 in *Evidence-Based Complementary and Alternative Medicine*, researchers from China compared the usefulness of acupuncture and hyaluronic acid injection versus the injection alone for people with knee osteoarthritis. The cohort consisted of 10 randomized controlled trials with a total of 998 subjects—470 men and 528 women. Of these, 501 received acupuncture therapy plus the injection, and 497 received only the injection. The researchers learned that the combination therapy was more effective than the injection alone. In fact, it significantly reduced pain more than the hyaluronic injection. Yet, the researchers underscored the fact that there was a great deal of heterogeneity among the included trials, and many had poor methodology. They also concluded that there is a need for better-designed trials with larger sample sizes in order to "overcome the limitations of the current study."[8]

Acupuncture May Help Women with the Pain Associated with Endometriosis

In a randomized clinical trial published in 2016 in *Complementary Therapies in Clinical Practice*, researchers from Brazil wanted to learn if acupuncture could help women with the problems, including pain, associated with endometriosis, or the presence of endometrial tissue outside the cavity of the uterus. The cohort consisted of 42 women with a positive diagnosis of endometriosis; they were divided into two groups. The women in one group received actual acupuncture therapy, and the women in the other group received placebo therapy—the needles were inserted 3 cm apart from the energy points. Both groups had five therapy sessions, each lasting an average of 40 minutes. When the intervention ended, the women in both groups had decreased chronic pelvic pain and dyspareunia. Yet, two months after the intervention ended, only the women in the actual acupuncture group continue to experience the improvements. The researchers concluded that "acupuncture confers beneficial and long-lasting effects, even 2 months after therapy."[9]

In a systematic review and meta-analysis published in 2017 in *PLoS ONE*, researchers from China and Gainesville, Florida (USA), evaluated 10 randomized controlled trials with 589 participants on the ability of acupuncture to relieve the pain associated with endometriosis. All of the studies were small; sample sizes ranged from 8 to 36 subjects per arm. At enrollment, the subjects were between 13 and 52 years of age. Nine of the trials were conducted in China; one took place in Boston, Massachusetts (USA). In all of the trials, the interventions were acupuncture, and the control interventions were placebo, Western medicine, and traditional Chinese medicine. The primary goal of the researchers was to assess the changes in pelvic pain not associated with menses or sexual activity. The researchers learned that acupuncture relieved endometriosis pain better than the other methods. Still, the researchers underscored the need for more studies. "To confirm this finding, additional studies with proper controls, blinding methods, and adequate sample sizes are needed."[10]

Acupuncture May Help People with Fibromyalgia

In a trial published in 2018 in the journal *Pain Medicine*, researchers from Portland, Oregon (USA), compared the use of group acupuncture to group education to treat subjects with fibromyalgia. (Fibromyalgia is a multisymptomatic disorder characterized by chronic widespread pain, fatigue, sleep and balance issues, cognitive impairment, depression, and anxiety.) The researchers, who worked at an academic health center in Portland, recruited 30 women with a mean age of 54 years who had moderate to severe levels of pain from fibromyalgia. Seventy-eight percent of the women reported having symptoms for more than 10 years. The women were then divided into two groups. Over a course of 10 weeks, the women in the acupuncture group ($n = 16$) received 20 treatments of group acupuncture for a total of 810 minutes; the women in the education group ($n = 14$) received group education over 10 weeks for a total of 861 minutes. There was a one-month post-treatment follow-up for both groups. Assessments were made at baseline, five weeks, 10 weeks, and during the follow-up. One subject in the acupuncture arm and two in the education arm did not complete the trial. The researchers found that the subjects in the acupuncture group experienced a statistically and clinically significant reduction in pain. Though the education group was taught by an experienced fibromyalgia researcher, the subjects in this group did not have similar improvements. The researchers concluded that people with fibromyalgia "who are otherwise not obtaining relief from the most common symptoms" should try acupuncture.[11]

Acupuncture and Reflexology May Help People Dealing with Chemotherapy-Induced Peripheral Neuropathy from Breast Cancer Treatment

In a retrospective analysis published in 2017 in the journal *Integrative Cancer Therapies*, researchers from Israel evaluated the ability of acupuncture and reflexology to help people dealing with chemotherapy-induced peripheral neuropathy from breast cancer treatment. The researchers began by reviewing the records of 30 consecutive female breast cancer patients who had received chemotherapy and also received acupuncture and reflexology treatments for chemotherapy-induced peripheral neuropathy. As the records of two patients were incomplete, the cohort had 28 patients. Twenty patients had sensory neuropathy, seven had motor neuropathy, and one had both sensory and motor neuropathy. Their median age was 44 years. The protocol included one to two weekly sessions of 20 minutes of acupuncture and 30 to 40 minutes of reflexology. No one experienced side effects from the acupuncture or reflexology. Periodic assessments were conducted, and only two subjects were still symptomatic at a 12-month evaluation. The researchers concluded that "the high rate of complete symptom resolution, long duration of response, and tolerability of the protocol, as reflected by the high completion rate, attest to the possible role of a joint protocol of acupuncture and reflexology in the treatment of CIPN [chemotherapy-induced peripheral neuropathy]."[12]

NOTES

1. Vickers, Andrew J., Emily A. Vertosick, George Lewith, et al. "Acupuncture for Chronic Pain: Update of an Individual Patient Data Meta-Analysis." *The Journal of Pain* 19, no. 5 (May 2018): 455–474.

2. Liu, Lizhou, Margot Skinner, Suzanne McDonough, et al. "Acupuncture for Low Back Pain: An Overview of Systematic Reviews." *Evidence-Based Complementary and Alternative Medicine* 2015 (2015): Article ID 328196.

3. Kizhakkeveettil, A., K. A. Rose, G. E. Kadar, and E. L. Hurwitz. "Integrative Acupuncture and Spinal Manipulative Therapy versus Either Alone for Low Back Pain: A Randomized Controlled Trial Feasibility Study." *Journal of Manipulative and Physiological Therapeutics* 40, no. 3 (March–April 2017): 201–213.

4. Makary, M. M., J. Lee, E. Lee, et al. "Phantom Acupuncture Induces Placebo Credibility and Vicarious Sensations: A Parallel fMRI Study of Low Back Pain Patients." *Scientific Reports* 8, no. 1 (January 17, 2018): 930–951.

5. Shetty, Geetha B., Balakrishna Shetty, and A. Mooventhan. "Efficacy of Acupuncture in the Management of Primary Dysmenorrhea: A Randomized Controlled Trial." *Journal of Acupuncture and Meridian Studies* 11, no. 4 (2018): 153–158.

6. Smith, C. A., M. Armour, X. Zhu, et al. "Acupuncture for Dysmenorrhoea." *Cochrane Database of Systematic Reviews* 18, no. 4 (April 2016): CD007854.

7. Ho, Lai Fun, Zhi Xiu Lin, Albert Wing Nang Leung, et al. "Efficacy of Abdominal Acupuncture for Neck Pain: A Randomized Controlled Trial." *PLoS ONE* 12, no. 7 (2017): e0181360.

8. Zheng, Yang, Xiangdong Duan, Shangfeng Qi, et al. "Acupuncture Therapy Plus Hyaluronic Acid Injection for Knee Osteoarthritis: A Meta-Analysis of Randomized Controlled Trials." *Evidence-Based Complementary and Alternative Medicine* 2020 (2020): Article ID 4034105.

9. de Sousa, T. R., B. C. de Sousa, K. Zomkowisk, et al. "The Effect of Acupuncture on Pain, Dyspareunia, and Quality of Life in Brazilian Women with Endometriosis: A Randomized Clinical Trial." *Complementary Therapies in Clinical Practice* 25 (2016): 114–121.

10. Xu, Yang, Wenli Zhao, Te Li, et al. "Effects of Acupuncture for the Treatment of Endometriosis-Related Pain: A Systematic Review and Meta-Analysis." *PLoS ONE* 12, no. 10 (2017): e0186616.

11. Mist, Scott D., and Kim Dupree Jones. "Randomized Controlled Trial of Acupuncture for Women with Fibromyalgia: Group Acupuncture with Traditional Chinese Medicine Diagnosis-Based Point Selection." *Pain Medicine* 19 (2018): 1862–1871.

12. Ben-Horin, Idan, Peretz Kahan, Larisa Ryvo, et al. "Acupuncture and Reflexology for Chemotherapy-Induced Peripheral Neuropathy in Breast Cancer." *Integrative Cancer Therapies* 16, no. 3 (2017): 258–262.

REFERENCES AND FURTHER READINGS

Ben-Horin, Idan, Peretz Kahan, Larisa Ryvo, et al. "Acupuncture and reflexology for Chemotherapy-Induced Peripheral Neuropathy in Breast Cancer." *Integrative Cancer Therapies* 16, no. 3 (2017): 258–262.

de Sousa, T. R., B. C. de Souza, Kamilla Zomkowisk, et al. "The Effect of Acupuncture on Pain, Dyspareunia, and Quality of Life in Brazilian Women with Endometriosis: A Randomized Clinical Trial." *Complementary Therapies in Clinical Practice* 25 (2016): 114–121.

Ho, Lai Fun, Zhi Xiu Lin, Albert Wing Nang Leung, et al. "Efficacy of Abdominal Acupuncture for Neck Pain: A Randomized Controlled Trial." *PLoS ONE* 12, no. 7 (2017): e0181360.

Kizhakkeveettil, A., K. A. Rose, G. E. Kadar, and E. L. Hurwitz. "Integrative Acupuncture and Spinal Manipulative Therapy versus Either Alone for Low Back Pain: A Randomized Controlled Trial Feasibility Study." *Journal of Manipulative and Physiological Therapeutics* 40, no. 3 (March–April 2017): 201–213.

Liu, Lizhou, Margot Skinner, Suzanne McDonough, et al. "Acupuncture for Low Back Pain: An Overview of Systematic Reviews." *Evidence-Based Complementary and Alternative Medicine* 2015 (2015): Article ID 328196.

Makary, M. M., J. Lee, E. Lee, et al. "Phantom Acupuncture Induces Placebo Credibility and Vicarious Sensations: A Parallel fMRI Study of Low Back Pain Patients." *Scientific Reports* 8, no. 1 (January 17, 2018): 930–951.

Mist, Scott D., and Kim Dupree Jones. "Randomized Controlled Trial of Acupuncture for Women with Fibromyalgia: Group Acupuncture with Traditional Chinese Medicine Diagnosis-Based Point Selection." *Pain Medicine* 19 (2018): 1862–1871.

Shetty, Geetha B., Balakrishna Shetty, and A. Mooventhan. "Efficacy of Acupuncture in the Management of Primary Dysmenorrhea: A Randomized Controlled Trial." *Journal of Acupuncture and Meridian Studies* 11, no. 4 (2018): 153–158.

Smith, C. A., M. Armour, X. Zhu, et al. "Acupuncture for Dysmenorrhoea." *Cochrane Database of Systematic Reviews* 18, no. 4 (April 2016): CD007854.

Vickers, Andrew J., Emily A. Vertosick, George Lewith, et al. "Acupuncture for Chronic Pain: Update of an Individual Patient Data Meta-Analysis." *The Journal of Pain* 19, no. 5 (My 2018): 455–474.

Xu, Yang, Wenli Zhao, Te Li, et al. "Effects of Acupuncture for the Treatment of Endometriosis-Related Pain: A Systematic Review and Meta-Analysis." *PLoS ONE* 12, no. 10 (2017): e0186616.

Yeganeh, Mohsen, Hamid Reza Baradaran, Mostafa Qorbani, et al. "The Effectiveness of Acupuncture, Acupressure, and Chiropractic Interventions on Treatment of Chronic Nonspecific Low Back Pain in Iran: A Systematic Review and Meta-Analysis." *Complementary Therapies in Clinical Practice* 27 (2017): 11–18.

Zheng, Yang, Xiangdong Duan, Shangfeng Qi, et al. "Acupuncture Therapy Plus Hyaluronic Acid Injection for Knee Osteoarthritis: A Meta-Analysis of Randomized Controlled Trials." *Evidence-Based Complementary and Alternative Medicine* 2020 (2020): Article ID 4034105.

Aromatherapy

INTRODUCTION

Aromatherapy is the use of essential oils from plants as a therapy to improve a physical, mental, or spiritual concern. Essential oils are the fragrant part of plants, often found under the surface of leaves, bark, or peel. The fragrance is released when the plant is crushed or a special steam process is used. Aromatherapy, which has been practiced for thousands of years, may be used in conjunction with other medical treatments, such as massage and acupuncture, or it may be used alone.

In most cases, essential oils should not be ingested; they may damage the liver or kidneys or interact with other medications. On the other hand, they may be massaged onto the skin, topically applied, or inhaled. When essential oils are massaged onto the skin or applied topically, they are absorbed into the body through the skin. Because they are so strong, essential oils must be combined with a carrier oil, such as sweet almond oil or olive oil, before they are massaged or applied. In general, a few drops of essential oils are added to an ounce of carrier oil. Using a diffuser containing spray, essential oils may evaporate into the air. The molecules then enter the nose or mouth and pass to the lungs and other parts of the body, especially the brain.

Essential oils are very concentrated. For example, it takes about 220 pounds of lavender flowers to make one pound of essential oil.

The National Association of Holistic Aromatherapy is the primary aromatherapy organization in the United States. Based in Seattle, Washington, it has about 4,000 members, most of whom are not licensed health professionals. Almost any health professional or para-health professional may study aromatherapy and include it in a workplace setting. The global market for all types of aromatherapy is huge; it is valued at well over one billion dollars.

ADMINISTRATION AND REGULATION

A visit to an aromatherapy provider will most likely begin with a history that includes questions about dietary intake and lifestyle. In addition to training in aromatherapy, the provider may well be licensed in another profession. For example, the aromatherapy provider may be a medical professional, such as a physician, nurse, physical therapist, or pharmacist; a complementary provider, such as an acupuncturist, naturopathic, or chiropractor; or a professional who integrates aromatherapy into an existing practice of massage therapy, Asian bodywork, esthetics, or herbal medicine. Practitioners may recommend a single or blended oil. The cost of aromatherapy varies widely, most notably by location and by the type of practitioner. In all probability, the costs associated with aromatherapy will not be covered by health insurance. However, it may be indirectly covered. For example, an insurer may pay for massage therapy, and if aromatherapy is used during the massage, then the insurer is paying for the service.

Aromatherapy providers tend to work in offices, spas, sports fitness facilities, and clinical settings. There are also a host of different online sites for obtaining aromatherapy information. For additional information, check the website of the National Association of Holistic Aromatherapy. Click onto their section on education.

The field of aromatherapy and aromatherapy training programs are currently unregulated and unlicensed. In addition, the Food and Drug Administration (FDA) does not control essential oils. As long as essential oils do not claim to treat a specific illness, the Food and Drug Administration is not involved in any essential oil administration.

Many individuals select their own essential oils, buying them online or in stores, and treat themselves at home. In these cases, people may know very little about essential oils, or the oils may be obtained from unreliable sources. This increases the potential for harm.

BENEFITS AND RISKS

A number of essential oils have been associated with pain reduction. Basil essential oil and lavender essential oil may relieve headaches and migraines. Lavender essential oil may reduce pain for people with osteoarthritis of the knee and reduce the pain of kidney stones. Black poppy essential oil is thought to be useful for muscle pains and bruises. When combined with ginger essential oil, it may reduce arthritis pain and improve flexibility. Peppermint essential oil is believed to reduce arthritis and knee pain. Marjoram essential oil is said to help low back pain and arthritis. Geranium essential oil has been found to reduce neuropathic pain. Clary sage essential oil and Roman essential oil are thought to reduce pain. Black pepper essential oil may relieve arthritis pain. Lemongrass essential oil may be useful for muscle pain. Black clove essential oil is a topical analgesic that is frequently used for toothaches. And rosemary essential oil may prevent muscle spasms.

In most cases, the highest potential for risk occurs when essential oils are ingested, which they may be in some formulations. Still, when combined with medications, the chemical compounds in essential oils may produce adverse effects. Likewise, essential oils may reduce the effectiveness of conventional medications or exacerbate health conditions. People who have allergies, hay fever, asthma, or skins conditions such as eczema or psoriasis should use all essential oils with extra care. People who have high blood pressure or epilepsy may be told to use extreme care or avoid essential oils. Side effects of essential oils include nausea, headaches, or allergic reactions. During the first trimester of pregnancy, aromatherapy may be a risk for the developing fetus.

RESEARCH FINDINGS

Aromatherapy Seems to Be Useful for Various Types of Pain

In a systematic review and meta-analysis published in 2016 in the journal *Pain Research and Treatment*, researchers from Los Angeles, California, Colton, California, and Cleveland, Ohio (USA), examined 12 studies, with 1,019 subjects, in which aromatherapy was used for pain management. All of the studies were published in English and measured pain on a visual analog scale (VAS). The studies included many types of pain, such as inflammatory pain, acute and chronic pain, postoperative pain, and obstetrical and gynecological pain. For each study, the researchers calculated the standardized mean difference of VAS pain between the treatment and control groups. The researchers learned that the reduction of pain experienced by subjects in the aromatherapy groups was statistically significant. The researchers concluded that their findings demonstrated "that aromatherapy should be considered a safe addition to current pain management procedures as no adverse effects were reported in any of the included studies."[1]

Aromatherapy Massage Appears Useful for Neuropathic Pain in People with Diabetes

In an open-label, randomized, controlled clinical trial published in the *Journal of Nursing Scholarship*, researchers from Turkey examined the ability of aromatherapy massage to help people with diabetes who suffer from neuropathic pain. The trial, which included 46 patients, was conducted in a university hospital endocrine outpatient clinic in Ankara, Turkey. The intervention group had 21 subjects, and the control group had 25; the mean ages of the patients in the intervention and control groups were 54.3 years and 57.2 years, respectively. The majority of the patients were female, and most of the patients in both groups were not receiving any treatment for their neuropathic pain. For four weeks, the subjects in the intervention group had aromatherapy massages three times per week. Data were collected during face-to-face interviews with the patients. The researchers learned that by the fourth week, the subjects in the intervention group experienced significant decreases in their neuropathic pain scores and improvements in their quality-of-life scores. However, since there was no follow-up, the researchers did not determine if the improvement was sustained over a period of time. Still, they concluded that "aromatherapy massage is a simple and effective nonpharmacological nursing intervention that can be used to manage neuropathic pain and improve QoL [quality of life] in patients with painful neuropathy."[2]

Geranium Aromatherapy Massage Seems to Help Premenstrual Syndrome

In a trial published in 2018 in the *International Journal of Preventive Medicine*, researchers from Iran evaluated the use of geranium aromatherapy massage for premenstrual syndrome. One hundred and twenty female university students (between 18 and 29 years) with premenstrual syndrome were randomly divided into three groups of 40: an aromatherapy massage group, a massage group, and a control group (no treatment). In the aromatherapy massage group, each female performed aromatherapy massage on herself for 30 minutes per week for 8 weeks. They used geranium 2 percent essential oil in almond carrier oil. In the massage alone group, the subjects performed massage with a sweet almond oil (placebo) for 30 minutes per week for eight weeks. The massages were performed using the effleurage technique in which there are circular strokes; each massage of the abdomen and arm regions used 8 ml of oil. The final analyses were conducted on 115 subjects. The aromatherapy massage group had 37 subjects, the massage group had 38 subjects, and the control group had 40 subjects. The researchers found that the geranium aromatherapy massage worked better at reducing premenstrual syndrome than the massage alone or the control. They concluded that "geranium aromatherapy massage is recommended for improving PMS symptoms as a complementary, low-cost, and noninvasive treatment."[3]

Aromatherapy Seems to Be Useful for Women Dealing with Primary Dysmenorrhea

In a meta-analysis published in 2017 in the journal *Complementary Therapies in Clinical Practice*, researchers from Turkey investigated the ability of aromatherapy to relieve the symptoms associated with primary dysmenorrhea, especially pain. The researchers found six randomized controlled trials with 362 subjects who met their criteria. In these trials, there were 184 subjects who had abdominal aromatherapy massage and 178 who were massaged with placebo oils. In five of the six trials, lavender essential oil was used, and lavender oil was found to have a pain-reducing effect in primary dysmenorrhea. However, lavender oil was mixed with another oil in three of the trials. When that occurred, the pain-reducing effect of the lavender oil was diminished. The researchers also found that aromatherapy massage with only lavender oil was superior to aromatherapy massage with only *Rosa damascene*. Furthermore, they concluded that "abdominal massage with essential oils is an effective complementary way to relieve pain in primary dysmenorrhea."[4]

In a systematic review and meta-analysis published in 2018 in the *Journal of Clinical Medicine*, researchers from Korea and Saud Arabia also examined the use of aromatherapy for primary dysmenorrhea. Their cohort consisted of 19 randomized controlled trials and quasi-randomized controlled trials. The trials, which originated from Iran, Korea, Turkey, Egypt, and Taiwan, almost exclusively tested inhalation and massage aromatherapy. Fifteen used a parallel design, and four employed a crossover design; all of the trials had a moderate risk of bias. In the two trials that assessed adverse effects, no adverse effects were reported. Yet, the researchers commented that the various studies had a lack of a standardized treatment, and there was extensive heterogeneity in ingredients, dose, and delivery methods between the trials. Still, the researchers determined that compared to the placebos, the trials found that aromatherapy offered "superior" treatment for the pain associated with primary dysmenorrhea. A subanalysis of inhalation aromatherapy was also found to be a "superior" treatment, whereas a subanalysis of aromatherapy massage "showed favorable effects." The researchers concluded that they found "a moderate level of evidence on the superiority of aromatherapy (inhalational, massage, or oral use) for pain reduction over placebo in primary dysmenorrhea."[5]

Aromatherapy with Rosa Damascene May Be Useful during the First Stage of Labor for Nulliparous Women

In a randomized, single-blind, clinical trial published in 2018 in the *Journal of Integrative Medicine*, researchers from Iran evaluated the ability of aromatherapy with *Rosa damascene* to help nulliparous women with the pain and anxiety associated with the first stage of labor. (A nulliparous woman has never given birth or has given birth to a child who was not able to survive outside the womb.) The initial cohort consisted of 116 women who were in labor at an Iranian maternity hospital; they were divided into two groups. The participants in the aromatherapy group received inhaled 0.08 ml of *Rosa damascene* essence every 30 minutes; the subjects in the control group received inhaled 0.08 ml of normal saline every 30 minutes. As six participants were excluded from the trial, the analyses were conducted on data from 110 women. The researchers found that during the first stage of labor, there was a significant difference in the levels of pain and anxiety between the intervention and control groups. At the same time, it had no effect on the babies' Apgar scores or the mothers' types of delivery. The researchers concluded that aromatherapy with *Rosa damascene* "is a convenient and effective method for pain and anxiety reduction during the first stage of labor."[6]

Aromatherapy May Be Useful in Reducing Labor Pain and Duration

In a meta-analysis published in 2019 in the journal *Women and Birth*, researchers from Taiwan evaluated the usefulness of aromatherapy for the pain associated with labor. The cohort consisted of 17 randomized, controlled trials in which women in labor were recruited upon arrival at a hospital. The trials were published between 2003 and 2018 and had sample sizes that ranged from 40 to 513 women. Twelve of the trials used acceptable randomization methods. Eight of the trials were single-blind, one was double-blind, one was without blinding, and seven had unclear blinding. In most of the trials, there was no loss to follow-up. The researchers learned that aromatherapy reduced labor pain during the dilation transition phase of the first stage of labor. In addition, aromatherapy reduced the duration of the second and third stages of labor, with a trend toward significance in the second stage. Still, while aromatherapy appears to be useful for labor, the researchers cautioned that it is still unclear "whether aromatherapy should be promoted as a major pain strategy" to help women cope with labor pain.[7]

Aromatherapy Seems to Be Useful for Knee Osteoarthritis

In a randomized, controlled trial published in 2019 in the *Japan Journal of Nursing Science*, researchers from Turkey evaluated the effects of aromatherapy massage on pain, function, and quality of life of elders with knee osteoarthritis. The cohort, which consisted of 90 elders, who resided in two nursing facilities in Bursa, Turkey, was divided into an aromatherapy massage group, a basic massage group, and a control group. (There was no difference in age, gender, education level, body mass index, and disease duration between the groups.) The subjects in both massage groups received a total of six massage sessions, twice a week for three weeks. In the aromatherapy group, the massages were performed using aromatic oils; in the basic massage group, the subjects were massaged with sunflower oil. The subjects in the control group had no massages. The main essential oils used were black seed oil, ginger, and rosemary. The researchers learned that aromatherapy massage improved pain and other problems associated with knee osteoarthritis in elders better than the basic massage. The researchers concluded that "aromatherapy massage performed in elderly patients with knee osteoarthritis reduced pain and improved functional status and quality of life."[8]

People with Neck Pain May Be Helped by Aromatherapy

In a trial published in 2014 in the *Journal of Alternative and Complementary Medicine*, researchers from Taiwan wanted to assess the efficacy of aromatherapy for neck pain. The cohort consisted of 60 subjects with a history of neck pain; 30 were randomly assigned to the intervention, and 30 were randomly assigned to the control group. For the intervention group, four essential oils—marjoram, black pepper, lavender, and peppermint—were mixed together and then mixed with an unscented cream. Each day, for four weeks, after showering or bathing, the subjects in the intervention group applied two teaspoons of the cream to the neck and upper trapezius muscles until fully absorbed. The subjects in the control group applied a cream without essential oils. The trial used four clinical and scientific assessments to evaluate the ability of aromatherapy to ease neck pain. At the end of the trial, the researchers observed that the intervention group had significant reductions in neck pain symptoms and increased range of motion. And, the researchers concluded that "essential oil cream may alleviate neck pain, improve neck range of motion, and be simply and conveniently self-applied."[9]

Aromatherapy Adverse Effects Do Not Appear to Be Uncommon

In a systematic review published in 2012 in the *International Journal of Risk & Safety in Medicine*, researchers from the United Kingdom evaluated evidence of adverse effects associated with aromatherapy. Forty-two primary reports, with 71 patients, met the inclusion criteria of the researchers. Whereas some of the articles were from the United States, scores of others were from countries throughout the world, including the United Kingdom, Australia, Germany, India, Italy, Austria, Canada, Belgium, France, New Zealand, and Turkey. Most often, the aromatherapy was applied to the skin. Adverse effects ranged from mild to severe; the subjects usually had a complete recovery, but there was one fatality. The duration of adverse effects ranged from 48 hours to one year. Six subjects required hospitalization, and in two cases, skin grafts were needed. Oral and topical steroids were the most common treatments. The most frequent adverse effects were skin irritation and dermatitis, and lavender, peppermint, tea tree oil, bergamot, laurel, and ylang-ylang were the essential oils that were most often responsible for problems. Because of these adverse effects, it is important to weigh the benefits of aromatherapy against the risks; the researchers commented that "it is questionable whether the benefits of aromatherapy outweigh the risks."[10]

There May Be Additional Problems with Aromatherapy

In an article published in 2016 in the journal *Dermatitis*, a dermatologist and medical student from Wisconsin (USA) outlined additional problems that may be associated with the use of essential oils. Aromatherapy products are used and sold in widely disparate settings, such as offices, salons, spas, markets, and hospitals; they are ubiquitous and available in a wide variety of online sites. At the same time, the authors noted that far more people are sensitive to essential oils than most people realize. For example, a study conducted in Germany found that slightly more than 4 percent of people who were tested reacted to at least one essential oil. Hence, people who are sensitive to essential oils may be unaware that they are being exposed to these products. Moreover, topically applied essential oils have repeatedly been identified as the cause of allergic contact dermatitis and photosensitization. In addition, the authors underscored the fact that essential oils "are under no formal regulation or standardization process." As a result, there is no way to ensure a consistent product. Also, as has been previously noted, the FDA does not play a role in the administration or control of aromatherapy. Conversely, within the European Union, "the quality of the herbal medicinal product must always be demonstrated." The dermatologist and medical student concluded that in the United States, "the perceived benignity of the botanical derived products may in fact be a misconception."[11]

NOTES

1. Lakhan, Shaheen E., Heather Sheafer, and Deborah Tepper. "The Effectiveness of Aromatherapy in Reducing Pain: A Systematic Review and Meta-Analysis." *Pain Research and Treatment* 2016 (2016): Article ID 8158693.

2. Gök Metin, Zehra, Ayse Arikan Donmez, Nur Izgu, et al. "Aromatherapy Massage for Neuropathic Pain and Quality of Life in Diabetic Patients." *Journal of Nursing Scholarship* 49, no. 4 (July 2017): 379–388.

3. Lotfipur-Rafsanjani, Seyede Maryam, Ali Ravari, Zohreh Ghorashi, et al. "Effects of Geranium Aromatherapy Massage on Premenstrual Syndrome: A Clinical Trial." *International Journal of Preventive Medicine* 9 (2018): 98–101.

4. Sut, Necdet, and Hatice Kahyaoglu-Sut. "Effect of Aromatherapy Massage on Pain in Primary Dysmenorrhea: A Meta-Analysis." *Complementary Therapies in Clinical Practice* 27 (2017): 5–10.

5. Lee, Myeong Soo, Hye Won Lee, Mohammed Khalil, et al. "Aromatherapy for Managing Pain in Primary Dysmenorrhea: A Systematic Review of Randomized Placebo-Controlled Trials." *Journal of Clinical Medicine* 7 (2018): 434–447.

6. Hamdamian, Sepideh, Soheila Nazarpour, Masoumeh Simbar, et al. "Effects of Aromatherapy with *Rosa damascena* on Nulliparous Women's Pain and Anxiety During First Stage of Labor." *Journal of Integrative Medicine* 16, no. 2 (March 2018): 120–125.

7. Chen, Shuo-Fei, Chia-Hui Wang, Pi-Tuan Chan, et al. "Labour Pain Control by Aromatherapy: A Mea-Analysis of Randomised Controlled Trials." *Women and Birth* 32 (2019): 327–335.

8. Pehlivan, Seda, and Ayfer Karadakovan. "Effects of Aromatherapy Massage on Pain, Functional State, and Quality of Life in an Elderly Individual with Knee Osteoarthritis." *Japan Journal of Nursing Science* 16, no. 4 (October 2019): 450–458.

9. Ou, Ming-Chiu, Yu-Fei Lee, Chih-Ching Li, and Shyi-Kuen Wu. "The Effectiveness of Essential Oils for Patients with Neck Pain: A Randomized Controlled Study." *Journal of Alternative and Complementary Medicine* 20, no. 10 (October 2014): 771–779.

10. Posadzki, Paul, Amani Alotaibi, and Edzard Ernst. "Adverse Effects of Aromatherapy: A Systematic Review of Case Reports and Case Series." *International Journal of Risk & Safety Medicine* 24, no. 3 (2012): 147–161.

11. Mortimer, Sarah, and Margo Reeder. "Botanicals in Dermatology: Essential Oils, Botanical Allergens, and Current Regulatory Practices." *Dermatitis* 27, no. 6 (November–December 2016): 317–324.

REFERENCES AND FURTHER READINGS

Chen, Shuo-Fei, Chia-Hui Wang, Pi-Tuan Chan, et al. "Labour Pain Control by Aromatherapy: A Meta-Analysis of Randomised Controlled Trials." *Women and Birth* 32 (2019): 327–335.

Gök Metin, Zehra, Ayse Arikan Donmez, Nur Izgu, et al. "Aromatherapy Massage for Neuropathic Pain and Quality of Life in Diabetic Patients." *Journal of Nursing Scholarship* 49, no. 4 (July 2017): 379–388.

Hamdamian, Sepideh, Soheila Nazarpour, Masoumeh Simbar, et al. "Effects of Aromatherapy with *Rosa damascena* on Nulliparous Women's Pain and Anxiety of Labor during First Stage of Labor." *Journal of Integrative Medicine* 16, no. 2 (March 2018): 120–125.

Lakhan, Shaheen E., Heather Sheafer, and Deborah Tepper. "The Effectiveness of Aromatherapy in Reducing Pain: A Systematic Review and Meta-Analysis." *Pain Research and Treatment* 2016 (2016): Article ID 8158693.

Lee, Myeong Soo, Hye Won Lee, Mohamed Khalil, et al. "Aromatherapy for Managing Pain in Primary Dysmenorrhea: A Systematic Review of Randomized Placebo-Controlled Trials." *Journal of Clinical Medicine* 7, no. 11 (2018): 434–447.

Lotfipur-Rafsanjani, Seyede Maryam, Ali Ravari, Zohreh Ghorashi, et al. "Effects of Geranium Aromatherapy Massage on Premenstrual Syndrome: A Clinical Trial." *International Journal of Preventive Medicine* 9 (2018): 98–101.

Mortimer, Sarah, and Margo Reeder. "Botanicals in Dermatology: Essential Oils, Botanical Allergens, and Current Regulatory Practices." *Dermatitis* 27, no. 6 (November–December 2016): 317–324.

Ou, Ming-Chiu, Yu-Fei Lee, Chih-Ching Li, and Shyi-Kuen Wu. "The Effectiveness of Essential Oils for Patients with Neck Pain: A Randomized Controlled Study." *Journal of Alternative and Complementary Medicine* 20, no. 10 (October 2014): 771–779.

Pehlivan, Seda, and Ayfer Karadakovan. "Effects of Aromatherapy Massage on Pain, Functional State, and Quality of Life in an Elderly Individual with Knee Osteoarthritis." *Japan Journal of Nursing Science* 16, no. 4 (October 2019): 450–458.

Posadzki, Paul, Amani Alotaibi, and Edzard Ernst. "Adverse Effects of Aromatherapy: A Systematic Review of Case Reports and Case Series." *International Journal of Risk & Safety in Medicine* 24 (2012): 147–161.

Sut, Necdet, and Hatice Kahyaoglu-Sut. "Effect of Aromatherapy Massage on Pain in Primary Dysmenorrhea: A Mata-Analysis." *Complementary Therapies in Clinical Practice* 27 (2017): 5–10.

Botox Injections

INTRODUCTION

Although Botox injections are primarily known for their ability to reduce facial wrinkles, especially in the forehead and around the eyes, they have been used successfully to lower levels of several types of pain. Botox injections use a toxin called onobotulinumtoxinA; it temporarily prevents a muscle from contracting, forcing the muscle to relax. OnobotulinumtoxinA is produced by the microbe that causes botulism, a type of food poisoning.

Specifically, Botox blocks the release of a substance called acetylcholine from the junction between a nerve and muscle. Normally, acetylcholine binds to its receptor at this junction and causes a muscle contraction. When Botox is injected to an area of chronic muscle spasm, acetylcholine is blocked, allowing the muscle to relax.

Botox was originally approved by the FDA in 1989 to treat severe muscle contractions caused by cervical dystonia. It was the first drug to use botulinum toxin. There are now other products, such as abobotulinumtoxinA (Dysport), rimabotlinumtoxinB (Myobloc), and incobotulinumtoxinA (Xeomin). They are each a little different from one another, and the dosages vary; they are not interchangeable.

While the use of Botox injections for cosmetic purposes is somewhat common, it is not clear how often Botox is incorporated into pain treatment. In addition, it is not known how many physicians have added Botox injections to their arsenal of pain treatments.

ADMINISTRATION AND REGULATION

Normally, Botox injections are administered in a physician's office. Most people feel no or very little discomfort from the procedure. However, some people request that their skin be numbed with topical anesthesia, ice, or vibration anesthesia, which uses massage, before the injections. Physicians use very tiny needles to inject very small amounts of Botox. The method, dosage, and frequency of injections are a function of the needs of the individual patient.

Botox injections for pain may or may not be covered by insurance. As Botox injections are not typical treatments for pain, at best, there may be partial coverage. If cost is an issue, before scheduling an appointment, check with your insurance provider. Insurers may also require that people suffering from various types of pain first try less expensive therapies. Botox injections for pain tend to be costly, especially if they are given over an extended period of time.

Botox injections may only be legally administered by licensed medical professionals. In order to perform this procedure, medical professionals must take and pass a Botox certification course.

Typically, Botox injections begin working about one to three days after treatment, but results may take as long as a week. Improvements should continue for three months or longer. Then the muscles will tend to become overactive, and more injections will probably be needed to achieve pain relief. That is why it is usually recommended to schedule injections four times a year.

BENEFITS AND RISKS

There are reports that Botox injections have successfully treated many conditions, including chronic back pain, chronic pelvic pain, osteoarthritis, rheumatoid arthritis, psoriatic arthritis, myofascial pain, and nerve pain. They appear to reduce the incidence of chronic migraines in people who experience this debilitating condition more than 15 days per month. Moreover, Botox injections may be useful for the previously noted cervical dystonia, a condition in which the neck muscles contract involuntarily, causing the head to twist or turn into an uncomfortable position.

When performed by an experienced physician, Botox injections are considered relatively safe. Still, because the doses used for pain are higher than those used for cosmetic purposes, there are some possible side effects and complications. These include pain, swelling or bruising at the injection site, muscle weakness, nausea, indigestion, and headache or flu-like symptoms. In rare instances, the toxin may spread in the body, which is a potential medical emergency. Symptoms of spread include muscle weakness, vision problems, trouble speaking or swallowing, breathing problems, and loss of bladder control. To help prevent the spread of Botox, do not rub or massage the treated area for 24 hours. Women who are pregnant or breastfeeding should avoid Botox injections, as should people who are allergic to cow's milk. Before having Botox injections, people who take muscle relaxants, sleeping aids, or allergy medications should share their medical history with their physician.

RESEARCH FINDINGS

Botox Injections Appear to Be Useful for Chronic Migraines

In an open-label, single-arm, prospective, five-headache-center clinical trial published in 2016 in *The Journal of Headache and Pain*, researchers from Greece tested the ability of Botox injections to help people dealing with chronic migraines. The researchers hoped to determine if Botox injections changed the mean number of monthly headache days, the severity of the headaches, and the use of medication. The cohort consisted of 119 subjects who had chronic migraines. All of the subjects were told to stop taking their oral migraine medication at least three months prior to study entry, and all the subjects were treated with Botox injections. The researchers planned to administer at least three courses of Botox injections to each subject. Eighty-one subjects completed the trial; there were 73 females and 8 males with a mean age of 43.5 years. The researchers learned that the subjects experienced significant improvement in all efficacy variables after three sessions or nine months of Botox injections. Between the first and third treatments, they had significant decreases in the mean headache days per month, significant decreases in days with peak intensity, and a significant change in the days that they used headache medication per month. There were few adverse effects, and none was serious. The researchers concluded that treatment with Botox injections "proved effective, safe and well tolerated in our setting."[1]

In a systematic review published in 2018 in the *Cochrane Database of Systematic Reviews*, researchers from the United Kingdom compared the use of Botox injections, active treatments, and placebos for the prevention or reduction in chronic and episodic migraines in adults. The researchers located 90 randomized, double-blind, controlled articles describing 28 trials that met their inclusion criteria. Twenty-one of the trials had fewer than 50 subjects per arm; 23 of the trials compared the use of Botox injections to a placebo. The researchers found that in chronic migraines, the injections reduced the number of migraine days per month by two days. Nonserious adverse effects appeared to be experienced by 60 out of every 100 subjects in the Botox group compared with 47 out of every 100 in the placebo group. The researchers were unable to determine if the injections were useful for episodic migraines; the quality of the limited evidence was very low. In the trials that compared Botox to other oral prophylactic medications for chronic or episodic migraines, there did not appear to be any differences in efficacy measures between the groups. The researchers concluded that "better reporting of outcome measures in published trials would provide a more complete evidence base on which to draw conclusions."[2]

The results of the Chronic Migraine OnabotulinumtoxinA Prolonged Efficacy Open Label (COMPEL) study were published in 2018 in the *Journal of Headache and Pain.* In this international, 35-center, prospective trial, researchers from Carlsbad, California and Irvine, California, Greensboro, North Carolina (USA), and Australia wanted to learn if Botox injections would help people dealing with chronic migraine headaches. The trial duration was 112 weeks and included a four-week baseline period and a 108-week open-label treatment intervention. During the baseline visit, demographics, medical history, headache features, and headache treatment history were recorded. There was also a physical examination. The initial cohort consisted of 716 men and women between the ages of 18 and 73 years; the mean age was 43 years. The vast majority—607 subjects—were female. At baseline, the subjects reported a mean of 22 headache days per every 28 days; of these, a mean of 18 were moderate to severe. Most of the subjects were using acute headache medications, and most of the subjects were overusing these medications. The subjects received a fixed dose of Botox injection every 12 weeks for nine treatment cycles. Slightly over half of the subjects, or 373 people, completed the trial. Assessments demonstrated that by the 24th week there was a 7.4 day reduction in headaches. By the 60th week, there was a 9.2 day reduction in headaches, and by the 108th week there was reduction of 10.7 headache days. The researchers concluded that the Botox injections were effective and well tolerated.[3]

Botox Injections Seem to Be Useful for People with Refractory Chronic Cluster Headaches

In a 28-week open-label, nonrandomized, single-center trial published in 2018 in the *Journal of Headache and Pain*, researchers from Austria noted that about 20 percent of people who suffer from cluster headaches experience recurrent attacks without periods of significant remission.

These people suffer from a medical problem known as refractory chronic cluster headaches. The cohort consisted of 17 male patients with an average age of 32 years; the men had been dealing with chronic cluster headaches for a mean of 6.6 years. The trial had a four-week pretreatment phase followed by a 24-week treatment phase. Headache frequency and duration were recorded daily. The first Botox injection was given one week after baseline, and a second injection was given during week 12. As Botox injections were administered as an add-on therapy, acute and prophylactic treatments were continued. The researchers learned that 10 of the patients received highly effective results; nine patients reported a more than 70 percent improvement in the number of minutes they experienced headaches. At week 24, the mean frequency of headache days dropped from 28.2 to 11.8. And, the intensity of attacks dropped significantly. While the researchers acknowledged that their results were "encouraging," they underscored the need for their findings to be confirmed in double-blind, randomized, controlled studies.[4]

Botox Injections May Play a Role in the Treatment of Knee Osteoarthritis

In a prospective, single-blinded, randomized, controlled clinical trial published in 2018 in the *Journal of Rehabilitation Medicine*, researchers from China and Forth Worth, Texas (USA) tested the ability of Botox injections followed by therapeutic exercise to help people dealing with knee osteoarthritis. The cohort consisted of 60 subjects with knee osteoarthritis; they ranged in age from 59 to 72 years, with a mean age of 65.9 years. The subjects were divided into three groups. The subjects in the first group received a saline injection; the subjects in the second groups received a Botox injection; and the subjects in the third group received a hyaluronate injection, a frequently employed treatment. (Hyaluronate, a major component of synovial fluid, acts as a lubricant and shock absorber.) Following injection, all the subjects participated in exercises that they performed 30 to 45 minutes per session, five times a week for eight weeks. Assessments were conducted at baseline and at the fourth and eighth week. All of the 26 males and 34 females completed the trial. The researchers found that subjects with knee osteoarthritis pain improved with both Botox and hyaluronate injections. However, Botox injections "combined with therapeutic exercises seems to be the more effective of these treatments, and [the injections] may provide clinicians with a new option for treatment of patients with knee OA [osteoarthritis]."[5]

It Is Not Clear if Botox Injections Are Useful for People with Temporomandibular Joint Disorders

In a systematic review published in 2015 in the *International Journal of Oral & Maxillofacial Surgery*, researchers from Taiwan, Boston, Massachusetts, and Baltimore, Maryland (USA), wanted to determine if Botox injections provided relief to people who suffer from temporomandibular joint disorders. The researchers included five relevant randomized controlled trials that met their criteria; these included 117 subjects with temporomandibular joint disorders. There were three parallel trials and two crossover trials. To avoid the carry-over effects of Botox injections, a washout period of at least three months was required. The subjects were most often females, and two studies included only females. The researchers found considerable variations in the study methods and several risks of bias. And there was a lack of consensus on the effects of Botox injections; it was unclear whether Botox injections had therapeutic benefits for temporomandibular joint disorders. The researchers concluded that "a more rigorous design of trials should be carried out in future studies."[6]

Botox Injections May or May Not Relieve the Pain Associated with Chronic Anal Fissures

In a retrospective trial published in 2017 in *Porto Biomedical Journal*, researchers based in Portugal evaluated the efficacy of Botox injections for the pain associated with chronic anal fissures. An anal fissure is a tear located in the distal section of the anal canal. The initial cohort consisted of 81 patients who had chronic anal fissures; they were recruited between January 2009 and December 2013. Forty-four patients were male; they had a mean age of 49.6 years. Using a numerical rating, levels of pain were assessed before treatment and four weeks after treatment. Most of the patients had previously used traditional types of treatment, such as consuming fiber products, soaking in sitz baths, and applying topical agents. None of these treatments healed the fissures. The researchers found that 23 patients (28.3%) did not respond to the Botox treatment. Of these, 19 eventually had surgery. So, while the Botox treatments helped many of the patients, a notable number did not benefit; "treatment failure in the long term is still significant."[7]

Botox Injections May Sometimes Be Useful for Chronic Functional Anorectal Pain

In an analysis published in 2019 in the journal *Techniques in Coloproctology*, researchers from the Netherlands searched their electronic database for patients who were treated between 2011 and 2016 with Botox injections for chronic functional anorectal pain. They found a total of 113 patients who met their criteria; of these, 42 percent were male. All of the injections, which were administered by four different surgeons, were given under either local or general anesthesia. Fifty-three patients had a good outcome; 23 patients had an initial good response but relapsed within three months; and 37 had a poor outcome. To achieve the good outcome, 29 patients needed only a single treatment, 11 needed a second treatment, and 13 needed three or more treatments. Although there were many people who did not receive any relief from the injections, many more did. The researchers concluded that Botox injections are "a safe and reasonably effective treatment for chronic functional anorectal pain."[8]

Botox Injections May Help People Suffering from Trigeminal Neuralgia

In a systematic review and meta-analysis published in 2016 in the *Journal of Headache and Pain*, researchers from Japan conducted an electronic search of randomized controlled trials on the use of Botox injections for trigeminal neuralgia, severe, sharp, stabbing electric shock-like pain in the face along the trigeminal nerve. (The largest of 12 cranial nerves, the main function of the trigeminal nerve is to transmit sensory information from the skin, sinuses, and mucous membranes. It also stimulates movement of jaw muscles.) The researchers located four trials with a total of 178 subjects that met their criteria. Ninety-nine of the subjects were in the Botox injections groups, and 79 were in placebo groups. Before treatment, the groups had no significant differences in their frequency of attacks and pain severity. Though there was no follow-up noted in one trial, the follow-up period in three of the trials ranged from 8 to 12 weeks. The amount of Botox injected, the route of injection, the number of injections, and the injection sites varied. The quality of the trials ranged from medium to high. The researchers learned that Botox injections were significantly better than the placebos for treating trigeminal neuralgia. When compared to placebos, the overall outcomes consistently favored Botox injections. While acknowledging that their analysis included only four trials, the researchers concluded that Botox injections may be "a promising alternative treatment option that might spare the need for surgical interventions for refractory cases of trigeminal neuralgia."[9]

Intravesical Botox Injections May Be Useful for People Dealing with Bladder Pain Syndrome/Interstitial Cystitis

In a systematic review and meta-analysis published in the journal *Medical Science Monitor*, researchers from China evaluated the usefulness of injecting Botox directly into the bladder to help people dealing with bladder pain syndrome/interstitial cystitis. The researchers found seven randomized controlled trials and one retrospective study that met their criteria; the studies had a total of 427 subjects, of whom 94 percent were female. Subjects in five of the randomized controlled trials and the retrospective study had failed to improve when they were given conventional treatments. The average follow-up time of the studies was 2.6 months, and the overall methodological quality of the included studies was moderate. One randomized controlled trial had a low risk of bias, five had a moderate risk of bias, and one had a high risk of bias. Still, the researchers determined that the Botox injections were associated with significant improvement in pelvic pain. The researchers emphasized the need for better-designed studies.[10]

Botox Injections and the More Recently Introduced Neuronox Are Equally Useful for Benign Essential Blepharospasm

In a split-face, prospective, randomized, controlled pilot trial published in 2019 in the *Korean Journal of Ophthalmology*, researchers from India tested the efficacy of Botox injections and Neuronox injections, which are structurally similar, to help people dealing with benign essential blepharospasm or the painful abnormal contractions of eye muscles. (The only difference between the two is that Botox is a vacuum-dried preparation, and Neuronox is a freeze-dried preparation.) The cohort consisted of 15 male and 9 female subjects (mean age of 52 years) with benign essential blepharospasm. All of the subjects received either Botox or Neuronox in the periorbital (around the eyes) region; the injection sites and doses were uniform. Three independent observers completed the toxin preparation, injection, and clinical evaluation. Neither the injectors nor the patients knew what was administered. Measurements were collected on several factors including improvement in the severity of the spasms. Grading was conducted at the preinjection visit and at the subsequent two-week and six-week follow-up visits. Specifically, the patients were asked which side of their face felt better than the other side. All 24 of the subjects indicated that the treatments had similar results on both sides of their faces. The researchers noted that the "drugs were equally effective."[11]

Botox Injections May Trigger Decreased Pulmonary Function

In a clinical correspondence published in 2018 in *Headache: The Journal of Head and Face Pain*, researchers from Rochester, Minnesota (USA), outlined the case of a 17-year-old female who first complained of subacute progressive headaches of the posterior head that radiated downward five years earlier, at the age of 12. According to the patient, the pain was constant and unchanging; she rated the pain 7 out of 10. In addition, upon standing, she experienced occasional double vision, nausea, and vertigo, and she reported photophobia, as well as a decline in memory recall and mental capacity. Until she turned 15, the symptoms were controlled with the medication topiramate. Then, she reported daily bifrontal headache pain that was rated 6 on a scale of 10 and "pulling rubber-band-like" pain on the right side of her face that she rated 7 out of 10. The pain started in the morning and worsened during the day. Increasing the dose of topiramate caused gastrointestinal side effects, and other medications failed to relieve the pain. Finally, her medical provider tried 24 months of Botox injections, which reduced the frequency of headaches dramatically, to once or twice a month. Moreover, the severity "decreased substantially." However, although her migraine symptoms improved, about six months after her first Botox treatment, the teen began having problems taking deep breaths of air, and she tired more easily during physically demanding activities. Pulmonary function tests revealed progressively declining pulmonary function. After the injections were discontinued, the teen experienced "mild improvement." Eight months after the injections were stopped, the researchers reported that the teen was "better able to tolerate more strenuous physical activities without respiratory fatigue."[12]

NOTES

1. Vikelis, Michail, Andreas A. Argyriou, Emmanouil V. Dermitzakis, et al. "Onabotulinumtoxin-A Treatment in Greek Patients with Chronic Migraine." *The Journal of Headache and Pain* 17 (2016): 84–88.

2. Herd, Clare P., Claire L. Tomlinson, Caroline Rick, et al. "Botulinum Toxins for the Prevention of Migraine in Adults." *Cochrane Database of Systematic Reviews* 6, no. 6 (June 25, 2018): CD011616.

3. Blumenfeld, Andrew M., Richard J. Stark, Marshall C. Freeman, et al. "Long-Term Study of the Efficacy and Safety of OnabotulinumtoxinA for the Prevention of Chronic Migraine: COMPEL Study." *The Journal of Headache and Pain* 19 (2018): 13–24.

4. Lampl, Christian, Mirjam Rudolph, and Elisabeth Bräutigam. "OnabotulinumtoxinA in the Treatment of Refractory Chronic Cluster Headache." *The Journal of Headache and Pain* 19 (2018): 45–50.

5. Bao, Xiao, Jie-Wen Tan, Michael Flyzik, et al. "Effect of Therapeutic Exercise on Knee Osteoarthritis after Intro-Articular Injection of Botulinum Toxin Type A, Hyaluronate or Saline: A Randomized Controlled Trial." *Journal of Rehabilitation Medicine* 50 (2018): 534–541.

6. Chen, Y-W., Y-W. Chiu, C-Y. Chen, and S-K. Chuang. "Botulin Toxin Therapy for Temporomandibular Joint Disorders: A Systematic Review of Randomized Controlled Trials." *International Journal of Oral & Maxillofacial Surgery* 44, no. 8 (August 2015): 1018–1026.

7. Amorim, Hugo, José Santoalha, Rui Cadilha, et al. "Botulinum Toxin Improves Pain in Chronic Anal Fissure." *Porto Biomedical Journal* 2, no. 6 (2017): 273–276.

8. Ocijevaar, R. E., R. J. F. Felt-Bersma, I. J. Han-Geurts, et al. "Botox Treatment in Patients with Chronic Functional Anorectal Pain: Experiences of a Tertiary Proctology Clinic." *Techniques in Coloproctology* 23 (2019): 239–244.

9. Morra, Mostafa Ebraheem, Ahmed Elgebaly, Ahmed Elmaraezy, et al. "Therapeutic Efficacy and Safety of Botulinum Toxin A Therapy in Trigeminal Neuralgia: A Systematic Review and Meta-Analysis of Randomized Controlled Trials." *The Journal of Headache and Pain* 17 (2016): 63–71.

10. Wang, Junpeng, Qiang Wang, Qinghui Wu, et al. "Intravesical Botulinum Toxin A Injections for Bladder Pain Syndrome/Interstitial Cystitis: A Systematic Review and Meta-Analysis of Controlled Studies." *Medical Science Monitor* 22 (2016): 3257–3267.

11. Sane, Sayali, Mohammad Javed Ali, and Milind N. Naik. "Comparison of Safety and Efficacy of Botox and Neuronox in the Management of Benign Essential Blepharospasm: A Split-Face Study." *Korean Journal of Ophthalmology* 33, no. 5 (2019): 430–435.

12. Oliver, Jeremie D., R. Paul Boesch, and Kenneth J. Mack. "Decreased Pulmonary Function during Botulinum Toxin A therapy for Chronic Migraines in a 17-Year-Old Female." *Headache: The Journal of Head and Face Pain* 58, no. 8 (September 2018): 1259–1261.

REFERENCES AND FURTHER READINGS

Amorim, Hugo, José Santoalha, Rui Cadilha, et al. "Botulinum Toxin Improves Pain in Chronic Anal Fissure." *Porto Biomedical Journal* 2, no. 6 (2017): 273–276.

Bao, Xiao, Jie-Wen Tan, Michael Flyzik, et al. "Effect of Therapeutic Exercise on Knee Osteoarthritis after Intra-Articular Injection of Botulinum Type A, Hyaluronate or Saline: A Randomized Controlled Trial." *Journal of Rehabilitation Medicine* 50 (2018): 534–541.

Blumenfeld, Andrew M., Richard J. Stark, Marshall C. Freeman, et al. "Long-Term Study of the Efficacy and Safety of OnabotulinumtoxinA for the Prevention of Chronic Migraine: COMPEL Study." *The Journal of Headache and Pain* 19 (2018): 13–24.

Chen, Y-W., Y-W. Chiu, C-Y. Chen, and S-K. Chuang. "Botulinum Toxin Therapy for Temporomandibular Joint Disorders: A Systematic Review of Randomized Controlled Trials." *International Journal of Oral & Maxillofacial Surgery* 44, no. 8 (August 2015): 1018–1026.

Herd, Clare P., Claire L. Tomlinson, Caroline Rick, et al. "Botulinum Toxins for the Prevention of Migraine in Adults." *Cochrane Database of Systematic Reviews* 6, no. 6 (June 25, 2018): CD011616.

Lampl, Christian, Mirjam Rudolph, and Elisabeth Bräutigam. "OnabotulinumtoxinA in the Treatment of Refractory Chronic Cluster Headache." *Journal of Headache and Pain* 19 (2018): 45–50.

Morra, Mostafa Ebrahem, Ahmed Elgebaly, Ahmed Elmaraezy, et al. "Therapeutic Efficacy and Safety of Botulinum Toxin A Therapy in Trigeminal Neuralgia: A Systematic Review and Meta-Analysis of Randomized Controlled Trials." *The Journal of Headache and Pain* 17 (2016): 63–71.

Oliver, Jeremie D., R. Paul Boesch, and Kenneth J. Mack. "Decreased Pulmonary Function During Botulinum Toxin A Therapy for Chronic Migraines in a 17-Year-Old Female." *Headache: The Journal of Head and Face Pain* 58, no. 8 (September 2018): 1259–1261.

Ooijevaar, R. E., R. J. F. Felt-Bersma, I. J. Han-Geurts, et al. "Botox Treatment in Patients with Chronic Functional Anorectal Pain: Experiences of a Tertiary Referral Proctology Clinic." *Techniques in Coloproctology* 23 (2019): 239–244.

Sane, Sayali, Mohammad Javed Ali, and Milind N. Naik. "Comparison of Safety and Efficacy of Botox and Neuronox in the Management of Benign Essential Blepharospasm: A Split-Face Study." *Korean Journal of Ophthalmology* 33, no. 5 (2019): 430–435.

Vikelis, Michail, Andreas A. Argyriou, Emmanouil V. Dermitzakis, et al. "Onabotulinumtoxin-A Treatment in Greek Patients with Chronic Migraine." *The Journal of Headache and Pain* 17 (2016): 84–88.

Wang, Junpeng, Qiang Wang, Qinghui Wu, et al. "Intravesical Botulinum Toxin A Injections for Bladder Pain Syndrome/Interstitial Cystitis: A Systematic Review and Meta-Analysis of Controlled Studies." *Medical Science Monitor* 22 (2016): 3257–3267.

Cannabis, Medical

INTRODUCTION

Also known as medical marijuana, medical cannabis has been used as a medicinal treatment for more than 3000 years. Although believed to be beneficial for many medical problems, in the United States, it is most-often thought to be a treatment for pain, especially chronic pain. It is not uncommon for people who fear addiction to opioids to turn to cannabis as an alternative.

Cannabis medicines contain cannabinoids, which are derived from the cannabis plant, including delta-9-tetrahydrocannabinol (THC), cannabidiol (CBD), or a combination of THC and CBD. Thus far, 568 unique molecules have been identified in cannabis; of these, more than 60 are cannabinoids or compounds that act on receptors in the body's endocannabinoid system (ECS), which plays a role in endogenous pain control. Some researchers believe that CBD interacts with a core component of the ECS, endocannabinoid receptors in the brain and immune system. Receptors are tiny particles attached to cells. They receive mostly chemical signals from different stimuli and help the cells respond. This response has pain-relieving and anti-inflammatory effects that reduce pain.

It is important to note that not all medical cannabis is the same. There are hundreds of different strains. THC is the most psychoactive cannabinoid found in cannabis and is primarily responsible for the elevated mood or "high" associated with cannabis. CBD does not support euphoria, but it is believed to be associated with reductions in inflammation and pain.

The first recorded use of medical cannabis may be traced to China. Later, it was introduced to Europe and to the United States in the 1600s. Though used for medical purposes, it gained popularity for recreational use in the 1930s and 1940s. It was then that states began passing laws against cannabis. In 1970, the Controlled Substance Act classified marijuana as a Schedule 1, making it illegal at the federal level.

It is impossible to know how many people use medical cannabis in the United States. It has been estimated that there are at least several million users.

ADMINISTRATION AND REGULATION

People who are considering the use of medical cannabis should begin with a discussion with their medical provider. While you do not need a prescription for medical cannabis, you do need a physician's recommendation. Not all medical providers are well-versed in this topic. In fact, many may feel uncomfortable discussing cannabis. Hence, some patients will require referrals to another physician. That physician will probably recommend the best ratio of THC to CBD to look for in a marijuana strain and may also suggest dosage and route of administration. Medical cannabis may be smoked, vaporized, taken under the tongue (sublingually), ingested, and used topically. People should bring their provider's written suggestions to a recommended dispensary. Experienced dispensary staff will provide additional guidance. Certain people may wish to apply for a state-issued formal medical marijuana card. This enables people who are stopped by law enforcement personnel to prove that they are using cannabis for a valid medical reason.

For people taking CBD alone, the amount is a function of their weight; the condition that is being treated; individual body chemistry; and the concentration of CBD in each pill, capsule, drop, or gummy. It is a good idea to ask the advice of a knowledgeable medical provider. If no such person is available, start with the smallest dose, such as 20 to 40 mg per day. If necessary, slowly increase the dosage by 5 mg per week until pain relief is obtained.

Doses of THC alone vary according to the type of THC. For example, people beginning to eat THC edibles should start with 1 to 2 mg THC. Gradually increase the dose by 1 mg every 24 hours, until pain relief is obtained. Similarly, with tinctures, it is best to begin with a TCH dose of 2 mg or less and increase the dose by 1 mg every 24 hours. When smoking flowers it is good to start with 10 percent THC or less.

People taking a combination of CBD and THC should usually begin with a one-on-one ratio, such as 7.5 mg of CBD and 7.5 mg of THC, three or four times per day. For pain relief, it might be necessary to increase the dose to 15 mg CBD and 15 mg THC.

Costs associated with medical cannabis products vary according to quality of the cannabis and the location where it is sold. The following are approximations. A gram of buds costs between $5 and $20; an ounce of buds costs between $200 and $400. More concentrated products, such as oils, which have higher levels of THC, cost between $20 and $60 per gram. Edible products tend to cost between $2 and $4 per dose, and concentrated liquids, called tinctures, are normally sold in one-ounce bottles for $15 to $50 per bottle. Currently, there are no health insurers in the United States that cover medical cannabis treatments.

Although the majority of states and the District of Columbia have legalized the medical use of cannabis, at present, medical and recreational cannabis is illegal under Federal law (via the Controlled Substance Act). (As was noted, at the Federal level, medical marijuana is classified as a Schedule 1 substance, and there are no recognized medical uses.) Physicians cannot prescribe medical cannabis. The states that have medical cannabis generally have amendments to protect patients and physicians from Federal laws. In many states with legalized cannabis, some type of testing is required. Yet, testing varies widely from state to state and may be limited to contamination tests or may include quantification of THC and CBD levels. It is evident that the consistency and quality of cannabis may differ from dispensary to dispensary and from state to state.

The majority of states with medical cannabis laws restrict the use to patients with certain medical conditions, such as cancer, HIV/AIDS, and multiple sclerosis. Still, more states are starting to include pain, a very common reason to use cannabis. The District of Columbia and California allow the use of cannabis for any condition that is not effectively treated by other means and that limits a person's ability to perform the activities of daily life.

Fourteen states do not permit the legal use of medical cannabis. They are Alabama, Georgia, Idaho, Indiana, Iowa, Kansas, Kentucky, Nebraska, North Carolina, South Carolina, Tennessee, Texas, Wisconsin, and Wyoming.

BENEFITS AND RISKS

There appears to be some evidence that cannabis is useful for several types of pain, especially chronic pain. Furthermore, there is some indication that cannabis may reduce opioid requirements for analgesia. Therefore, people with chronic pain who use cannabis must reduce or stop their intake of opioids. Cannabis may also be useful for migraines, Parkinson's disease, multiple sclerosis, fibromyalgia, rheumatoid arthritis, and lupus. (The actual conditions approved for treatment vary from state to state.)

Cannabis is known to have a few potential side effects, which are more likely to occur in novice users. These include paranoia, panic attacks, and a feeling of deep uneasiness or dissatisfaction (dysphoria). As a result, it is best to start with a low dose. Moreover, the regular use of cannabis may result in increased insurance premiums, and people who work in jobs where there is drug testing may place their jobs at risk, especially with employers who do not recognize the need for medical cannabis. And although medical cannabis is not thought to be physically addictive, it may well be psychologically addictive. Some people may struggle to stop using cannabis, even after the pain has resolved.

CBD may have a few side effects. These include fatigue, diarrhea, and changes in appetite and weight. Further, CBD may interact with some over-the-counter medicines, prescription medicines, and dietary supplements. People who take any medicine or supplement with a "grapefruit warning" should not take CBD. They may interfere with enzymes that are crucial to drug metabolism. CBD may increase the risk of liver toxicity. As they do not enter the bloodstream, it is assumed that topical CBD products do not have these risks.

Side effects of THC tend to occur when it is taken in excessive amounts, which obviously varies from person to person. Hence, it is best to start with smaller amounts of THC. For inhalation forms of THC, wait 15 minutes between puffs; for edible forms of THC, wait two hours before ingesting more. These side effects include dry or bloodshot eyes, dry mouth, hypothermia/shivering, fast heartbeat, impaired coordination, impaired thinking/concentration/learning, difficulty sleeping, dizziness/vertigo, nausea and vomiting, anxiety or panic attack, and paranoia. In rare instances, excessive intake of THC may result in psychotic symptoms, such as delusions and hallucinations, cardiac injury, and seizures.

RESEARCH FINDINGS

Many People Believe Cannabis Is Useful for Pain and It May Reduce the Need for Opioids and Other Medications for Pain

In a study published in 2019 in the *Journal of Psychoactive Drugs*, researchers from the Bronx, New York City, and Miami, Florida (USA), conducted a survey from August to October 2016 at two retail stores within a single cannabis dispensary located in Colorado. Of the 1,000 adult customer respondents, who were all at least 21 years old, 90 percent were under the age of 50 years, with 42 percent women and 66 percent reporting white, non-Hispanic race/ethnicity. Sixty-five percent indicated they used cannabis to relieve pain, and 74 percent said that they used cannabis to promote sleep. Among the respondents using cannabis for pain, 80 percent noted that it was very or extremely helpful, and the vast majority of those who used over-the-counter or opioid medications were able to reduce their intake or stop taking them. Among respondents taking over-the-counter medications, 82 percent said that they reduced or stopped these drugs. Among respondents taking opioids, 88 percent reduced or stopped them. The researchers concluded that "adult use cannabis laws may broaden access to cannabis for the purpose of symptoms relief."[1]

Then Again, the Use of Cannabinoids May or May Not Lower the Intake of Opioids for Pain Relief

In a systematic review and meta-analysis published in 2017 in the journal *Neuropsychopharmacology*, researchers from Australia and Canada examined the opioid-sparing effects of cannabinoids (any group of closely related compounds which include cannabinol and the active constituents of cannabis). The researchers found 19 preclinical studies and 9 clinical studies that met their criteria. Seventeen of the 19 preclinical studies demonstrated that combining a cannabinoid with an opioid has a synergistic effect on analgesia. A meta-analysis of six of the preclinical studies found that the use of a cannabinol enabled patients to use less opioid medication. Because the studies were so different, no meta-analysis could be conducted of the clinical studies. Further, only three randomized trials had high-quality evidence. Two studies had moderate-quality evidence, and four studies had low- or very-low-quality evidence. None of the high-quality studies provided evidence of an opioid-sparing effect. The only study that did was deemed to be of a very low quality. Commenting on their findings, the researchers noted that although the outcomes of preclinical studies are often similar to clinical studies, preclinical studies "may over-represent effects." The researchers concluded that "it remains to be seen if these promising preclinical and observational findings can be replicated in large, well-designed clinical studies."[2]

Cannabis May Be Useful for Neuropathic Pain, but It Appears to Have Limited Use for Other Types of Pain

In a systematic review published in 2017 in the *Annals of Internal Medicine*, researchers from Portland, Oregon (USA) examined the use of plant-based cannabis preparations for treating chronic pain and any potential harmful effects. The researchers located 27 chronic pain trials that met their criteria. The sources of the pain included neuropathic pain, multiple sclerosis, cancer, rheumatoid arthritis, fibromyalgia, and abdominal pain from problems such as chronic pancreatitis and abdominal surgery. Further, they found 11 systematic reviews and 32 primary studies of potential harm from cannabis use. The researchers found low-level evidence that cannabis may alleviate neuropathic pain but insufficient evidence for other types of pain. Most of the studies were small and had methodological flaws, and as they tended to be short in duration, the long-term effects were unclear. Interestingly, the use of cannabis was associated with an increased risk of motor vehicle accidents, psychotic symptoms, and short-term cognitive impairment. The researchers commented that "virtually no conclusive information exists about the benefits of cannabis in chronic pain populations."[3]

Some People Are More Likely Than Others to Treat Their Pain with Cannabis

In a study published in 2020 in the journal *Advances in Therapy*, researchers from Massachusetts, New Jersey, Illinois, and Ohio (USA) wanted to learn about the demographic characteristics of the people who use cannabis to treat their chronic pain. The researchers used data from 2011 to 2015 obtained from the National Inpatient Sample (NIS), which is publicly available. (The NIS is one of the Healthcare Cost and Utilization Projects databases sponsored by the Agency for Healthcare Research and Quality. It is based on data extracted from 7 to 8 million hospital stays.) The researchers included chemical dependency treatment facilities, long-term acute care hospitals, short-term rehabilitation facilities, and psychiatric hospitals. The researchers identified 10.3 million patients with chronic pain. Of these, 247,949 used cannabis. The yearly prevalence of cannabis used increased from 2.4 percent in 2011 to 3.9 percent in 2015. The highest proportion of patients using cannabis were in the 45 to 64 age range; the lowest were the elderly, people 84 years or older. More males than females used cannabis, and the lowest income quartile had the highest proportion of cannabis use. The cannabis users tended to be white. Trauma patients had the highest use of cannabis, and patients with failed back surgery syndrome had the lowest. Overall, the researchers learned that chronic pain patients are increasing their use of cannabis. At the same time, the rates of use among opioid users were "downtrending simultaneously."[4]

Cannabis May Be Useful for Fibromyalgia Syndrome

In a retrospective clinical trial published in 2021 in the *Journal of Cannabis Research*, a researcher from Italy evaluated the use of cannabis for the symptoms associated with fibromyalgia syndrome, including pain. Data from patient files were obtained between June 1, 2016, and October 31, 2018. The cohort consisted of 38 patients (36 women and 2 men) who did not respond sufficiently well to, or had adverse effects from, conventional treatments for fibromyalgia syndrome. Their median age was 56 years. Thirty, 18, and 12 patients continued cannabis therapy for 1, 3, and 12 months, respectively. The cannabis was administered as an adjunct therapy, and the baseline therapy was slowly decreased or interrupted as patients had better pain management. The starting dose of milled flowers was 50 or 100 mg twice per day. The doses could be increased by the physician as needed. The researchers learned that about half of the patients reported that cannabis reduced their pain, with 34.2 percent deciding to continue their treatment for a year. And about half had adverse events, such as "mental confusion," leading to the interruption of cannabis treatment. But, this confusion tended to stop in longer courses of therapy. Other side effects included dizziness, nausea/vomiting, and restlessness/ irritation, but none of these side effects was considered "serious." The researchers underscored the need for more studies on the medical use of cannabis. "Further studies are warranted to confirm these findings."[5]

Inhaled Cannabis Appears to Be Useful for Neuropathic Pain

In an individual patient meta-analysis published in 2015 in the *Journal of Pain*, researchers from New York, California, and Quebec wanted to learn if inhaled cannabis would be useful for patients with neuropathic pain, a persistent problem seen in about one in 40 adults. The researchers located five randomized, placebo-controlled, double-blind studies with 178 subjects and 405 observations that met their criteria. Four used a crossover design, and one study had a parallel design. Duration of follow-up varied from hours to weeks, and withdrawals due to adverse events were rare. One case of a serious adverse event leading to withdrawal occurred in a placebo group. Other reported mild side effects included anxiety, dizziness, disorientation, concentration problems, headache, dry eyes, burning sensation, and numbness. One study found short-term declines in attention, psychomotor performance, and learning and memory in those taking the highest dose. Longer-term side effects were not addressed. The researchers determined that inhaled cannabis resulted in short-term reductions in chronic neuropathic pain for one in every five or six subjects. "This effect in chronic painful neuropathy is consistent across diverse etiologies, all hitherto resistant to available treatments."[6]

Inhaled Cannabis May Help People with Headaches and Migraines

In a study published in 2020 in the *Journal of Pain*, researchers from Washington State University in Pullman, Washington (USA), investigated the use of inhaled cannabis for headaches and migraines. Data were obtained from Strainpoint, a free medical cannabis app that provides people with the ability to track changes in symptom severity as a function of different doses and strains of cannabis. Users of this app, begin by entering basic demographic information as well as their medical conditions and symptoms. Then, people open the app when they are about to use cannabis, and enter the relevant information. The researchers' analyses included data from 1,306 cannabis users who used the app a total of 12,293 times to tract changes in headache severity and from 653 users who used the app 7,441 times to tract changes in migraine severity. The researchers found significant reductions—almost 50 percent—in headache and migraine severity after cannabis use. Men had larger reductions than women. The researchers noted that their sample probably "over-represents" people who find cannabis useful for the headaches and migraines. Those who do not find it useful would probably discontinue using cannabis and the app. In addition, those who repeatedly use cannabis may develop a tolerance. The researchers underscored the need for "future double-blind, placebo-controlled clinical trials."[7]

Cannabis May or May Not Be Useful for Orthopedic Pain

In a systematic review published in 2019 in the *Canadian Journal of Surgery*, researchers from Canada, the Netherlands, and Spain wanted to determine if cannabis would help people with pain from the orthopedic conditions of post-trauma pain, postsurgery pain, back pain, and arthritis. The researchers identified 33 orthopedic studies, including 21 primary studies and 12 reviews. These included 5 randomized, controlled trials, one nonrandomized intervention study, 8 case reports/case series, 6 surveys, one qualitative study, and 12 systematic reviews. Of the 12 systematic reviews, 9 included randomized controlled trials, 2 included non randomized studies, and one review had an unclear design. Study quality was generally low to moderate. Six of the studies had a control group, and 15 were noncontrolled. The studies had a good deal of heterogeneity in methodologies, drugs and protocols of administration, frequencies, populations, and outcomes. As a result, no meta-analysis was conducted. Still, study conclusions tended to be mixed in controlled studies and positive in noncontrolled studies. In addition, studies that used higher doses of cannabis were more likely to reduce pain, but they had greater potential to trigger harmful effects. The researchers concluded that there is insufficient evidence to know whether or not the use of cannabis relieves orthopedic-related pain. "Although most of the existing evidence suggests that medical cannabis use is effective, this efficacy has been demonstrated only when either there is no comparator or cannabis is compared to a placebo. Studies using an active comparator have not demonstrated the efficacy of cannabis use."[8]

NOTES

1. Bachhuber, Marcus, Julia Arnsten, and Gwen Wurm. "Use of Cannabis to Relieve Pain and Promote Sleep by Customers at an Adult Use Dispensary." *Journal of Psychoactive Drugs* 51, no. 5 (2019): 400–404.

2. Nielson, Suzanne, Pamela Sabioni, Jose M. Trigo, et al. "Opioid-Sparing Effects of Cannabinoids: A Systematic Review and Meta-Analysis." *Neuropsychopharmacology* 42 (2017): 1752–1765.

3. Nugent, Shannon M., Benjamin J. Morasco, Maya E. O'Neil, et al. "The Effects of Cannabis Among Adults with Chronic Pain and an Overview of General Harms: A Systematic Review." *Annals of Internal Medicine* 167, no. 5 (September 5, 2017): 319–331.

4. Orhurhu, Vwaire, Ivan Urits, Mayowa Olusunmade, et al. "Cannabis Use in Hospitalized Patients with Chronic Pain." *Advances in Therapy* 37 (2020): 3571–3583.

5. Mazza, Manuela. "Medical Cannabis for the Treatment of Fibromyalgia Syndrome: A Retrospective, Open-Label Case Series." *Journal of Cannabis Research* 3, no. 4 (February 17, 2021): NA.

6. Andreae, Michael H., George M. Carter, Naum Shaparin, et al. "Inhaled Cannabis for Chronic Neuropathic Pain: An Individual Patient Data Meta-Analysis." *Journal of Pain* 16, no. 12 (December 2015): 1221–1232.

7. Cuttler, Carrie, Alexander Spradlin, Michael J. Cleveland, et al. "Short- and Long-Term Effects of Cannabis on Headache and Migraine." *Journal of Pain* 21, no. 5–6 (May/June 2020): 722–730.

8. Madden, Kim, Annie George, Niek J. van der Hoek, et al. "Cannabis for Pain in Orthopedics: A Systematic Review Focusing on Study Methodology." *Canadian Journal of Surgery* 62, no. 6 (December 1, 2019): 369–380.

REFERENCES AND FURTHER READINGS

Andreae, Michael H., George M. Carter, Nuam Shaparin, et al. "Inhaled Cannabis for Chronic Neuropathic Pain: An Individual Patient Data Meta-Analysis." *Journal of Pain* 16, no. 12 (December 2015): 1221–1232.

Bachhuber, Marcus, Julia H. Arnsten, and Gwen Wurm. "Use of Cannabis to Relieve Pain and Promote Sleep by Customers at an Adult Use Dispensary." *Journal of Psychoactive Drugs* 51, no. 5 (2019): 400–404.

Cuttler, Carrie, Alexander Spradlin, Michael J. Cleveland, et al. "Short- and Long-Term Effects of Cannabis on Headache and Migraine." *Journal of Pain* 21, no. 5–6 (May/June 2020): 722–730.

Madden, Kim, Annie George, Niek J. van der Hoek, et al. "Cannabis for Pain in Orthopedics: A Systematic Review Focusing on study Methodology." *Canadian Journal of Surgery* 62, no. 6 (December 1, 2019): 369–380.

Mazza, Manuela. "Medical Cannabis for the Treatment of Fibromyalgia Syndrome: A Retrospective, Open-Label Case Series." *Journal of Cannabis Research* 3, no. 4 (February 17, 2021): NA.

Nielson, Suzanne, Pamela Sabioni, Jose M. Trigo, et al. "Opioid-Sparing Effect of Cannabinoids: A Systematic Review and Meta-Analysis." *Neuropsychopharmacology* 42 (2017): 1752–1765.

Nugent, Shannon M., Benjamin J. Morasco, Maya E. O'Neil, et al. "The Effects of Cannabis Among Adults with Chronic Pain and an Overview of General Harms: A Systematic Review." *Annals of Internal Medicine* 167, no. 5 (September 5, 2017): 319–331.

Orhurhu, Vwaire, Ivan Uritis, Mayowa Olusunmade, et al. "Cannabis Use in Hospitalized Patients with Chronic Pain." *Advances in Therapy* 37 (2020): 3571–3583.

Chiropractic

INTRODUCTION

A licensed health-care profession, chiropractic focuses on disorders of the musculoskeletal system and the nervous system as well as the body's ability to heal itself. Normally, treatments involve manual therapy, including spinal manipulation and nutrition counseling and exercise. The manual treatment methods include stretching and pressure placed on specific joints, delivered by hand with a quick, gentle thrust. Although other parts of the body may be treated, the manipulations are usually directed to the spine. The goal of spinal manipulation, which is also known as chiropractic adjustment, is to restore joint mobility that has been hampered by tissue injury, thus relieving pain and muscle tightness and allowing tissues to heal. Chiropractors provide acute, chronic, and preventive care. It is important to note that adjustments may result in the release of a gas bubble between the joints, which creates a popping sound. There is no reason to be concerned about the pops.

There are more than 70,000 chiropractors in the United States; it has been estimated that every year, they treat more than 35 million adults and children. In an article published in 2017 in the journal *Chiropractic & Manual Therapies*, researchers based in Canada conducted a systematic review of aspects of the chiropractic profession. They learned that globally, the median 12-month utilization of chiropractic services was 9.1 percent. Most patients visiting chiropractors were female, with a median age of 43.4 years, and employed. The most common reasons for a chiropractic visit were low back pain, neck pain, and extremity problems. Four out of five people who visit a chiropractor received spinal manipulation. However, other common practices include soft tissue therapy and formal patient education.[1]

The chiropractic profession is a relatively new addition to the health-care field. It began in 1895, when Daniel David Palmer adjusted the spine of a deaf janitor and claimed that the janitor's hearing was restored. Two years later, in 1897, Palmer founded the Palmer School of Cure, now known as the Palmer School of Chiropractic, in Davenport, Iowa. He taught his methods to the first generation of chiropractors. Though types of manipulation had been used for thousands of years, this was the first organized scientific approach. The name "chiropractic" comes from the Greek words cheir (hand) and prakto (done), or "done by hand." Today, chiropractors frequently work in conjunction with other medical providers, such as medical doctors and physical therapists.[2]

ADMINISTRATION AND REGULATION

Appointments with a chiropractor begin with an interview and a health history review, followed by a clinical examination and perhaps some laboratory testing, diagnostic imaging, or other interventions. At that point, the chiropractor normally has a working diagnosis and treatment plan, which he or she discusses with the patient.

Although some chiropractors work in physician offices, most work in their own office settings, clinics, or hospitals. During an acute medical problem, a chiropractor may advise a patient to come two or three times per week for several weeks. After that problem improves, adjustments will be less frequent. Many people visit chiropractors once or twice a month to maintain their health and prevent problems from recurring. In 2019, the average cost of an adjustment in the United States was $115. But fees vary widely, and adjustments may well be covered, at least in part, by health insurance.

To do their work, chiropractors use a variety of manipulations and tools. Manipulations include direct thrust technique, spinal mobilization, myofascial release, muscle energy technique, indirect positional technique, articulatory, cervical spine manipulation, and functional technique. The best-known tool is the chiropractic table, but there are others. An activator adjustment tool sends a low amount of force into the back, and an electronic impulse-adjusting instrument allows the chiropractor to use greater painless force to treat back problems. Also, a pro adjustor is a tool that works with software to test an area before an adjustment. It helps determine the exact amount of adjustment needed.

In the United States, in order to practice chiropractic medicine, men and women must earn a Doctor of Chiropractic (D.C.) degree, pass the National Board of Chiropractic Examiners test, and have a state license. All of the states require chiropractors to take continuing education courses, and many states require them to pass a test on state-specific laws. To enroll in a four-year chiropractic program, students must have completed at least three years of undergraduate study, including premedical courses. Chiropractic programs are accredited by the Council on Chiropractic Education, which is recognized as an accrediting agency by the U.S. Secretary of Education. Chiropractic education includes classes in basic sciences, such as anatomy and physiology, and supervised clinical experience. Some chiropractors complete postgraduate training and specialize in areas such as radiology, rehabilitation, and neurology. To maintain their license, chiropractors must earn continuing education credits through state-approved programs. Though costs vary widely, chiropractic is usually covered or partially covered by health insurance. Some health plans require a referral to a chiropractor. Before visiting a chiropractor, it is a good idea to check your health plan coverage and requirements.

BENEFITS AND RISKS

Chiropractic primarily treats musculoskeletal complaints such as back pain, neck pain, pain in the joints of the arms or legs, and headaches. With these problems, which are all very common, chiropractic may become the primary method of treatment. But, there are many other potential benefits of chiropractic. Treatments may tighten loose muscles and loosen tight muscles. They may decrease the degeneration of joints and connective tissues and improve the circulation of blood and the nervous system. In addition, chiropractic may strengthen the body's immunity and increase energy and vitality while improving sleep.

Chiropractic adjustments rarely cause any pain or discomfort. Still, some people experience mild soreness or aching after an adjustment session. These usually resolve within a day or two. There are reports of an association between high-velocity upper neck manipulation and a certain kind of uncommon stroke. It is believed that this occurs spontaneously in people who have preexisting arterial disease; it is exceedingly rare.

RESEARCH FINDINGS

People Who Use Chiropractic Treatment for Low Back Pain Have a Lower Risk of Adverse Drug Events Than Nonusers

In a study published in 2018 in the *Journal of Manipulative and Physiological Therapeutics*, researchers from California and New Hampshire (United States) examined the potential association between utilization of chiropractic services for a primary diagnosis of low back pain and the likelihood of an adverse drug event, such as overdoses, medication errors, or adverse or allergic reactions. The researchers used a retrospective cohort design to analyze health insurance claims data from the state of New Hampshire. The data source consisted of all the payer claims databases administered by the Department of Health and Human Services of the state of New Hampshire. In total, there were 19,150 participants included in the study; they were almost evenly divided between recipients and nonrecipients of chiropractic services. While the groups did not differ by sex, they did differ by age. The group that received chiropractic care had a larger proportion of young adults. Also, the nonrecipients had a significantly inferior health status. The researchers learned that the risk of an adverse drug event was significantly lower among recipients of chiropractor services, as compared with those who have not used these services. In fact, "the adjusted likelihood of an ADE [adverse drug event] occurring in an outpatient setting within 12 months was 51 percent lower among recipients of chiropractic services." Still, the researchers commented that before the establishment of a causal relationship, future research needs to include larger and more variable datasets.[3]

Chiropractic Spinal Manipulation May Help People with Chronic Low Back Pain

In a systematic review and meta-analysis published in 2019 in the journal *BMJ*, researchers from the Netherlands and Denmark assessed the benefits and harms of spinal manipulative therapy for the treatment of chronic low back pain. The researchers initially identified 47 published randomized controlled trials with 9211 subjects that met their criteria. On average, the subjects were between the ages of 35 and 60 years. Most of the trials compared spinal manipulation with other recommended therapies. Fifteen of the trials were conducted in the United States, and seven were conducted in the United Kingdom. The other countries were Finland, Australia, Italy, Sweden, Denmark, Egypt, India, Belgium, Spain, Switzerland, the Netherlands, Greece, Turkey, Pakistan, and Tunisia. All of the trials, except the one from Tunisia, were published in English. Study sample sizes ranged from 21 to 1,334. The researchers learned that when treating chronic low back pain in adults, spinal manipulative therapy had "similar outcomes" to recommended therapies for short, intermediate, and long-term pain relief as well as improvements in function. And when compared to nonrecommended therapies or sham, spinal manipulative therapy had better short-term improvement. "SMT [spinal manipulative therapy] produces similar effects to recommended therapies for chronic low back pain, whereas SMT seems to be better than non-recommended interventions for improvement in function in the short-term." Furthermore, adverse events and serious adverse events associated with spinal manipulation appeared to be rare.[4]

Spinal Manipulative Therapy May Benefit People with Acute Low Back Pain

In a systematic review and meta-analysis published in 2017 in *JAMA*, researchers from several locations in the United States (based in Los Angeles, California) wanted to learn if spinal manipulative therapy benefited people with acute low back pain. The cohort consisted of 26 randomized clinical trials. Spinal manipulative therapy was provided by physical therapists, chiropractors, medical doctors, and osteopathic physicians. Some studies employed multiple disciplines; all of the studies were conducted in ambulatory or outpatient settings. Whereas 12 studies were classified as high quality, 14 were classified as low quality. Fifteen randomized controlled trials, with 1,711 subjects, provided "moderate-quality evidence" that spinal manipulative therapy has a statistically significant association with improvements in pain. And 12 randomized controlled trials, with 1,381 subjects, produced "moderate-quality evidence" that spinal manipulative therapy had a statistically significant association with improvement in function. The researchers determined that the use of spinal manipulative therapy for acute low back pain was associated with a statistically significant but modest benefit in pain and function at up to six weeks. The three trials that reported the most benefit used clinical criteria to select patients who were more likely to benefit. Still, it is important to note that "minor transient adverse events such as increased pain, muscle stiffness, and headaches were reported 50% to 67% of the time."[5]

When Added to Usual Medical Care, Chiropractic Care May Benefit People with Low Back Pain

In a six-week, three-site, "pragmatic" comparative effectiveness clinical trial published in 2018 in the journal *JAMA Network Open*, researchers from Davenport, Iowa, Dallas, Texas, Silver Spring, Maryland, and Santa Monica, California (USA), wanted to determine if adding chiropractic care to usual medical treatments offered better relief than the use of only the usual medical care. The trial was conducted at two large military centers in major metropolitan areas and one smaller hospital at a military training site. Subjects were active duty U.S. service members between the ages of 18 and 50 years, with a mean age of 30.9 years, who had low back pain from a musculoskeletal source. A total of 750 subjects were enrolled; there were 250 subjects at each site. About one-fourth of the subjects were female, and about one-third were nonwhite. Almost 6 percent of the subjects reported the current use of narcotic analgesics, and 53.1 percent took nonsteroidal, anti-inflammatory drugs for pain. Close to 60 percent had never been treated with chiropractic care. The cohort was divided into two groups of 375 subjects. The subjects received either the usual medical care for low back pain or that care combined with chiropractic care. During the trial, the subjects in the chiropractic group could have as many as 12 chiropractic visits. The primary chiropractic procedure was spinal manipulative therapy in the low back and adjacent areas. There were 19 adverse effects in the subjects receiving usual medical care; of these, 12 consisted of muscle or joint stiffness. There were 43 adverse effects in the subjects receiving both types of care; of these, 38 were described as muscle or joint stiffness. The researchers learned that the subjects who had usual medical care combined with chiropractic care had better short-term moderate improvements in pain intensity and disability, and they were more satisfied that those who only received the usual medical care. At the same time, the combination care "demonstrated a low risk of harm, and led to high patient satisfaction and perceived improvement in active-duty military personnel." The findings support the inclusion of chiropractic in the treatment of low back pain.[6]

People with Chronic Low Back Pain and Chronic Neck Pain Who Seek Chiropractic Care Have Some Common Characteristics, and They Seem Satisfied with Their Outcomes

In a study published in 2018 in the *Journal of Manipulative and Physiological Therapies*, researchers from Santa Monica and Los Angeles, California, and Pittsburgh, Pennsylvania (USA), examined data collected from chiropractic patients with chronic low back pain and chronic neck pain. Data were collected from subjects from clinics located in California, Florida, Minnesota, New York, Oregon, and Texas, all in the United States. A total of 6,342 patients from 125 clinics completed a prescreening questionnaire.

After eliminations, 2,829 subjects were eligible for the study, and 2,014 started and completed the baseline survey. While 1,159 subjects had both chronic low back pain and chronic neck pain, 518 had chronic low back pain, and 347 had chronic neck pain. The researchers learned that their subjects tended to be "highly-educated non-Hispanic, white females" who had at least partial chiropractic insurance coverage. Most sought chiropractic treatment after trying other types of care. Generally, they had been visiting chiropractors for years for their ongoing pain, and they consistently had high levels of satisfaction with their chiropractic care; they successfully managed their chronic low back pain, chronic neck pain, or both. The researchers concluded that their findings demonstrated that chiropractors may play an expanded role in treating chronic pain in the future. There is a "need to find effective nonpharmacologic alternatives for chronic pain."[7]

When Compared to Other Treatments for Spine Pain, Chiropractic May or May Not Be Cost Effective

In a systematic review published in 2015 in the journal *BMC Health Services Research*, researchers based in Winchester, Massachusetts, but also from Santa Ana, Irvine, and Los Angeles, California (all in the United States) and a location in Ontario, Canada, compared the costs associated with several types of spine pain treatments provided by health-care professionals. Their cohort consisted of 25 studies, all of which were conducted in the United States and published between 1993 and 2015. Twelve of the studies were from private health plans, six were from worker's compensation plans, and seven examined clinical outcomes. Most often, chiropractic care was compared to treatment from a medical physician. The researchers learned that in the United States the cost of care "may be somewhat lower" when spinal pain is managed with chiropractic care. However, the researchers added that "the methods used in these studies differed widely, limiting their interpretation and generalizability."[8]

Chiropractic May or May Not Be Useful for Cervicogenic Headaches

In a 17-month, prospective, three-armed, single-blind, placebo-controlled, randomized trial published in 2017 in the journal *BMC Research Notes*, researchers from Norway and Australia wanted to determine if chiropractic would help people suffering from debilitating cervicogenic headaches, which develop in the neck but are felt in the head. These headaches do not tend to respond to pharmacological interventions, and, in an attempt to obtain some relief, people often overuse their medications. The cohort consisted of 19 subjects—5 men and 14 women—with cervicogenic headaches, diagnosed by a neurologist. Participants received actual chiropractic treatments or sham chiropractic treatments or no chiropractic treatments. Twelve subjects completed the entire trial; four subjects were in each intervention. The researchers learned that subjects in the chiropractic and placebo groups had improvements in headache frequency. Headache frequency was reduced in the chiropractic group at all time points; the frequency was reduced at, 6 and 12 months' follow-up in the placebo group. During the entire study, the subjects in the control group remained unchanged. The researchers noted that their findings indicated "that manual-therapy might be a safe treatment option for participants with cervicogenic headache." However, because of the small sample size of this trial, "data need to be confirmed in a randomized controlled trial with sufficient sample size and statistical power."[9]

The Risk of Injury from Chiropractic Spinal Manipulation in Elderly Adults Appears to Be Low

In a retrospective study published in 2015 in the journal *Spine*, researchers from Lebanon, New Hampshire, and Whittier, California (USA), evaluated the risk of injury to the head, neck, or trunk from chiropractic spinal manipulation in elders enrolled in Part B Medicare. All of the elders had a neuromuscular complaint and were between the ages of 66 and 99 years; they represented a population "particularly vulnerable to traumatic injury." The researchers found 7,448,430 Medicare B beneficiaries who had either a primary care or chiropractic office visit for a neuromuscular problem in 2007. After the researchers excluded subjects who saw both types of providers or had a recent history of trauma, there were 6,669,603 subjects in the study sample. The primary care cohort consisted of 5,669,032 subjects, more than five times as large as the chiropractic cohort, which was 1,000,571. Yet, the number of primary care office visits (13,536,595) exceeded the number of chiropractic office visits (10,532,213) by 29 percent. By chance, the chiropractic cohort was younger, predominantly white and female, healthier than the primary care cohort, and had fewer numbers of chronic conditions. The researchers found that the adjusted risk of injury in the chiropractic cohort was lower than the primary care cohort. The cumulative probability of injury in the chiropractic cohort was

40 injury incidents per 100,000 subjects, as compared to 153 incidents per 100,000 subjects in the primary care cohort. The likelihood of injury was higher in subjects with certain conditions, such as osteoporosis or a coagulation defect. The researchers concluded that among this cohort of elders the "risk of injury to the head, neck or trunk within seven days was 76% lower among subjects with a chiropractic office visit as compared to those who saw a primary care physician."[10]

Though Children and Teens Have Frequent Musculoskeletal Complaints, They Rarely Utilize Chiropractic Care

In a data analysis published in 2018 in the *Journal of Manipulative and Physiological Therapeutics*, researchers from Austin, Texas (USA), noted that children and teens frequently have musculoskeletal complaints, such as neck and low back pain. In fact, one three-year Danish study found the prevalence of spine pain among children and teens between the ages of 8 and 15 years to be 55.5 percent. The researchers used data from 9,734 respondents to the 2012 National Health Interview Survey to investigate the utilization of chiropractic care during the previous 12 months. The researchers found that overall utilization of chiropractic care by children and teens was 3 percent. Utilization was higher among subjects between the ages of 12 and 17 years than those between the ages of 4 and 11 years. White children and teens were more likely than nonwhite children to use chiropractic care, and children and teens from the Midwest and West were more likely to seek this treatment option. The researchers concluded that "considerations should be made to explore the reasons for underutilization in the minority groups, increase supply of chiropractic services in underutilized areas, and bolster interprofessional relationships and referrals among CIH [complementary and integrative health] providers."[11]

NOTES

1. Beliveau, Peter J. H., Jessica J. Wong, Deborah A. Sutton, et al. "The Chiropractic Profession: A Scoping Review of Utilization Rates, Reasons for Seeking Care, Patient Profiles, and Care Provided." *Chiropractic & Manual Therapies* 25 (2017): 35–51.

2. American Chiropractic Association website. https://wwwacatoday .org.

3. Whedon, James M., Andrew W. J. Toler, Justin M. Goehl, and Louis A. Kazal. "Association between Utilization of Chiropractic Services for Treatment of Low Back Pain and Risk of Adverse Drug Events." *Journal of Manipulative and Physiological Therapeutics* 41 (2018): 383–388.

4. Rubinstein, Sidney M., Annemarie de Zoete, Marienke van Middelkoop, et al. "Benefits and Harms of Spinal Manipulative Therapy for the Treatment of Chronic Low Back Pain: Systematic Review and Meta-Analysis of Randomised Controlled Trials." *BMJ* 364 (2019): 1689.

5. Paige, Neil M., Isomi M. Miake-Lye, Marika Suttorp Booth, et al. "Association of Spinal Manipulative Therapy with Clinical Benefit and Harm for Acute Low Back Pain." *JAMA* 317, no. 14 (April 11, 2017): 1451–1460.

6. Goertz, Christine M., Cynthia R. Long, Robert D. Vining, et al. "Effect of Usual Medical Care Plus Chiropractic Care vs Usual Medical Care Alone on Pain and Disability among U.S. Service Members with Low Back Pain: A Comparative Effectiveness Clinical Trial." *JAMA Network Open* 1, no. 1 (2018): e180105.

7. Herman, Patricia M., Mallika Kommareddi, Melony E. Sorbero, et al. "Characteristics of Chiropractic Patients Being Treated for Chronic Low Back Pain and Neck Pain." *Journal of Manipulative and Physiological Therapies* 41 (2018): 445–455.

8. Dagenais, Simon, O'Dane Brady, Scott Haldeman, and Pran Manga. "A Systematic Review Comparing the Costs of Chiropractic Care to Other Interventions for Spine Pain in the United States." *BMC Health Services Research* 15 (2015): 474–494.

9. Chaibi, Aleksander, Heidi Knackstedt, Peter J. Tuchin, and Michael Bjørn Russell. "Chiropractic Spinal Manipulative Therapy for Cervicogenic Headache: A Single-Blinded, Placebo, Randomized Controlled Trial." *BMC Research Notes* 10 (2017): 310–317.

10. Whedon, James M., Todd A. MacKenzie, Reed B. Phillips, and Jon D. Lurie. "Risk of traumatic Injury Associated with Chiropractic Spinal Manipulation in Medicare Part B Beneficiaries Aged 66–99." *Spine* 40, no. 4 (February 2015): 264–270.

11. Peng, Trent, Baojiang Chen, and Kelley Pettee Gabriel. "Utilization of Chiropractic Care in U.S. Children and Adolescents: A Cross-Sectional Study of the 2012 National Health Interview Survey." *Journal of Manipulative and Physiological Therapeutics* 41, no. 9 (November/December 2018): 725–733.

REFERENCES AND FURTHER READINGS

Beliveau, Peter J. H., Jessica J. Wong, Deborah A. Sutton, et al. "The Chiropractic Profession: A Scoping Review of Utilization Rates, Reasons for Seeking Care, Patient Profiles, and Care Provided." *Chiropractic & Manual Therapies* 25 (2017): 35–51.

Chaibi, Aleksander, Heidi Knackstedt, Peter J. Tuchin, and Bjørn Russell. "Chiropractic Spinal Manipulative Therapy for Cervicogenic Headache: A Single-Blinded, Placebo, Randomized, Controlled Trial." *BMC Research Notes* 10 (2017): 310–317.

Dagenais, Simon, O'Dane Brady, Scott Haldeman, and Pran Manga. "A Systematic Review Comparing the Costs of Chiropractic Care to Other Interventions for Spine Pain in the United States." *BMC Health Services Research* 15 (2015): 474–494.

Goertz, Christine M., Cynthia R. Long, Robert D. Vining, et al. "Effect of Usual Medical Care Plus Chiropractic Care vs Usual Medical Care Alone on Pain and Disability among U.S. Service Members with Low Back Pain: A Comparative Effectiveness Clinical Trial." *JAMA Network Open* 1, no. 1 (2018): e180105.

Herman, Patricia M., Mallika Kommareddi, Melony E. Sorbero, et al. "Characteristics of Chiropractic Patients Being Treated for Chronic Low Back Pain and Neck Pain." *Journal of Manipulative and Physiological Therapeutics* 41 (2018): 445–455.

Paige, Neil M., Isomi M. Maike-Lye, Marika Suttorp Booth, et al. "Association of Spinal Manipulative Therapy with Clinical Benefit with Harm for Acute Low Back Pain." *JAMA* 317, no. 14 (April 11, 2017): 1451–1460.

Peng, Trent, Baojiang Chen, and Kelly Pettee Gabriel. "Utilization of Chiropractic Care in US Children and Adolescents: A Cross-Sectional Study of the 2012 National Health Interview Survey." *Journal of Manipulative and Physiological Therapeutics* 41, no. 9 (November/December 2018): 725–733.

Rubinstein, Sidney M., Annemarie de Zoete, Marienke van Middelkoop, et al. "Benefits and Harms of Spinal Manipulative Therapy for the Treatment of Chronic Low Back Pain: Systematic Review and Meta-Analysis of Randomised Controlled Trials." *BMJ* 364 (2019): 1689.

Whedon, James M., Todd A. Mackenzie, Reed B. Phillips, and Jon D. Lurie. "Risk of Traumatic Injury Associated with Chiropractic

Spinal Manipulation in Medicare Part B Beneficiaries Aged 66 to 99 Years." *Spine* 40, no. 4 (February 2015): 264–270.

Whedon, James M., Andrew W. J. Toler, Justin M. Goehl, and Louis A. Kazal. "Association between Utilization of Chiropractic Services for Treatment of Low Back Pain and Risk of Adverse Drug Events." *Journal of Manipulative and Physiological Therapeutics* 41 (2018): 383–388.

Cognitive Behavioral Therapy

INTRODUCTION

Unlike some forms of psychological therapy that may continue for indefinite periods of time, cognitive behavioral therapy (CBT) is a practical, hands-on, "solutions-oriented" type of therapy that focuses on modifying dysfunctional emotions, behaviors, and thoughts by directly addressing these negative and irrational assumptions. According to cognitive behavioral therapy, thoughts and perceptions influence behavior. When negative and erroneous thoughts and perceptions are substituted with positive and correct validations, behaviors will alter. People learn to reframe their negative thoughts and put their pain in perspective.

Cognitive behavioral therapy focuses on the present, not childhood events and experiences. It emphasizes a quick identification of problems and their solutions. The number of sessions is usually limited, often between 5 and 20, and they tend to be somewhat structured. While cognitive behavioral therapy is thought to be useful for various psychological problems, such as depression and anxiety, it is also believed to help people manage pain.

Aaron Beck, a psychiatrist who was disillusioned with Freudian psychoanalysis, founded cognitive behavioral therapy in the 1960s. He supported a more empirical type of therapy. CBT also has roots in rational emotive behavioral therapy, founded by Albert Ellis, a psychologist.

ADMINISTRATION AND REGULATION

You need to locate a therapist who is not only skilled in cognitive behavioral therapy but who has also used the therapy for pain management. Check with your medical provider, insurance plan, or any other trusted source. Your employer, who may have other employees dealing with pain issues, may even have suggestions. People with health insurance should check the mental health coverage that it offers.

Providers with varied backgrounds may be skilled in cognitive behavioral therapy. Physicians who specialize in mental health are usually psychiatrists. In all probability, they have trained in CBT. But, people who have earned master's or doctoral degrees in psychological counseling may be skilled in this therapy as well. There are no reliable statistics on the number of therapists that practice cognitive behavioral therapy. It is known to be widely used.

Cognitive behavior therapy may be conducted one-on-one or in groups with family members and other people with the same issues, such as pain. During the first few sessions, the therapist will ask about your medical history and your pain. Time will be devoted to pain education, how pain arises in the body, and multiple factors that influence the perception of pain. The goal is to begin to see yourself as a well person with pain and to decrease the preoccupation with pain and with the stress it creates The first sessions are an opportunity to attempt to determine if the therapist is a good match for you and will help you better manage your pain. Be sure to ask the therapist to estimate the number of appointments you may need. After a few sessions, if you are not beginning to make at least some initial progress, you may wish to search for a new therapist.

Therapists are taught cognitive behavior therapy during their academic training or in a specialized program. Today, there are many online offerings. Costs associated with cognitive behavioral therapy are a function of the type of practitioner. Therapy with a psychiatrist will cost more than with a master's level therapist. Health insurance usually covers at least part of the costs. It is important to see a therapist who has met certification and licensing requirements.

BENEFITS AND RISKS

Cognitive behavioral therapy is most often used for psychological problems, such as anxiety, depression, and eating disorders. However, because pain management has a clear emotional component, cognitive behavioral therapy has the potential to improve pain and general well-being. People who are demoralized by their pain may benefit from help with chronic stress, managing symptoms, reducing anxiety, and an improved ability to move forward and function.

For most people, there is little risk associated with cognitive behavioral therapy. However, because the process explores some painful experiences and feelings, people may feel uncomfortable, upset, angry, and emotionally and physically fatigued. Working with a skilled therapist should reduce the risks.

RESEARCH FINDINGS

Cognitive Behavioral Therapy May Help Some People with Chronic Pain

In a review published in 2016 in the *Western Journal of Nursing Research*, researchers from Ann Arbor Michigan and Birmingham, Alabama (USA), wanted to learn more about the usefulness of cognitive behavioral therapy for chronic pain. The cohort consisted of 35 randomized, controlled trials published between 2009 and 2015 that reported on CBT interventions in adults with chronic pain. The sample sizes ranged from 20 to 442 subjects, and the mean ages of the subjects ranged from 39.57 to 74.59 years. The most frequently studied medical problem was chronic back or neck pain. That was followed by pain of mixed etiology and fibromyalgia. There were no studies on cancer-related pain and only two studies on military veterans with chronic pain. The most frequently study duration was 6 to 10 weeks, and most of the trials followed subjects for 6 months. The total amount of time spent on cognitive behavioral therapy training in each of the studies was usually 6 to 10 hours. The researchers learned that 43 percent of the trials reported positive effects on pain intensity. According to the researchers, this lower percentage may be a function of study design. For example, pain intensity as the primary outcome was the goal of only eight studies. Furthermore, 17 studies compared CBT with another active intervention, which was not a true control group. Interestingly, cognitive behavioral therapy online training for pain was as useful as in-person individual or group therapy. The researchers observed that "further studies are needed to examine the long-term efficacy of CBT for pain intensity in individuals with chronic pain."[1]

Cognitive Behavioral Therapy May Help Adults with Chronic Back Pain

In a randomized, interviewer-blind, controlled trial published in 2016 in *JAMA*, researchers from Washington State (USA) evaluated the use of cognitive behavioral therapy, mindfulness-based stress reduction, or usual care for treating people with chronic back pain. The cohort consisted of 342 adults between the ages of 20 and 70 years with chronic low back pain; the average duration of the back pain was 7.3 years. One hundred thirteen were assigned to cognitive behavioral therapy; 116 were assigned to mindfulness-based stress reduction; and 113 were assigned to usual care. The CBT and mindfulness training were delivered in eight weekly two-hour groups. The researchers found that at 26 weeks the subjects in the two intervention groups had higher amounts of clinically meaningful improvements than those in the usual care group. Although relief was slightly higher in the mindfulness group, the subjects in both groups had greater improvements in pain and functional limitations. There were no meaningful differences in outcomes between the groups. Hence, cognitive behavioral therapy may well be a useful tool in the relief of pain.[2]

The Differences in Results between Cognitive Behavioral Therapy and Mindfulness-Based Stress Reduction May Be Greater Than the Previous Study Indicates

In a randomized trial published in 2017 in the journal *Spine*, researchers from Seattle Washington (USA) examined the usefulness and cost-effectiveness of cognitive behavior therapy, mindfulness-based stress reduction, and usual care for low back pain. The initial cohort consisted of 342 adults, between the ages of 20 and 70 years, with chronic low back pain, who were treated at the Group Health Cooperative, a large health plan in Washington State. One hundred and thirteen subjects received cognitive behavioral therapy; 116 received mindfulness-based stress reduction; and 113 received the usual care. The subjects in both intervention groups received their therapies in groups of 10 to 12 participants two hours per week for eight weeks. The mindfulness program also included a six-hour retreat. All of the instructors were experienced in their areas of expertise. Clinical outcomes were assessed by telephone at baseline, and 4, 8, 26, and 52 weeks. Both interventions were found to be cost-effective treatments for low back pain. However, the mindfulness program was better than the cognitive behavioral treatments. "These findings suggest that MBSR [mindfulness-based stress reduction], and to a lesser extent CGT, may provide cost-effective treatment for CLBP [chronic low back pain] for payers and society."[3]

Some People with Chronic Pain Benefit More Than Others from Cognitive Behavioral Therapy

In a multisite, randomized, controlled trial published in 2016 in the journal *Pain*, researchers from several locations in the United States but based in Los Angeles, California, wanted to determine who benefits most from the use of cognitive behavior therapy for chronic pain. The cohort consisted of 256 people from community practices in New York, Virginia, and North Carolina who had chronic pain from hip or knee osteoarthritis; the subjects were placed in a CBT group or a usual care group. At baseline, the subjects in both groups were not significantly different on demographic and health variables. The 10-session therapy was delivered by trained nurse practitioners in community primary care and rheumatology offices; the goal of the therapy was to teach and promote the use of cognitive behavioral pain management skills. A variety of assessments were conducted on the subjects in both of the groups. The researchers found that some subjects had substantially better responses to the cognitive behavioral therapy than others. There were five significant moderators for outcomes; these were pain coping style, patient expectation for treatment response, radiographically assessed disease severity, age, and education. Subjects with interpersonal problems associated with pain tended not to benefit from the treatment. In addition, only subjects who at baseline had moderate and high expectations of the therapy improved, and those with moderate to high osteoarthritis disease demonstrated stronger responses to therapy. Finally, in contrast to the younger and less educated subjects, the oldest and most educated subjects had stronger responses to the therapy. The researchers commented that "the ability to identify patients who might respond best to behavioral approaches may be particularly useful to clinicians working with patients who fail to respond adequately to biological approaches."[4]

Cognitive Behavioral Therapy May Help in the Recovery from Total Knee Arthroplasty

In a parallel-group, randomized, controlled pilot trial published in 2018 in the *Journal of Arthroplasty*, researchers from China explained that it is not uncommon for patients who have had total knee arthroplastic surgery to experience kinesiophobia, the fear of pain associated with moving the knee. That fear may reduce the effectiveness of rehabilitation and hamper the overall recovery. Could cognitive behavioral therapy reduce this fear?

The initial cohort consisted of 100 patients who had the surgery and were highly fearful of moving their knees. Half were assigned to participate in a four-week, individually tailored, 30-minute cognitive behavioral program; the other half received standard care and served as controls. Data were collected before the intervention, four weeks after the intervention, and six months after the treatment ended. The researchers learned that the program based on CBT was superior to standard care in reducing kinesiophobia as well as "pain catastrophizing" and knee pain intensity. It also enhanced knee functioning. And these positive results were still evident at the six-month follow-up. The researchers concluded that "future studies are needed to evaluate the effects of a CBT program on kinesiophobia at different time points."[5]

The Use of Cognitive Behavioral Therapy for Subacute Low Back Pain Has Not Been Sufficiently Studied

In a systematic review published in 2018 in the journal *Current Pain and Headache Reports*, researchers from Boston, Massachusetts, and Providence, Rhode Island (USA), wanted to learn if cognitive behavior therapy would help people dealing with subacute low back pain, defined by the researchers as pain having a 7- to 12-week duration (before chronic low back pain develops). The researchers located six prospective randomized, controlled trials that met their criteria, such as having at least 30 subjects and published in 1997 or later. The studies varied widely in their sample sizes, precise definition of subacute low back pain, nature of cognitive behavioral therapy interventions, and outcome measures. Five of the studies found significant improvements associated with CBT, but the studies differed so dramatically that it was hard to make any comparisons. The researchers underscored the need for more research on the topic. "Given the widespread attention now being given to the US opioid epidemic, there is an urgent need for effective non-pharmacologic pain treatments."[6]

Internet-Delivered Cognitive Behavioral Therapy May, Possibly, Help Manage Pain in Children, Adolescents, and Adults

In a systematic review and meta-analysis published in 2018 in the journal *Medicine*, researchers from China evaluated the ability of internet-delivered cognitive behavioral therapy to help children and teens dealing with chronic pain. Four trials met the inclusion criteria; of the 404 subjects, 208 received internet-delivered cognitive behavioral therapy and 196 were controls. The subjects were between the ages of 11 and 17 years. All of the trials were conducted in the USA and were published in English. Even though the sample size was small, the researchers observed small to moderate reductions in pain, compared to pretreatment, in the subjects in the intervention groups. Yet, they cautioned that "although the overall quality of the studies was high, we are still not confident in yielding strong conclusions."[7]

In a trial published in 2013 in *Pain*, researchers examined the ability of a clinician guided internet-delivered CBT program, known as "Pain Course," to manage chronic pain and emotional well-being in adults. Sixty-two adults with chronic pain were randomized to either an eight-week treatment group conducted by a clinical psychologist or a waitlist control group. The volunteers came from every state and territory in Australia, and they had a variety of different pain conditions for an average of 7.36 years. More than 41 percent reported pain in three or more locations. Twenty-nine subjects in the treatment group completed the five sessions, and then the waitlist subjects were provided access to the course. Both groups completed questionnaires at pretreatment and post-treatment, but only the treatment group completed a questionnaire at a three-month follow-up. The researchers determined that the subjects in the treatment group reported significant improvements on measures of average pain ratings, disability, depression, and anxiety, and they sustained these improvements at the follow-up. The researchers concluded that "the outcomes of the Treatment Group were superior to those of the Control group." Also, "the emerging data support the potential of ICBT [Internet cognitive behavioral therapy] to reduce barriers to effective psychological treatment for people with chronic pain."[8]

Internet Cognitive Behavioral Therapy May Be Useful for Teens with Functional Abdominal Pain or Functional Dyspepsia

In an open, uncontrolled pilot trial published in 2019 in the journal *Behavior Therapy*, researchers from Sweden examined the feasibility and efficacy of an online cognitive behavioral therapy program for teens dealing with functional abdominal pain or functional dyspepsia (indigestion).

They all had weekly abdominal pain for at least two months. The initial cohort consisted of 20 female and 11 male adolescents between the ages of 13 and 17 years from all over Sweden; they participated in the program with one of their parents. The CBT consisted of 10 weekly online modules, which focused on abdominal symptoms, delivered by three clinical psychologists, with substantial child and adolescent CBT experience. To help them support their teens, the parents received five modules. For example, in one module, parents were taught to increase the focus on things that work well and reduce the focus on abdominal problems. The teens completed an average of 7.2 modules. Assessments were conducted before treatment began, after treatment ended, and during a six-month follow-up. The researchers learned that the teens had significant reductions in pain intensity. There were clinically significant changes in 17 of the participants at post-treatment and at the six-month follow-up. The researchers noted that "the intervention was feasible and acceptable, as well as potentially efficacious in reducing pain intensity, GI symptoms, avoidant behavior, fear of symptoms, and quality of life with large within-group effect sizes."[9]

When Combined with Neuromuscular Training Cognitive Behavioral Therapy May Play a Role in the Treatment of Juvenile Fibromyalgia

In a two-arm, randomized, controlled trial published in 2018 in the *Journal of Pain*, researchers from Cincinnati, Ohio (USA) evaluated the ability of cognitive behavioral therapy combined with neuromuscular training to reduce pain and disability in children with juvenile fibromyalgia. The cohort consisted of 40 teens between the ages of 12 and 18 years with juvenile fibromyalgia. They received either eight weeks of group cognitive behavior therapy alone or eight weeks of group cognitive behavior therapy combined with neuromuscular training, a program known as Fibromyalgia Integrative Training for Teens, or FIT Teens. Groups consisted of four or five teens; there were two one-and-a-half-hour sessions per week. Parents attended 6 of the 16 sessions; during these sessions, the parents were introduced to the coping skills and exercises that their children were learning. Assessments were conducted at baseline, post-treatment, and at a three-month follow-up. Thirty-six subjects (90% female) completed the trial. The subjects in the combination program had significantly better decreases in pain than the subjects in the cognitive behavioral program. The teens in the combination program also showed significant improvements in disability, primarily in pain reduction, but that progress was no longer evident at the follow-up. The researchers concluded "that the FIT Teens intervention provides added benefits beyond CBT in the treatment of JFM, particularly in pain reduction."[10]

Cognitive Behavioral Therapy Did Not Provide Pain Relief to Children with Juvenile Idiopathic Arthritis

In a study published in 2015 in the journal *Pediatric Rheumatology*, researchers from Denmark wanted to learn if cognitive behavior therapy would offer some relief to children dealing with juvenile idiopathic arthritis. In total, there were 15 girls and 4 boys with a mean age of 11.7 years. Nine children with juvenile idiopathic arthritis were given six 120-minute sessions of group cognitive behavior therapy, and 10 were placed in a waitlist control group. The sessions, which also included family members, took place in three different cities in western Denmark. Children and parents completed questionnaires before the sessions began and after they ended, and the children completed a one-week daily pain diary the week following completion of the questionnaires. Families on the waitlist completed questionnaires and pain diaries on three occasions, including one after they finally participated in their own sessions. Assessments of pain and other factors were conducted. Eighteen families finished the entire intervention. Twelve families attended all six sessions, four families missed one session, and two families missed two sessions. Though the children and parents were satisfied with the interventions and found them to be credible, the children did not experience reductions in their pain. Still, the participants in the intervention had "increased quality of life and improvements in adaptive pain cognitions." It is important to note that the children in the intervention group had a small but insignificant increase in disease activity, and the children in the waitlist group had a small but insignificant decrease in disease activity. "Conclusions on the strength of efficacy require further research in a large, randomized, controlled trial."[11]

NOTES

1. Knoerl, Robert, Ellen M. Lavoie Smith, and James Weisberg. "Chronic Pain and Cognitive Behavioral Therapy: An Integrative Review." *Western Journal of Nursing Research* 38, no. 5 (May 2016): 596–628.

2. Cherkin, Daniel C., Karen J. Sherman, Benjamin H. Balderson, et al. "Effects of Mindfulness-Based Stress Reduction vs Cognitive-Behavioral Therapy and Usual Care on Back Pain and Functional Limitations among Adults with Chronic Low Back Pain: A Randomized Clinical Trial." *JAMA* 315, no. 12 (March 22, 2016): 1240–1249.

3. Herman, Patricia M., Melissa L. Anderson, Karen J. Sherman, et al. "Cost-Effectiveness of Mindfulness-Based Stress Reduction vs Cognitive Behavioral Therapy or Usual Care Among Adults with Chronic Low-Back Pain." *Spine* 42, no. 20 (October 15, 2017): 1511–1520.

4. Broderick, Joan E., Francis J. Keefe, Stefan Schneider, et al. "Cognitive Behavioral Therapy for Chronic Pain is Effective, but for Whom?" *Pain* 157, no. 9 (September 2016): 2115–2123.

5. Cai, Libai, Huanhuan Gao, Huiping Xu, et al. "Does a Program Based on Cognitive Behavioral Therapy Affect Kinesiophobia in Patients following Total Knee Arthroplasty? A Randomized, Controlled Trial with a 6-Month Follow-Up." *The Journal of Arthroplasty* 33, no. 3 (March 2018): 704–710.

6. Mariano, Timothy Y., Richard D. Urman, Catherine A. Hutchinson, et al. "Cognitive Behavioral Therapy (CBT) for Subacute Low Back Pain: A Systematic Review." *Current Pain and Headache Reports* 22, no. 3 (February 2018): 15–21.

7. Tang, Wen-Xin, Lu-Feng Zhang, Yan-Qiu, and Zhi-Song. "Efficacy of Internet-Delivered Cognitive-Behavioral Therapy for the Management of Chronic Pain in Children and Adolescents: A Systematic Review and Meta-Analysis." *Medicine* 97 (2018): 36–46.

8. Dear, Blake F., Nick TItov, Kathryn Nicholson Perry, et al. "The *Pain Course*: A Randomised Controlled Trial of a Clinician-Guided Internet-Delivered Cognitive Behaviour Therapy Program for Managing Chronic Pain and Emotional Well-Being." *Pain* 154, no. 6 (June 2013): 942–950.

9. Bonnert, Marianne, Ola Olén, Maria Lalouni, et al. "Internet-Delivered Exposure-Based Cognitive-Behavioral Therapy for Adolescents with Functional Abdominal Pain or Functional Dyspepsia: A Feasibility Study." *Behavior Therapy* 50 (2019): 1177–1188.

10. Kashikar-Zuck, Susmita, William R. Black, Megan Pfeiffer, et al. "Pilot Randomized Trial of Integrated Cognitive-Behavioral Therapy and Neuromuscular Training for Juvenile Fibromyalgia: The FIT Teens Program." *Journal of Pain* 19, no. 9 (September 2018): 1049–1062.

11. Lomholt, Johanne Jeppesen, Mikael Thastum, Anne Estmann Christensen, et al. "Cognitive Behavioral Group Intervention for Pain and

Well-Being in Children with Juvenile Idiopathic Arthritis: A Study of Feasibility and Preliminary Efficacy." *Pediatric Rheumatology* 13 (2015): 35–44.

REFERENCES AND FURTHER READINGS

Bonnert, Marianne, Ola Olén, Maria Lalouni, et al. "Internet-Delivered Exposure-Based Cognitive-Behavioral Therapy for Adolescents with Functional Abdominal Pain or Functional Dyspepsia: A Feasibility Study." *Behavior Therapy* 50 (2019): 177–188.

Broderick, Joan E., Francis J. Keefe, Stefan Schneider, et al. "Cognitive Behavioral Therapy for Chronic Pain IS Effective, but for Whom?" *Pain* 157, no. 9 (September 2016): 2115–2123.

Cai, Libai, Huanhuan Gao, Huiping Xu, et al. "Does a Program Based on Cognitive Behavioral Therapy Affect Kinesiophobia in Patients following Total Knee Arthroplasty? A Randomized, Controlled Trial with a 6-Month Follow-Up." *The Journal of Arthroplasty* 33 (2018): 704–710.

Cherkin, Daniel C., Karen J. Sherman, Benjamin H. Balderson, et al. "Effects of Mindfulness-Based Stress Reduction vs Cognitive-Behavioral Therapy and Usual Care in Back Pain and Functional Limitations among Adults with Chronic Back Pain: A Randomized Clinical Trial." *JAMA* 315, no. 12 (March 22, 2016): 1240–1249.

Dear, Blake F., Nick Titov, Kathryn Nicholson Perry, et al. "The *Pain Course*: A Randomised Controlled Trial of a Clinician-Guided Internet-Delivered Cognitive Behaviour Therapy Program for Managing Chronic Pain and Emotional Well-Being." *Pain* 154, no. 6 (June 2013): 942–950.

Herman, Patricia M., Melissa L. Anderson, Karen J. Sherman, et al. "Cost-Effectiveness of Mindfulness-Based Stress Reduction vs Cognitive Behavioral Therapy or Usual Care among Adults with Chronic Low-Back Pain." *Spine* 42, no. 20 (October 15, 2017): 1511–1520.

Kashikar-Zuck, Susmita, William R. Black, Megan Pfeiffer, et al. "Pilot Randomized Trial of Integrated Cognitive-Behavioral Therapy and Neuromuscular Training for Juvenile Fibromyalgia: The FIT Teens Program." *Journal of Pain* 19, no. 9 (September 2018): 1049–1062.

Knoerl, Robert, Ellen M. Lavoie, and James Weisberg. "Chronic Pain and Cognitive Behavioral Therapy: An Integrative Review." *Western Journal of Nursing Research* 38, no. 5 (May 2016): 596–628.

Lomholt, Johanne Jeppesen, Mikael Thastum, Anne Estmann Christensen, et al. "Cognitive Behavioral Group Intervention for Pain and Well-Being in Children with Juvenile Idiopathic Arthritis: A Study of Feasibility and Preliminary Efficacy." *Pediatric Rheumatology* 13 (2015): 35–44.

Mariano, Timothy Y., Richard D. Urman, Catherine A. Hutchison, et al. "Cognitive Behavioral therapy (CBD) for Subacute Low Back Pain: A Systematic Review." *Current Pain and Headache Reports* 22, no. 3 (February 2018): 15–21.

Tang, Wen-Xin, Lu-Feng Zhang, Yan-Qiu Ai, and Zhi-Song Li. "Efficacy of Internet-Delivered Cognitive-Behavioral Therapy for the Management of Chronic Pain in Children and Adolescents: A Systematic Review and Meta-Analysis." *Medicine* 97 (2018): 36–46.

Cold and Heat Therapy

INTRODUCTION

People have been using cold and heat therapy to treat pain for centuries. Treating pain with cold or heat applications may be effective for a wide variety of medical problems, and it is readily available and affordable. It is important to know when to use cold therapy, when to use hot therapy, and when to alternate between the two.

When cold therapy, which is also known as cryotherapy, is applied to the body, the blood vessels contract. That process, which is called vasoconstriction, causes reductions in circulation and a reduction in inflammation and swelling, especially around a joint or tendon. Cold therapy may also reduce nerve activity, which relieves pain, and, like a local anesthetic, it numbs sore tissues and slows the pain messages transmitted to the brain. When the cold is removed, the veins expand, a process known as vasodilation. As blood vessels expand, circulation improves, and the blood brings nutrients to aid the injured tissues. Improved circulation may eliminate the buildup of lactic acid and waste, which may occur after some types of exercise.

By increasing the temperature, heat therapy or thermotherapy improves circulation and blood flow to a particular area. In so doing, it soothes discomfort, heals damaged tissue, and increases muscle flexibility.

Heat therapy tends to be more effective than cold therapy at treating the chronic muscle pain and sore joints of arthritis. Heat therapy may help people dealing with osteoarthritis, strains and sprains, tendonitis, and pain or spasms in the neck or back. It may be used to warm muscles and tissues before exercise.

In general, cold therapy is used for acute injuries or pain, inflammation, and swelling. Hot therapy is used for muscle pain or stiffness. Alternating cold and heat may be useful for osteoarthritis and exercise-induced injury, especially in elite athletes.

ADMINISTRATION AND REGULATION

The most frequent types of cold therapy include ice packs, frozen gel packs, coolant sprays, ice massage, and ice baths. Other types of cold therapy include cryostretching, which uses cold to reduce muscle spasms during stretching; cryokinetics, which combines cold treatment with active exercise and may be useful for ligament sprains; and whole-body cold therapy chambers.

For home use, an ice pack wrapped in a towel should be applied to the affected area within 48 hours of an injury. One may also use a water bottle filled with cold water, pads that may be frozen in the freezer, or an ice bath. Even frozen peas are a good option, as is a plastic bag filled with ice. Unless they are being used for massage, frozen items should never be applied directly to the skin. It is best to apply cold therapy for shorter periods of time, several times a day. Ten to 15 minutes is just about right; to prevent skin or nerve damage, it should be used for no more than 20 minutes. If possible, while applying cold therapy, it is a good idea to elevate the affected area.

There are many different types of heat therapy products that are sold in pharmacies, large retail outlets such as Target and Costco, and online. Products range from electrical heating pads to hot-water bottles to hot compresses to heat wraps to pads that may be heated in a microwave. Heat packs may be dry or moist. Dry heat may be applied for up to eight hours; moist heat may be applied for up to two hours. However, less serious pain may only require shorter applications, such as 20 minutes.

It is well known that cold and heat are frequently used to treat pain, both at home and in therapeutic settings. In general, it is a free or relatively inexpensive means of treatment, especially in the home setting.

BENEFITS AND RISKS

The goal of both cold and heat therapy is to reduce pain and improve function. Cold therapy should also reduce swelling, which tends to be useful for pain.

People may easily use cold and heat therapy at home. At-home cold therapy may be useful for a recent injury, gout, strains, and tendonitis. People who suffer from migraines should consider a cold cloth or mask on the forehead. At-home heat therapy should help low back pain, shoulder pain, knee pain, sore muscles, joint pain, menstrual pain, osteoarthritis strains, tendonitis, neck pain, and headaches.

When not used properly, cold therapy may cause damage to skin, tissues, or nerves. If two days of cold therapy have not resulted in improvements, a medical provider should be consulted.

People with sensory disorders, such as sometimes occurs in diabetes, should not use cold therapy at home. They may be unable to ascertain if the cold is causing damage. People with heart disease should not use cold therapy without the approval of a medical provider. Cold therapy should not be applied to stiff muscles or joints, and it should not be used on people with poor circulation.

With heat therapy, only warm heat should be used. Hot heat should be avoided as heat that is too hot may burn the skin. People with localized infections should not use heat therapy; it may increase the risk of the infection spreading. If intense swelling occurs, stop the heat therapy immediately. Heat therapy should not be used if the skin is hot, red, or inflamed; if the person has dermatitis or an open wound; if the area is numb; or if the person lacks the ability to sense heat, as in peripheral neuropathy. People with high blood pressure or heart disease should check with their healthcare provider before using heat therapy.

RESEARCH FINDINGS

Heat Therapy and Home Exercise Are Useful for People with Knee Osteoarthritis

In a randomized, controlled trial published in 2019 in the *International Journal of Nursing Practice*, researchers from Turkey examined the use of heat and home exercise for people with knee osteoarthritis. The trial, which was conducted between January 2014 and February 2015, had 62 subjects who had bilateral knee osteoarthritis for at least six months. Most of the subjects, with an average age of 57.8 years, had stage 2 knee osteoarthritis, and the pain affected their normal daily activities. Fifteen subjects used heat applications; they applied heat packs to their knees for 20 minutes twice each day, morning and evening, five days a week for four weeks. Fifteen subjects were told to do seven different muscle strengthening exercises for 10 minutes twice each day, morning and evening, five days per week for four weeks. Fifteen subjects were told to complete the recommended exercises for 10 minutes twice each day, morning and evening, five days per week for four weeks; this was followed by heat applied to both knees for 20 minutes. No specific practices were recommended for the 17 subjects in the control group. The researchers found that all of the interventions significantly reduced levels of pain. The researchers commented that their findings "demonstrated that the use of both heat and exercises, separately or in combination, have a positive effect on pain and function level."[1]

A Computer Controlled Cooling Device May Be More Beneficial after Primary Total Knee Arthroplasty Than the Usual Cold Therapy

In a prospective, randomized, single-blinded, comparative, and controlled trial published in 2018 in the journal *International Orthopaedics*, researchers from Austria and the Netherlands tested the efficacy and safety of a new cryotherapy device in patients having unilateral, primary total knee arthroplasty and compared it to the conventional standard cold therapy regimen. The trial was conducted between December 2011 and April 2013 at the Department of Orthopaedic Surgery of the Medical University of Graz in Austria. The cohort consisted of 97 patients; there were 53 females and 44 males. All of the patients, who were between the ages of 55 and 90 years, suffered from severe degenerative end-stage osteoarthritis of the knee joint. For six days after their surgery, they were treated with the new device, which has a continuous cold flow for varied periods of time (cTreatment®), or the standard cold therapy protocol (cold pack applications three times a day). (During the day before the surgery, the cTreatment patients also received a one-hour treatment.) There were 46 patients in the new device group and 51 patients in the standard care group. Periodic assessments were conducted. Eight of the patients were excluded from the final analyses. While both types of cold therapy provided pain relief, the researchers determined that the cTreatment provided better pain relief, particularly on the fourth and sixth postoperative days, "but all of these results did not reach statistical significance."[2]

Local Cold Application Appears to Benefit People with Fibromyalgia Pain

In an one-group, pre-test/post-test, pre-experimental model trial published in 2017 in the *International Journal of Rheumatic Disease*, researchers from Turkey evaluated the ability of cold therapy to help people dealing with the pain associated with fibromyalgia. The cohort consisted of 55 female patients, with an average age of 33.2 years and length of disease duration of 3.2 years, who were treated at the rheumatology outpatient clinic in a hospital located in Erzurum, Turkey. The patients were all asked on which side (left or right) they felt more pain. Cold gel packs, which had been in a freezer for at least 4 hours, were then applied for 10 minutes to the trapezius muscle (top of back) on the side where they had more pain. Pain measurements were taken at baseline and 10 minutes after the application ended and 1½ hours later. The next day, 24 hours after the application, the patients again visited the clinic and pain measurements were taken. The researchers learned that during all three post-application assessments, the cold therapy resulted in significant reductions in pain. Though the researchers noted that the study had some limitations, such as the lack of a control group, their findings nevertheless "contribute significantly to science because it suggests a new method of controlled pain" in people with fibromyalgia.[3]

Heat Therapy May Play a Role in the Relief of Nonspecific Neck Pain

In a randomized, controlled trial published in 2017 in the *Journal of Back and Musculoskeletal Rehabilitation*, researchers from Henderson, Nevada (USA) and Jordan and Korea wanted to determine if the use of heat therapy and ibuprofen between physical therapy appointments would help people with chronic neck pain. The initial cohort consisted of 92 subjects between the ages of 18 and 70 years who were neck pain patients at an outpatient physical therapy center in Southern California. The subjects were divided into four groups. Thirty-one of the subjects used low levels of continuous heat before home exercise; 30 subjects used ibuprofen and low levels of continuous heat before home exercise; 15 subjects used a sham wrap and an ibuprofen placebo before home exercise, and 16 had no heat or ibuprofen before home exercise. All of the subjects had one hour of conventional physical therapy twice a week for two weeks. The subjects were given logs to record their daily adherence to the protocol and their levels of pain. Periodic assessments were taken. Seventy-two subjects were included in the final analyses. The researcher learned that there was a significant reduction in subjective pain in all of the groups. Low levels of continuous heat combined with ibuprofen resulted in a greater reduction in pain than the heat alone. The reduction in pain in the placebo and control groups was significantly less than in the intervention groups. According to the researchers, "it is of interest that most patients that dropped out were in the control and placebo groups stating that they needed to get pain relief."[4]

Alternating Cold and Heat May Improve Function, but It Does Not Reduce Heel Pain

In a trial published in 2016 in the journal *The Foot*, researchers from India and Australia tested the use of alternating cold and heat to treat heel pain. The cohort consisted of 20 subjects. While everyone received the usual naturopathic physiotherapy care, 10 subjects were assigned to cold and hot compresses, and 10 received therapeutic ultrasound, which has been proven to have no effect beyond placebo. Alternating compresses is one of the most common types of treatment in naturopathic medicine. All of the subjects completed the 7 days of treatments. The subjects tended to be in their mid to late 40s, and there were 15 females and 5 males. The researchers observed no significant difference in pain levels between the two groups. However, the subjects in the compresses group did have significant improvements in functioning. The researchers noted that "the use of numerous therapies and practices in treatment may make it difficult to observe which aspects of care resulted in clinical improvements."[5]

Cold Therapy Does Not Sufficiently Reduce the Pain Associated with Chest Tube Removal

In a prospective, randomized clinical trial published in 2019 in the journal *Complementary Therapies in Clinical Practice*, researchers from Turkey compared the usefulness of cold therapy to music therapy, lidocaine spray, and no additional treatment for helping with the removal of chest tubes. Many people have described the removal of chest tubes as painful and anxiety provoking. The pain is said to be brief but intense—a burning feeling. The initial cohort consisted of 120 patients with chest tubes who were being treated, between March 2016 and September 2017, at the cardiovascular surgery unit in a private hospital in Ordu, Turkey. The patients were assigned to one of four groups—gel pack cold therapy, music therapy, lidocaine spray, and control. There were 30 patients in each group. The chest tubes were removed by the same general practitioner; the same charge nurse noted outcomes. Pain assessments were conducted 10 minutes before chest tube removals, immediately after the removals, and 20 minutes later. The patients in all four groups reported "unacceptably high pain ratings" immediately after the chest tube removal. And after 20 minutes, the patients in the cold therapy group did not exhibit significant differences in pain. The researchers concluded that "it is important for nurses to adequately address pain and anxiety with pharmacological and non-pharmacological approaches before the procedure." It may be necessary to administer pharmacological and non-pharmacological approaches combined.[6]

Heat Therapy May Provide Some Relief for Dysmenorrhea, the Pain Associated with Menstruation

In an analysis published in 2018 in the journal *Scientific Reports*, researchers from Korea examined the usefulness of heat therapy for the pain associated with menstruation. Apparently, heat therapy is a common method—estimates are between 36.5 and 50 percent—to deal with this type of pain. The researchers included six randomized controlled trials in a qualitative analysis; all of the trials were published in peer-reviewed journals. Four of the studies used a heating device, such as a patch or wrap, and two studies used a ceramic belt emitting far-infrared radiation. Two of these studies were conducted in the United States; the others were conducted in Iran, Korea, Taiwan, and Turkey. Three randomized controlled trials were included in the meta-analysis. The researchers learned that heat therapy decreased menstrual pain in women with primary dysmenorrhea. Still, it is important to note that their analyses included only a few trials with small sample sizes. The researchers concluded that "rigorous high-quality trials are still needed to provide robust evidence."[7]

In a systematic review published in 2016 in *Complementary Therapies in Clinical Practice*, researchers from Nigeria and the United Kingdom reviewed studies that examined the use of heat therapy or TENS to relieve primary dysmenorrhea. (TENS stands for "transcutaneous electrical nerve stimulation." It is the electrical stimulation of the skin to relieve pain by interfering with the neural transmission of signals from underlying pain receptors.) The cohort consisted of three studies on heat and six on TENS. Sample sizes ranged from 21 to 147 subjects, and the age of the subjects ranged from 12 to 41 years. The methodological quality of the trials ranged from low to high. The researchers learned that both heat therapy and TENS may significantly reduce the pain associated with dysmenorrhea. However, they cautioned that "higher quality trials are needed to assess the effectiveness of these interventions for the treatment of menstrual pain."[8]

Cold and Heat Pack May or May Not Be Useful for Neck and Back Strain

In a single-center, prospective, randomized controlled trial published in 2010 in the journal *American Emergency Medicine*, researchers from Stony Brook, New York (USA), compared the pain-relieving effect of cold and heat for pain from back and neck strains. Research assistants in a university-based emergency department identified 60 patients presenting with back or neck pain from a minor injury that occurred within the previous 24 hours. Sixty-four percent were Caucasian, 12 percent were Black or African American, 10 percent were Hispanic, and 8.5 percent were Asian. Sixty-one percent reported low back pain, 27 percent had neck pain, and 12 percent had upper back pain. All of the subjects received 400 mg oral ibuprofen and either 30 minutes of a cold pack application (n=29) or 30 minutes of the application of an electric heating pad set on high (n=31). Assessments were conducted before and after the cold/hot application. The researchers found no differences in pain scores between the cold and hot groups both before and after the treatments. Though statistically significant, the reductions did not result in clinically significant reductions in pain. According to the researchers, "it is possible that pain relief is mainly the result of ibuprofen therapy."[9]

Both Cold and Heat Appear to Have a Limited Use for Pain

In a clinical trial published in 2017 in the *Journal of Clinical Nursing*, researchers from Turkey investigated the use of self-administered superficial local cold and hot applications for pain in people with primary knee arthritis in both knees. The cohort consisted of 96 subjects with newly diagnosed primary knee osteoarthritis; the subjects were placed in a cold application group, a heat application group, or a control group. There were 32 subjects in each group; the mean age of all the subjects was 63.12 years. The majority—81.3 percent—were females. For three weeks, the subjects self-administered cold or heat applications, twice each day. The subjects in the control group received standard care. The researchers learned that subjects in both treatment groups experienced reductions in pain; no such reduction was seen in the subjects in the control group. But these reductions were not statistically significant, and they were not sufficiently strong to observe a notable difference between the groups. Moreover, two weeks after the study ended, the subjects in both treatment groups had higher levels of pain, indicating that the effects decrease after the treatments end. The researchers concluded that the cold and heat applications provided "mild" improvements in pain, functional status, and life quality, "but this improvement was not at a level that would create a difference between the groups."[10]

Cold Compression Therapy Does Not Appear to Be Any Better Than Cold Pack Therapy Following Shoulder Arthroscopic Surgery

In a trial published in 2016 in the journal *Knee Surgery, Sports Traumatology, Arthroscopy*, researchers from Germany wanted to learn if cold pack therapy or cold compression therapy would be useful after shoulder arthroscopy surgery. The cohort consisted of 52 patients (31 males and 21 females) with a mean age of 53 years; they all had arthroscopy surgery of the glenohumeral joint (shoulder). After the surgery, which was performed by the same shoulder surgeon, they were randomly assigned to the experimental group of cold compression bandages or the control group of cold packs. For the cold compression therapy, the researchers used a commercially available compression product; for the cold pack, they used a common, readily available cold pack, which was covered with a cloth to protect the skin. Patients were told to apply the cold pack for 15 to 20 minutes per hour and to remove it if they experienced any discomfort. Baseline measurements were taken upon hospital admission. Outcome measurements were taken 2, 8, and 24 hours after the surgery. Only one patient did not complete the treatment. The researchers learned that the cold compression therapy did not relieve more pain than the cold packs. The researchers concluded that "no recommendation can be made with respect to the question whether cold compression therapy or cold therapy after arthroscopic surgery of the should should be preferred."[11]

NOTES

1. Karadağ, Songül, Sultan Taşci, Nurhan Doğan, et al. "Application of Heat and a Home Exercise Program for Pain and Function Levels in Patients with Knee Osteoarthritis: A Randomized Controlled Trial." *International Journal of Nursing Practice* 25, no. 5 (October 2019): e12772.

2. Sadoghi, Patrick, Sandro Hasenhütl, Gerald Gruber, et al. "Impact of a New Cryotherapy Device on Early Rehabilitation after Primary Total Knee Arthroplasty (TKA): A Prospective Randomised Controlled Trial." *International Orthopaedics* 42, no. 6 (June 2018): 1265–1273.

3. Yillmaz, Naside, and Emine Kiyak. "The Effects of Local Cold Application on Fibromyalgia Pain." *International Journal of Rheumatic Diseases* 20, no. 8 (August 2017): 929–934.

4. Petrofsky, Jerrold S., Michael Laymon, Faris Alshammari, et al. "Use of Low Level of Continuous Heat and Ibuprofen as an Adjunct to Physical therapy Improves Pain Relief, Range of Motion and the Compliance for Home Exercise in Patients with Nonspecific Neck Pain: A Randomized Controlled Trial." *Journal of Back and Musculoskeletal Rehabilitation* 30, no. 4 (2017): 889–896.

5. Arankalle, Dhananjay, Jon Wardle, and Pradeep M. K. Nair. "Alternate Hot and Cold Application in the Management of Heel Pain: A Pilot Study." *The Foot* 29 (December 2016): 25–28.

6. Aktaş, Y. Y., and N. Karabulut. "The Use of Cold Therapy, Music Therapy and Lidocaine Spray for Reducing Pain and Anxiety following Chest Tube Removal." *Complementary Therapies in Clinical Practice* 34 (February 2019): 179–184.

7. Jo, Junyoung, and Sun Haeng Lee. "Heat Therapy for Primary Dysmenorrhea: A Systematic Review and Meta-Analysis of Its Effects on Pain Relief and Quality of Life." *Scientific Reports* 8, no. 1 (November 2, 2018): 16252.

8. Igwea, Sylvester Emeka, Chidinma Samantha Tabansi-Ochuogu, and Ukachukwu Okoroafor Abaraogu. "TENS and Heat Therapy for Pain Relief and Quality of Life Improvement in Individuals with Primary Dysmenorrhea: A Systematic Review." *Complementary Therapies in Clinical Practice* 24 (August 2016): 86–91.

9. Garra, Gregory, Adam J. Singer, Richard Leno, et al. "Heat or Cold Packs for Neck and Back Strain: A Randomized Controlled Trial of Efficacy." *Academic Emergency Medicine* 17, no. 5 (May 2010): 484–489.

10. Aciksoz, Semra, Aygul Akyuz, and Servet Tunay. "The Effect of Self-Administered Superficial Local Hot and Cold Application Methods on Pain, Functional Status and Quality of Life in Primary Knee Osteoarthritis Patients." *Journal of Clinical Nursing* 26, no. 23–24 (December 2017): 5179–5190.

11. Alfuth, Martin, Marion Strietzel, Tim Vogler, et al. "Cold versus Cold Compression Therapy after Shoulder Arthroscopy: A Prospective

Randomized Clinical Trial." *Knee Surgery, Sports Traumatology* 24, no. 7 (July 2016): 2209–2215.

REFERENCES AND FURTHER READINGS

Aciksoz, Semra, Aygul Akyuz, and Servet Tunay. "The Effect of Self-Administered Superficial Local Hot and Cold Application Methods on Pain, Functional Status and Quality of Life in Primary Osteoarthritis Patients." *Journal of Clinical Nursing* 26, no. 23–24 (December 2017): 5179–5190.

Aktaş, Y. Y., and N. Karabulut. "The Use of Cold Therapy, Music Therapy and Lidocaine Spray for Reducing Pain and Anxiety following Chest Tube Removal." *Complementary Therapies in Clinical Practice* 34 (February 2019): 179–184.

Alfuth, Martin, Marion Strietzel, Tim Vogler, et al. "Cold versus Cold Compression Therapy after Shoulder Arthroscopy: A Prospective Randomized Controlled Trial." *Knee Surgery, Sports Traumatology, Arthroscopy* 24, no. 7 (July 2016): 2209–2215.

Arankalle, Dhananjay, Jon Wardle, and Pradeep M. K. Nair. "Alternate Hot and Cold Application in the Management of Heel Pain: A Pilot Study." *The Foot* 29 (December 2016): 25–28.

Garra, Gregory, Adam J. Singer, Richard Leno, et al. "Heat or Cold Packs for Neck and Back Strain: A Randomized Controlled Trial of Efficacy." *Academic Emergency Medicine* 17, no. 5 (May 2010): 484–489.

Igwea, Sylvester Emeka, Chidinma Samantha Tabansi-Ochuogu, and Ukachukwu Okoroafor Abaraogu. "TENS and Heat Therapy for Pain Relief and Quality of Life Improvement in Individuals with Primary Dysmenorrhea: A Systematic Review." *Complementary Therapies in Clinical Practice* 24 (August 2016): 86–91.

Jo, Junyoung, and Sun Haeng Lee. "Heat Therapy for Primary Dysmenorrhea: A Systematic Review and Meta-Analysis of Its Effects on Pain Relief and Quality of Life." *Scientific Reports* 8, no. 1 (November 2, 2018): 16252.

Karadağ, Songül, Sultan Taşci, Nurhan Doğan, et al. "Application of Heat and a Home Exercise Program for Pain and Function Levels in Patients with Knee Osteoarthritis: A Randomized Controlled Trial." *International Journal of Nursing Practice* 25, no. 5 (October 2019): e12772.

Petrofsky, Jerrold, Michael Laymon, Faris Alshammari, et al. "Use of Low Level of Continuous Eat and Ibuprofen as an Adjunct to Physical

Therapy Improves Pain Relief, Range of Motion and the Compliance for Home Exercise in Patients with Nonspecific Neck Pain: A Randomized Controlled Trial." *Journal of Back and Musculoskeletal Rehabilitation* 30, no. 4 (2017): 889–896.

Sadoghi, Patrick, Sandro Hasenhütl, Gerald Gruber, et al. "Impact of a New Cryotherapy Device on Early Rehabilitation after Primary Total Knee Arthroplasty (TKA): A Prospective Randomised Controlled Trial." *International Orthopaedics* 42, no. 6 (June 2018): 1265–1273.

Yilmaz, Naside and Emine Kiyak. "The Effects of Local Cold Application on Fibromyalgia Pain." *International Journal of Rheumatic Diseases* 20, no. 8 (August 2017): 929–934.

Corticosteroids

INTRODUCTION

Also known as steroids, corticosteroids are a class of synthetic drugs that lower inflammation in the body while simultaneously reducing the activity of the body's immune system. They ease swelling, itching, redness, and allergic reactions. Corticosteroids decrease the pressure on nerve endings, relieving pain.

Some of the best-known steroids are cortisone, hydrocortisone, prednisone, prednisolone, dexamethasone, and betamethasone. While they are known to be effective and fast-acting, making them useful for treating sudden, severe symptoms, they also have a host of side effects, which limit their use. Because of these side effects, medical providers often prescribe other medications before prescribing corticosteroids. Taking lower dosages over shorter periods of time may reduce the risk of these side effects.

Corticosteroids mimic the effects of cortisol, which is produced in the adrenal glands. Medical providers prescribe corticosteroids to either increase the action of specific hormones above a normal level or return them to a normal level. The increases in hormonal activity suppress the immune system, which activates inflammation in the body. The process of suppressing immune system activity reduces inflammation.

The first use of corticosteroids may be traced to 1948, when a patient at the Mayo Clinic who had debilitating rheumatoid arthritis was treated by rheumatologists with an experimental injectable steroid. In 1950, cortisone was the first corticosteroid approved for use in the United States.

ADMINISTRATION AND REGULATION

Corticosteroid use may be systemic or localized. Systemic corticosteroids may be administered through tablet or capsule medications, an intravenous injection, or with a needle injected into a joint or muscle. Localized corticosteroids may be applied via skin creams, gels, and ointments; nasal or mouth sprays; eye drops or eardrops; and inhalers that target the lungs. It is best to take the lowest dose possible for the shortest period of time. Prices on the various corticosteroids vary widely.

Topical medications with low levels of steroids may be sold over the counter. Like all prescription medications, corticosteroids with higher doses are regulated by the FDA. Health providers with patients on these medications must monitor them carefully.

BENEFITS AND RISKS

Medical providers prescribe corticosteroids for problems such as asthma, arthritis, eczema, lupus, hay fever, hives, chronic obstructive pulmonary disease (COPD), inflammatory bowel diseases (such as Crohn's disease and ulcerative colitis), psoriasis, multiple sclerosis, and allergies. They reduce the inflammation associated with these illnesses. Corticosteroids may help people suffering from Addison's disease, an illness in which the body makes insufficient amounts of cortisol, a hormone naturally produced by the body's adrenal glands. As they suppress the immune system, corticosteroids may help prevent rejection in people with organ transplants.

Although side effects may occur with all types of steroids, they are most likely to occur with the oral forms. Side effects from oral steroids include acne, blurred vision, water retention, increased appetite and weight gain, difficulty sleeping, gastritis, mood changes and mood swings, confusion, behavior changes, glaucoma, thin skin, easy bruising, high blood pressure, muscle weakness, increased growth of body hair, susceptibility to infection, worsening of diabetes, delayed wound healing, stomach ulcers, Cushing's syndrome, osteoporosis, depression, and stunted growth in children. Side effects from injected steroids include loss of skin color, insomnia, high blood sugar, temporary skin thinning, intense pain at injection site, insomnia, high blood sugar, and facial flushing. Side effects from topical steroids include thin skin, acne, and red skin lesions. And side effects from inhaled corticosteroids include cough, sore throat, difficulty speaking, minor nosebleeds, and oral thrush (fungal infection in the mouth). These side effects are caused when some of the drug lingers in the mouth and throat instead of traveling to the lungs. This risk may be reduced by rinsing or gargling with water after taking all the medication and spitting out any water that remains in the mouth.

Side effects of steroids are more likely to occur when they are used at higher doses for longer periods of time. When used for a few days to a few weeks, there may be no or minimal side effects. Older people are at increased risk for high blood pressure and osteoporosis; children may have stunted growth; and breastfeeding moms may pass the steroids to their babies. Taking corticosteroids for longer periods of time may increase the risk of cataracts, high blood sugar levels and diabetes, infection from common bacteria and viruses, osteoporosis, suppressed adrenal-gland hormone production, thin skin with higher rates of bruising, and slowed wound healing.

Corticosteroids may interact with medications used for a number of medical concerns, such as HIV/AIDS, herpes simplex infection of the eye; tuberculosis; diabetes; intestinal problems; glaucoma; high blood pressure; fungal infections; diseases of the heart, liver, thyroid, or kidney; and medications used during recent surgery or serious injury. People taking steroids need to avoid grapefruit juice.

When combined with corticosteroids, certain live vaccines, such as those for measles, mumps, and rubella, may have dangerous interactions. Other vaccines, such as those for flu and pneumonia, may not work properly in a person taking high doses of a corticosteroid.

If corticosteroid medicine is suddenly discontinued or reduced too quickly, withdrawal symptoms may occur. These include muscle, bone, and joint pain; nausea; weight loss; and headaches.

Although pregnant women may take corticosteroids, they should be considered a medicine of last resort. Whenever possible, medical providers tend to avoid prescribing them to women who are known to be pregnant.

RESEARCH FINDINGS

Corticosteroids Help Manage Postoperative Endodontic Pain

In a systematic review and meta-analysis published in 2018 in the *Journal of Endodontics*, researchers from Iran evaluated the effectiveness of corticosteroids on postoperative endodontic pain. The researchers identified 18 randomized clinical trials with 1,088 subjects who met their criteria; the trials compared the use of corticosteroids to the use of a placebo. All of the subjects were over the age of 15 years and had primary root canal surgery. Pain intensity scores were taken several times after surgery. The researchers learned that during the first 24 hours following surgery, the administration of corticosteroids significantly lowered pain scores. It is important to note that patients in the various trials were given different types of corticosteroids. The corticosteroids used were dexamethasone, betamethasone, prednisolone, triamcinolone, methylprednisolone, and meticortelone. Thus, there was notable heterogeneity between the trials. Most of the drugs were administered orally, but some drugs were administered in other ways, such as by injection into the muscle or ligament. Also, the sample sizes tended to be relatively small. The researchers learned that pain scores reported 6, 12, and 24 hours after the surgery were all significantly lower in the subjects taking corticosteroids than in the subjects on placebos. The researchers concluded that "corticosteroids had a postoperative pain-reducing effect in endodontic patients."[1]

Steroid Injections Seem to Be Very Helpful for the Pain Associated with Adhesive Capsulitis of the Shoulder

In a systematic review and meta-analysis published in 2016 in the journal *Medicine*, researchers from China compared the efficacy and safety of steroid injections to physiotherapy for the treatment of adhesive capsulitis of the shoulder, also known as "frozen shoulder." The researchers identified nine randomized controlled trials with 453 patients that met their criteria; 227 patients received steroid injections, and 226 received physiotherapy. In one study, the patients received the injections three times per week. In another study, the patients received no more than three injections per week. In seven studies, the patients received only one injection. The researchers learned that both steroid injections and physiotherapy had similar results in improving pain, function, and passive rotation, and the injection was as safe as the physiotherapy. Further, shoulder disability was improved by week six or seven, and the improvements continued up to 24 to 26 weeks after the intervention. Because a single injection is so easily administered, the researchers suggested that the injection is preferable over physiotherapy, which requires "several sessions with different modalities, adding financial burden to patients and decreasing compliance." And, they concluded that "one steroid injection might be the 1st choice for ACS [adhesive capsulitis of the shoulder]."[2]

However, Maybe the Injections Do Not Work as Well in People with Diabetes

In a randomized, two-parallel group trial published in 2020 in the *Journal of Shoulder and Elbow Surgery*, researchers from Egypt compared the effectiveness of ultrasound-guided, low-dose, intra-articular steroid injections to radical extracorporeal shock-wave therapy (rESWT) for improving frozen shoulder pain, function, and range of motion in people with controlled type 2 diabetes. The cohort consisted of 103 people with diabetes and frozen shoulder diagnoses; there were 79 women and 24 men. The mean age was 55.87 years in the rESWT group and 57.96 years in the steroid group. Symptom duration ranged from 6 to 30 months in both groups. During a 12-week period of time, 52 subjects received four sessions of rESWT, one week apart, with 2,000 impulses per session, and 51 subjects had a single ultrasound-guided low-dose intra-articular steroid injection of 20 mg triamcinolone acetonide. The application of rESWT was associated with mild to moderate pain immediately after the treatment in about one-third of the subjects, and the pain stopped within a day or two. No other adverse events were reported. While both types of treatment offered pain relief, the subjects in the rESWT group experienced more improvement in pain, function, and range of motion than the subjects in the single injection group. "Therefore, rESWT might be considered a safe alternative to steroid injections in diabetic patients with should AC [adhesive capsulitis]."[3]

Corticosteroid Injections May or May Not Provide Some Short-Term Help for People with Plantar Fasciitis

In a systematic review and meta-analysis published in 2019 in the journal *BMC Musculoskeletal Disorders*, researchers from Australia wanted to learn if corticosteroid injections would help people suffering from plantar fasciitis or plantar heel pain. The researchers included 47 trials with 2,989 subjects that met their criteria; 65.1 percent of the subjects were female with a mean age of 46.5 years. In all of the trials, corticosteroid injections were compared to another type of treatment, such as autologous blood injections, foot orthotics, platelet-rich plasma, dry needling, or a placebo. The mean group size was 28. Eight different types of corticosteroids were used, with methylprednisone acetate the most common. Most trials mixed corticosteroid with a local anesthetic, and lidocaine was the most common. The researchers found low quality evidence that corticosteroids were more effective than autologous blood injections and foot orthotics for up to 6 weeks. For periods of time greater than 12 weeks, the researchers noted very low-quality evidence that platelet-rich plasma and dry needling were more effective than corticosteroids. However, corticosteroid injections were not more effective than placebo injections for reducing pain or improving function. They both had similar results. The researchers deemed that finding "notable."[4]

Corticosteroids Seem to Be Useful for People Having Knee Arthroplasty Surgery

In a systematic review and meta-analysis published in 2021 in the journal *Knee Surgery, Sports Traumatology, Arthroscopy*, researchers from Switzerland and Italy examined the benefits and risks of perioperative steroid supplementation in total knee arthroplasty. The researchers reviewed total knee arthroplasty surgery, with or without steroids, in terms of pain, inflammatory response, length of hospitalization, and complications. The researchers found 20 randomized controlled trials that met their criteria; there were a total of 1,830 subjects. Fifteen of the trials had a two-arm design, and five had a three-arm design. Intravenous steroids were used in 12 studies, and local steroids were used in eight studies. The risk of bias was low in 11 trials; there was concern about bias in 9 of the trials. The researchers determined that steroid use was associated with lower perioperative pain, but only until the fourth day after surgery. The drugs reduced the length of hospitalization without increasing the incidence of short-term and midterm complications. In fact, when steroids were used, one out of every two patients had a one-day reduction in hospital stay. In addition, steroid use decreased nausea, vomiting, and the use of opioid medication. Patients on steroids had lower inflammation markers, and their range of motion was better. To these researchers, the perioperative use of steroids for knee arthroplasty surgery had a number of clear benefits and resulted in better outcomes.[5]

Intravenous Corticosteroids Help with Pain Management after Total Knee or Hip Arthroplasty

In a systematic review and meta-analysis published in 2018 in the journal *Pain Practice*, researchers from China investigated the ability of corticosteroids to help with the management of pain following total knee or hip arthroplasty surgery. Pain is a major concern for people undergoing these types of surgeries. Surgeons want to control pain but also limit the amount of opioids they prescribe. The researchers located 14 randomized controlled trials with

1,023 patients who met their criteria. There were 542 patients in corticosteroids groups and 481 patients in control groups. The researchers determined that intravenous steroids significantly reduced postoperative pain, both at rest and with activity, during the first 24 hours after the surgery. But, this statistical difference was gone 48 hours after surgery. Patients on steroids used significantly fewer opioid medications, but their hospital stays were not significantly shortened. The researchers wrote that "corticosteroids may be a reasonable choice and a promising method to control postoperative pain."[6]

Adding Corticosteroids to Local Anesthetics May Not Improve Pain Relief

In a systematic review and meta-analysis published in 2020 in the *British Journal of Anaesthesia*, researchers from Canada and Brazil assessed the benefits and safety of adding steroids to local anesthetics to treat chronic noncancer pain. The researchers located 73 trials that met their criteria. Of these, 69 were included in the meta-analysis. The studies involved different types of injections for chronic pain conditions. The researchers determined that only one in every 13 subjects may achieve some added pain relief from the addition of corticosteroids. In a separate analysis, in which minor changes were made, that figure changed from one in 13 to one in 22. According to the researchers, the decrease in pain scores was less than clinically meaningful. There were no differences in physical functioning, global improvement or satisfaction, or quality of life. The researchers noted that findings "do not support the hypothesis that addition of steroids may prolong pain relief or that higher doses of steroids are associated with better success." They further concluded that there is minimal benefit for adding steroids to local anesthetics. At the same time, adding steroids increases the chances of harm. The number of injections should be limited, and high doses should be avoided.[7]

Corticosteroid Knee Injections May Help People with Knee Osteoarthritis, but Not as Much as Platelet-Rich Plasma Injections

In a prospective, randomized, controlled trial published in 2019 in the journal *Orthopäde*, researchers from China compared the efficacy of three different intra-articular injections—corticosteroid, platelet-rich plasma, and hyaluronic acid—for knee osteoarthritis. The cohort consisted of 120 patients, all between the ages of 40 and 65 years, with early stage knee osteoarthritis. Sixty-five patients were men, and 55 were women. The patients were divided into three groups, according to the type of intra-articular injections they received. Patient questionnaires were completed prior to the first injection and then at 3, 6, 9, and 12-month follow-ups. No patients were lost or excluded during the follow-up period. A few patients in each group reported short periods of pain, nausea, and dizziness. Although the patients in all three groups experienced improvements in pain, the best results were seen with the platelet-rich plasma injections. The researchers commented that platelet-rich plasma injections were far better than corticosteroids and hyaluronic acid injections "in reducing pain and recovering physical function in the long term."[8]

Then Again, Intra-Articular Injections of Triamcinolone May Not Be Useful for Knee Osteoarthritis Pain

In a two-year, randomized, placebo-controlled, double-blind trial published in 2017 in the journal *JAMA*, researchers from Boston, Massachusetts (USA), compared the efficacy of intra-articular triamcinolone, a steroid, to saline for the pain associated with knee osteoarthritis. The trial, which was conducted between June 2011 and January 2015, initially included 140 subjects with knee osteoarthritis; all of the subjects were at least 45 years old. For two years, 70 subjects received intra-articular injections of 40 mg triamcinolone acetonide and 70 subjects received saline injections every three months; the injections were administered every three months. The researchers assessed levels of pain as well as cartilage loss, articular structural damage, and physical function. The subjects had MRI scans at baseline, after 12 months, and at the end of the trial. Fifty-nine subjects in the intervention group and 60 in the saline group completed the trial. Though the treatment subjects experienced more cartilage loss than the saline subjects, there were no statistical differences between the groups in levels of pain. The researchers concluded that their findings "do not support this treatment for patients with symptomatic knee osteoarthritis."[9]

Corticosteroids May Offer Relief to People with Metastatic Bone Cancer

In an analysis published in 2017 in the journal *Current Opinion in Supportive and Palliative Care*, researchers from Canada and Brazil noted that corticosteroids are frequently used in the palliative care setting. In fact, over 50 percent of palliative patients are treated with these medications. In many instances, the figures are probably much higher. The researchers wanted to learn if these treatments would help people dealing with metastatic bone cancer. They found 12 articles that met their criteria. Corticosteroids appeared to be used for three main reasons. The first indication was for patients with uncontrolled bone pain; the corticosteroids were used as adjuvant analgesics. The second indication was for the management of pain following palliative radiotherapy. The third indication was for specific cancer types, including hormone driven cancer such as breast and prostate. Reports of adverse events were not consistently documented in the studies. Rates of relief from pain ranged from 30 to 70 percent; pain relief was usually considered moderate. The researchers commented that "the risk of developing adverse effects should be carefully considered prior to therapy initiation on a case-by-case basis."[10]

Corticosteroids May Not Be as Useful for Cancer Pain as Many People Believe

In an analysis published in 2015 in the *Cochrane Database of Systematic Reviews*, researchers from Australia reviewed the use of corticosteroids for the management of cancer-related pain. The researchers found 15 randomized or prospective controlled trials, with 1926 subjects, that met their criteria. The trials ranged in size from 20 to 598 subjects; all of the trials had patients who were over 18 years and were dealing with cancer-related pain. Most trials compared corticosteroids, especially dexamethasone, to standard therapy. Adverse events were poorly documented. The various studies had a lack of standardized measurements; the use of different agents, dosages, and comparisons; and various routes of drug delivery. The researchers were unable to conduct a subgroup analysis according to the type of cancer, and they commented that the quality of the evidence was limited by the risk of bias, small sample sizes, attrition, and missing data from enrolled subjects. The researchers wrote that they found only weak evidence that corticosteroids are useful for pain control in cancer patients. Yet, some studies did find significant pain relief, if only for a relatively short period of time. "This could be important for patients with poor clinical status."[11]

Corticosteroids May or May Not Be Useful for Acute Gout

In a systematic review and meta-analysis published in 2017 in the journal *Steroids*, researchers from China examined the usefulness of steroids for treating acute gout. (A type of arthritis, gout is characterized by sudden, severe attacks of pain, swelling, redness, and tenderness in one or more joints, most often in the big toe.) The researchers located seven randomized controlled trials with 929 subjects that met their criteria. Sample sizes ranged from 60 to 376, and mean ages ranged from 44.1 to 65.0 years. In all of the trials, the vast majority of the subjects were males. The researchers learned that corticosteroids had "analgesic efficacy" for the pain associated with gout. Still, the researchers were unable to determine if steroids were better than nonsteroidal medications for treating gout. The trials that they reviewed failed to provide "sufficient or precise evidence that corticosteroids are superior to non-corticosteroids in pain relief for acute gout patients." However, corticosteroids may well be better than non-corticosteroids in reducing tenderness and swelling. It should be noted that in most of the trials, the diagnoses were based on clinical symptoms, not joint aspirations. The researchers underscored the need for more studies.[12]

Long-Term Systemic Use of Corticosteroids Is Associated with a Number of Problems

In a systematic review of the literature published in 2017 in the journal *Clinical Therapeutics*, researchers from Boston, Massachusetts, and Hampton, New Jersey (USA), wanted to learn more about some of the problems associated with the long-term systemic use of corticosteroids. The researcher found 32 articles that met their criteria. Of these, 75 percent focused on autoimmune disease, asthma, or lung disease. Fourteen of the included articles were database analyses. There were also six simulations, six clinical trials, three systematic literature reviews, two patient surveys, and one chart review. The articles included oral, parenteral, and inhaled corticosteroids. Twenty-seven articles were published between 2007 and 2013, and five were published between 2014 and 2016. From the articles, the researchers learned that many medical problems are associated with the long-term, systemic use of corticosteroids. The most commonly cited medical problems were hypertension and bone fracture. Other problems included cataracts, gastrointestinal concerns, myocardial infarction and other cardiac conditions, type 2 diabetes mellitus, hyperglycemia, and metabolic issues. People who moved from a higher to a lower daily dose were able to reduce the incidence or avoid some medical problems. Still, the researchers noted that long-term users of corticosteroids may experience "numerous" adverse events, "suggesting a need for further research to fill current data gaps, as well as a potential need for alternative treatment options."[13]

NOTES

1. Shamszadeh, Sayna, Armin Shirvani, Mohammad Jafar Eghbal, and Saeed Asgary. "Efficacy of Corticosteroids on Postoperative Endodontic Pain: A Systematic Review and Meta-Analysis." *Journal of Endodontics* 44, no. 7 (July 2018): 1057–1065.

2. Suj, Yaying, Shuai Lu, Peng Zhang, et al. "Steroid Injection versus Physiotherapy for Patients with Adhesive Capsulitis of the Shoulder: A PRIMSA Systematic Review and Meta-Analysis of Randomized Controlled Trials." *Medicine* 95, no. 20 (2016): e3469.

3. El Naggar, T. E. D., A. I. E. Maaty, and A. E. Mohamed. "Effectiveness of Radial Extracorporeal Shock-Wave Therapy Versus Ultrasound-Guided Low-Dose Intra-Articular Steroid Injection in Improving Should Pain, Function, and Range of Motion in Diabetic Patients with Shoulder Adhesive Capsulitis." *Journal of Shoulder and Elbow Surgery* 29, no. 7 (July 2020): 1300–1309.

4. Whittaker, Glen A., Shannon E. Munteanu, Hylton B. Menz, et al. "Corticosteroid Injection for Plantar Heel Pain: A Systematic Review and Meta-Analysis." *BMC Musculoskeletal Disorders* 20 (2019): 378.

5. Davide Previtali, Gioegio Di Llaura Frattura, Giuseppe Filardo, et al. "Peri-Operative Steroids Reduce Pain, Inflammatory Response and Hospitalisation Length following Knee Arthroplasty Without Increased Risk of Acute Complications: A Meta-Analysis." *Knee Surgery, Sports Traumatology, Arthroscopy* 29, no. 1 (January 2021): 59–81.

6. Li, Donghai, Changde Wang, Zhouyuan Yang, and Pengde Kang. "Effect of Intravenous Corticosteroids on Pain Management and Early Rehabilitation in Patients Undergoing Total Knee or Hip Arthroplasty: A Meta-Analysis of Randomized Controlled Trials." *Pain Practice* 18, no. 4 (April 2018): 487–499.

7. Shanthanna, Harsha, Jason Busse, Li Wang, et al. "Addition of Corticosteroids to Local Anaesthetics for Chronic Non-Cancer Pain Injections: A Systemic Review and Meta-Analysis of Randomised Controlled Trials." *British Journal of Anaesthesia* 125, no. 5 (November 2020): 779–801.

8. Huang, Yong, Xiaolu Liu, Xinliang Xu, and Junbin Liu. "Intra-Articular Injections of Platelet-Rich Plasma, Hyaluronic Acid or Corticosteroids for

Knee Osteoarthritis: A Prospective Randomized Controlled Study." *Orthopäde* 48, no. 3 (March 2019): 239–247.

9. McAlindon, Timothy E., Michael P. LaValley, William F. Harvey, et al. "Effect of Intro-Articular Triamcinolone vs Saline on Knee Cartilage Volume and Pain in Patients with Knee Osteoarthritis: A Randomized Clinical Trial." *JAMA* 317, no. 19 (2017): 1967–1975.

10. Lim, Fiona M. Y., Adam Bobrowski, Arnav Agarwal, and Mauricio F. Silva. "Use of Corticosteroids for Pain Control in Cancer Patients with Bone Metastases: A Comprehensive Literature Review." *Current Opinion in Supportive and Palliative Care* 11, no. 2 (June 2017): 78–87.

11. Haywood, Alison, Phillip Good, Sohil Khan, et al. "Corticosteroids for the Management of Cancer-Related Pain in Adults." *Cochrane Database of Systematic Reviews* 24, no. 4 (April 2015): CD010756.

12. Liu, Xinliang, Dehong Sun, Xiaosong Ma, et al. "Benefit-Risk of Corticosteroids in Acute Gout Patients: An Updated Meta-Analysis and Economic Evaluation." *Steroids* 128 (December 2017): 89–94.

13. Rice, J. Bradford, Alan G. White, Lauren M. Scarpati, et al. "Long-Term Systemic Corticosteroid Exposure: A Systematic Literature Review." *Clinical Therapeutics* 39 (2017): 2216–2229.

REFERENCES AND FURTHER READINGS

El Naggar, T. E. D. M., A. I. E. Maaty, and A. E. Mohamed. "Effectiveness of Radical Extracorporeal Shock-Wave Therapy versus Ultrasound-Guided Low-Dose Intra-Articular Steroid Injection in Improving Should Pain, Function, and Range of Motion in Diabetic Patients with Should Adhesive Capsulitis." *Journal of Shoulder and Elbow Surgery* 29, no. 7 (July 2020): 1300–1309.

Haywood, Alison, Phillip Good, Sohil Khan, et al. "Corticosteroids for the Management of Cancer-Related Pain in Adults." *Cochrane Database of Systematic Reviews* 24, no. 4 (April 2015): CD010756.

Huang, Yong, Xiaolu Liu, Xinliang Xu, and Junbin Liu. "Intro-Articular Injections of Platelet-Rich Plasma, Hyaluronic Acid or Corticosteroids for Knee Osteoarthritis: A Prospective Randomized Controlled Study." *Orthopäde* 48, no. 3 (March 2019): 239–247.

Li, Donghai, Changde Wang, Zhouyuan, and Pengde Kang. "Effect of Intravenous Corticosteroids on Pain Management and Early Rehabilitation in Patients Undergoing Total Knee or Hip Arthroplasty:

A Meta-Analysis of Randomized Controlled Trials." *Pain Practice* 18, no. 4 (April 2018): 487–499.

Lim, Fiona M. Y., Adam Bobrowski, Arnav Agarwal, and Mauricio F. Silva. "Use of Corticosteroids for Pain Control in Cancer Patients with Bone Metastases: A Comprehensive Literature Review." *Current Opinion in Supportive and Palliative Care* 11, no. 2 (June 2017): 78–87.

Liu, Xinliang, Dehong Sun, Xiaosong Ma, et al. "Benefit-Risk of Corticosteroids in Acute Gout Patients: An Updated Meta-Analysis and Economic Evaluation." *Steroids* 128 (December 2017): 89–94.

McAlindon, Timothy E., Michael P. LaValley, William F. Harvey, et al. "Effect of Intra-Articular Triamcinolone vs Saline on Knee Cartilage Volume and Pain in Patients with Knee Osteoarthritis: A Randomized Clinical Trial." *JAMA* 317, no. 19 (2017): 1967–1975.

Mohammad, Hasan R., Thomas W. Hamilton, Louise Strickland, et al. "Perioperative Adjuvant Corticosteroids for Postoperative Analgesia in Knee Arthrosplasty: A Meta-Analysis of 1,396 Knees." *Acta Orthopaedica* 89, no. 1 (2018): 71–76.

Previtali, Davide, Giorgio Di Laura Frattura, Giuseppe Filardo, et al. "Peri-Operative Steroids Reduce Pain, Inflammatory Response and Hospitalisation Length following Knee Arthroplasty Without Increased Risk of Acute Complications: A Meta-Analysis." *Knee Surgery, Sports Traumatology, Arthroscopy* 29, no. 1 (January 2021): 59–81.

Rice, J. Bradford, Alan G. White, Lauren M. Scarpati, et al. "Long-Term Systemic Corticosteroid Exposure: A Systematic Literature Review." *Clinical Therapeutics* 39 (2017): 2216–2229.

Shamszadeh, Sayna, Armin Shirvani, Mohammad Jafar Eghbal, and Saeed Asgary. "Efficacy of Corticosteroids on Postoperative Endodontic Pain: A Systematic Review and Meta-Analysis." *Journal of Endodontics* 44, no. 7 (July 2018): 1057–1065.

Shanthanna, Harsha, Jason Busse, Li Wang, et al. "Addition of Corticosteroids to Local Anaesthetics for Chronic Non-Cancer Pain Injections: A Systematic review and Meta-Analysis of Randomised Controlled Trials." *British Journal of Anaesthesia* 125, no. 5 (November 2020): 779–801.

Sun, Yaying, Shuai Lu, Peng Zhang, et al. "Steroid Injection versus Physiotherapy for Patients with Adhesive Capulitis of the Shoulder: A

PRIMSA Systematic Review and Meta-Analysis of Randomized Controlled Trials." *Medicine* 95, no. 20 (2016): e3469.

Wang, Wei, Mingmin Shi, Chenhe Zhou, et al. "Effectiveness of Corticosteroid Injection In Adhesive Capsulitis of Shoulder: A Meta-Analysis." *Medicine* 96, no. 28 (July 2017): e7529.

Whittaker, Glen A., Shannon E. Munteanu, Hylton B. Menz, et al. "Corticosteroid Injection for Plantar Heel Pain: A Systematic Review and Meta-Analysis." *BMC Musculoskeletal Disorders* 20 (2019): 378.

Craniosacral Therapy

INTRODUCTION

Also known as CST, craniosacral therapy, which may be written as CranioSacraal, is a type of bodywork that relieves compression in the bones of the head, the sacrum or a triangular bone in the lower back, and the spinal column. "Cranio" refers to the bony part of the head known as the cranium, and "sacral" refers to the sacrum, or bottom of the spine.

The craniosacral system extends from the head down to the sacrum and coccyx. It consists of the dura mater membrane, which surrounds the brain and spinal cord, the cerebrospinal fluid, the skull bones that are attached to the membranes, and the joints and sutures that interconnect these bones.

During CST, which is a noninvasive hands-on therapy, practitioners use gentle pressure on the head, neck, and back to relieve the stress and pain caused by compression. It is believed that this gentle manipulation of the bones in the skull, spine, and pelvis normalize the flow of cerebrospinal fluid in the central nervous system. This removes blockages and enhances the body's ability to heal.

After extensive scientific studies from 1975 to 1983 at Michigan State University, CST was pioneered and developed by osteopathic physician John E. Upledger. Upledger was drawn to the work of an earlier physician, William Sutherland, who had explored the concept that the bones of the skull were structured to allow for movement.

ADMINISTRATION AND REGULATION

Many osteopaths, chiropractors, physical therapists, and massage therapists use craniosacral therapy as part of their normal treatments. Upon arrival at an appointment dressed in comfortable clothing, be prepared to review your symptoms and preexisting conditions. Most likely, you will lie down on your back on a massage table, and the practitioner will begin at your head, feet, or near the middle of your body. For about 45 to 90 minutes, the practitioner will gently press or reposition you to normalize the flow of cerebrospinal fluids and may use tissue-release methods while supporting a limb. Practitioners use a gentle touch—no more than five grams, which is about the weight of a nickel. In so doing, they release restrictions in the soft tissues that surround the central nervous system. During a session, you may experience deep relaxation, sensing pulsations, numbing sensations, and hot or cold feelings. Sometimes, people fall asleep. Practitioners maintain that CST may be a stand-alone treatment or combined with other therapies.

Practitioners typically use a number of different procedures. These include compression-decompression of temporomandibular joint (TMJ), decompression of temporal fascia, compression-decompression of spheno-basilar joint, parietal lift, frontal lift, scapular waist release, and pelvic diaphragm release. The quiet intervals between the manipulations are known as "still points." They happen every three or four minutes and last up to one minute.

At present, craniosacral therapy education is not regulated at the state or federal level. However, many states regulate the practice of massage therapy and bodywork. Craniosacral therapy practitioners may obtain a voluntary Registered Craniosacral Therapist certification from the Biodynamic Craniosacral Therapy Association of North America.

At present, there are no reliable statistics on the numbers of craniosacral practitioners and how frequently CST is incorporated into practices. In all probability, the costs associated with craniosacral therapy are a function of the practitioner who is providing the care. Hence, treatment from a physical therapist will tend to cost more than treatment from a massage therapist. However, it is more likely that an insurer will cover a physical therapy session than a visit with a massage therapist.

BENEFITS AND RISKS

Because craniosacral therapy is thought to relieve compression in the head, neck, and back, it may soothe pain and release emotional and physical stress and tension. In addition, it is believed to improve cranial mobility and ease or release restrictions of the head, neck, and nerves. Craniosacral therapy may be a component of the treatment of a wide variety of medical problems. These include chronic back and neck pain, central nervous system disorders, migraines and headaches, scoliosis, TMJ syndrome, orthopedic problems, and fibromyalgia. However, CST is also considered a means to boost the immune system and prevent health issues.

The most common risk associated with craniosacral therapy is mild discomfort following treatment. Generally, the discomfort fades within a day. People with certain conditions should not have craniosacral therapy. These include severe bleeding disorders, a diagnosed aneurysm, and a history of recent head injuries.

RESEARCH FINDINGS

Craniosacral Therapy Appears to Have Some Overall Benefits, Including Relieving Pain

In a frequently cited study published in 2011 in the *Journal of Alternative and Complementary Medicine*, researchers from the United Kingdom examined the records of 157 patients treated with craniosacral therapy. The patients ranged in age from neonates to 68 years. Seventy-three patients were treated by 10 different practitioners, and 84 patients were treated by a single practitioner working within the National Health Service. Seventy-four patients reported a noticeable improvement in their main problem; 67 percent reported a valuable improvement in their general well-being or a second health problem. The researchers determined that craniosacral therapy was particularly useful for certain pain problems, such as headaches, migraines, and neck and back pain. Seventy percent of the patients taking medication decreased or discontinued their use. Furthermore, during the six months following craniosacral treatment, the patients' average general practitioner consultation rate dropped by 60 percent. According to the researchers, the patients' responses indicated that craniosacral therapy may "help patients manage their problems and gain an improvement in their general well-being."[1]

Craniosacral Therapy Appears to Be Useful for Chronic Pain

In a systematic review and meta-analysis published early in 2020 in the journal *BMC Musculoskeletal Disorders*, researchers from Germany, Australia, and Sweden reviewed the ability of craniosacral therapy to help people dealing with chronic pain. Ten randomized controlled trials with 681 subjects met their criteria. The subjects had back and neck pain, migraines, headaches, fibromyalgia, epicondylitis, and pelvic girdle pain. The trials were conducted in the United States, Spain, Germany, Iceland, Poland, and Sweden. Sample sizes ranged from 20 to 123, with a median size of 62. The median age of the total sample was 43.4 years. The trials provided between one and 50 CST treatments, with a median number of 7 treatments within a maximum of 25 weeks. The researchers learned that craniosacral therapy resulted in significant small to medium improvements in pain intensity, functional disability, and physical quality of life. In addition, there were no reports of adverse events. Though they acknowledged the need for more studies, the researchers commented that "the summarized evidence suggested robust short-term efficacy and comparative effectiveness of CST on pain intensity and functional disability." Moreover, "longer-term effects seem plausible as well."[2]

Craniosacral Therapy Seems to Help People with Chronic Low Back Pain

In a single-blind, randomized, controlled clinical trial published in 2016 in the *Journal of Alternative and Complementary Medicine*, researchers from Spain investigated the use of craniosacral therapy for people with chronic low back pain. The cohort consisted of 64 men and women, with a mean age of 50 years, who had chronic nonspecific lower back pain for at least three months. The subjects were assigned to 10 sessions of craniosacral therapy or 10 sessions of traditional massage. Two experienced therapists administered all of the treatments, and all of the subjects attended a physical therapy clinic once per week for 10 weeks. Assessments were conducted before the first treatment session, at the end of the interventions, and one month after the last treatment session. The researchers found that the subjects in both groups had statistically similar reductions in disability, pain intensity, and spinal mobility immediately after the interventions and during the follow-up. However, subjects who had craniosacral therapy reported experiencing better improvements in pain intensity. Interestingly, the researchers noted that because they did not have a control group, "it cannot be determined whether the improvements seen in both groups can be attributed to the interventions or simply the passage of time."[3]

In a clinical trial published in 2014 in the journal *Ortopedia Traumatologia Rehabilitacja*, researchers from Poland randomly placed 55 people, between the ages of 24 and 47 years with nonspecific low back pain, in one of two groups. The 27 subjects in one group were treated with craniosacral therapy, and the 28 subjects in the other group were treated with trigger point therapy. Each subject took part in three sessions at three- to four-day intervals; each session lasted for about 30 minutes. All of the subjects were asked not to alter their normal daily activities. Pain severity assessments were conducted before and immediately after treatments. The researchers learned that both therapies were significantly effective in reducing the intensity and frequency of pain. However, neither therapy significantly influenced spine mobility. The researchers concluded that "craniosacral therapy and trigger point therapy are effective in the treatment of patients with non-specific lumbosacral pain."[4]

Craniosacral Therapy Is Probably Useful for Chronic Neck Pain

In a randomized, controlled, parallel-design trial published in 2016 in the *Clinical Journal of Pain*, researchers from Germany and Australia investigated the use of craniosacral therapy for chronic neck pain. The initial cohort consisted of 54 subjects who had been dealing with chronic neck pain for a mean of 9.6 years. They ranged in age from 19 to 65 years, with a mean age of 44.6 years. More than 80 percent were female; most of the subjects had used a variety of pharmacological and nonpharmacological treatments. The subjects, who were all white, received eight weekly sessions of craniosacral therapy or a light-touch sham treatment, which was specifically designed not to be effective. Assessments were conducted at baseline, after the eighth treatment, and three months later, at week 20. The subjects were treated by one of four licensed physiotherapists with advanced CST qualifications and with an average of six years of clinical practice. No serious adverse events were reported. When compared to the subjects in the sham group, the researchers learned that the subjects who had craniosacral therapy treatments had significant and clinically relevant reductions in pain intensity directly after the treatment period and at the three-month follow-up. Likewise, the treatments may improve functional disability and quality of life for up to three months after the intervention. "Particularly in chronic and recurrent neck pain, CST may be a worthwhile treatment option in addition to standard medical care."[5]

Craniosacral Therapy May Help People Suffering from Migraines

In a trial published in 2013 in the journal *Complementary Therapies in Clinical Practice*, researchers from Iceland wanted to learn if craniosacral therapy would be useful for people suffering from migraines. The initial cohort consisted of 18 women and 2 men, between the ages of 20 and 50 years, who had at least two migraine attacks per month. All of the subjects received six craniosacral treatments during a four-week period of time, and they all answered the Short-Form Headache Impact Test (HIT-6) four times. (This questionnaire is used to assess the effects of headaches or migraines on health and well-being.) The subjects were divided into two groups. The subjects in Group A answered the questionnaire before the first treatment and then after the next three treatments. The subjects in Group B answered the questionnaire before the first and second treatments, after the third treatment, and four weeks after the fourth treatment. The mean age for Group A was 37.4 years, and the mean age for Group B was 37.9 years; there were no significant differences between the groups. The researchers noted that after only a few treatments, the subjects in both groups experienced significant reductions in pain. The researchers concluded that although more research on the topic is needed, "craniosacral therapy could be considered as a potential therapy for migraine sufferers with the aim of improving quality of life."[6]

Craniosacral Therapy Seems to Help People with Cervicogenic Headaches

In a trial published in 2017 in the journal *MOJ Yoga & Physical Therapy*, researchers from India hypothesized that craniosacral therapy would be useful for people with cervicogenic headaches or headaches that arise primarily from dysfunction in the three upper cervical segments. These types of headaches are known to be debilitating, and the medications to treat them have numerous side effects. Forty-nine people met the selection criteria for the trial; 71 percent were females. The subject received three sessions (on alternative days per week) for three weeks, thus a total of nine sessions. The subjects maintained a headache diary from the first visit until their interventions ended. During the course of the study, the 49 subjects contributed 121 diary entries. The researchers found that craniosacral therapy was an effective treatment for cervicogenic headaches.[7]

Craniosacral Therapy Seems to Help How People with Fibromyalgia Perceive Their Pain

In a double-blind, longitudinal, clinical trial published in 2011 in the journal *Evidence-Based Complementary and Alternative Medicine*, researchers from Spain wanted to learn if craniosacral therapy would help people with the symptoms associated with fibromyalgia, such as pain, anxiety, and depression. The initial cohort consisted of 104 people who were diagnosed with fibromyalgia. Twenty-one subjects were being treated with muscle relaxants, 32 with antidepressants, 46 with anxiolytics, 59 with anti-inflammatories, 36 with corticoids, and 84 with analgesics. The subjects were randomly assigned to a craniosacral therapy group or a simulated treatment group with a disconnected ultrasound; there were no differences in baseline demographic characteristics between the two groups. The subjects in the intervention group had two weekly sessions of one hour; the subjects in the placebo group had two weekly 30-minute sessions of sham ultrasound treatment. During that 25-week trial, 9 subjects withdrew from the intervention group, and 11 withdrew from the placebo group. As a result, 81 women and 3 men, between the ages of 34 and 63 years, were included in the final analyses. The researchers learned that by the end of the study, the subjects in the intervention group had significant improvement in a number of fibromyalgia symptoms, including pain. The researchers concluded that their findings demonstrated "that craniosacral therapy improves the quality of life of patients with fibromyalgia, reducing their perception of pain and fatigue and improving their night rest and mood, with an increase in physical function."[8]

Craniosacral Therapy May or May Not Ease Pelvic Girdle Pain in Pregnant Women

In a randomized, multicenter, single-blind controlled trial published in 2013 in the journal *Acta Obstetricia Gynecologica*, researchers from Sweden wanted to learn if craniosacral therapy would ease the pain of pregnant women suffering from pelvic girdle pain, which affects according to the researchers about 30 percent of pregnant women. The initial cohort consisted of 123 pregnant women with pelvic girdle pain who were treated in a university hospital, a private clinic and 26 maternity care centers in Gothenburg, Sweden. The women, who were generally healthy, were pregnant with a single fetus between 12 and 29 gestational weeks. Sixty women received the standard care, including an elastic pelvic belt and specific exercises, and 63 women received the standard care and craniosacral therapy. The craniosacral therapy sessions lasted for 45 minutes and were held once weekly for two weeks, and then every second week for six weeks. Two therapists with 14 to 16 years of experience gave the craniosacral therapy treatments. Though no serious adverse events were reported, ten women in each group reported treatment-related disadvantages. The main finding of the trial was that the women receiving craniosacral therapy had reduced intensity of morning pain and less functional deterioration. There were no differences in the evening pain and the need for sick leave. The researchers commented that the effects were small and clinically questionable. At the same time, significantly more women in the intervention group had fewer symptoms and found treatment helpful. The researchers observed that "conclusions should be drawn carefully."[9]

More Studies on Craniosacral Therapy Are Needed

In a systematic review published in 2012 in the journal *Complementary Therapies in Medicine*, researchers from the United Kingdom examined the clinical benefits of craniosacral therapy on well-being and pain. Seven studies met their criteria; of these, three were randomized controlled trials, and four were observational, with two studies reporting data before and after the intervention and two studies using retrospective surveys to retrieve outcome data. The three randomized controlled studies had a "strong-quality" rating, while the four observational studies varied in their quality. Sample sizes ranged from 23 to 92 subjects in the randomized controlled trials and from 9 to 130 subjects in the observational studies. The follow-up periods, treatment frequency, and duration of studies varied extensively. The researchers found that the craniosacral treatments were generally associated with improvements in well-being and pain. Only two of the studies reported on the safety of craniosacral therapy, and they found no negative effects on either the children or the adults. The researchers noted that their main finding was the fact that there are so few studies on the effectiveness of craniosacral therapy on pathological conditions. The researchers concluded that "the current moderate quality of the studies and scarcity of available data indicates that further research into this area is needed."[10]

NOTES

1. Harrison, Rachel E., and John S. Page. "Multipractitioner Upledger CranioSacral Therapy: Descriptive Outcome Study 2007–2009." *Journal of Alternative and Complementary Medicine* 17, no. 1 (2011): 13–17.

2. Haller, Heidemarie, Romy Lauche, Tobias Sundberg, et al. "Craniosacral Therapy for Chronic Pain: A Systematic Review and Meta-Analysis of Randomized Controlled Trials." *BMC Musculoskeletal Disorders* 21, no. 1 (January 2020): 1–14.

3. Castro-Sánchez, A. M., I. C. Lara-Palomo, G. A. Matarán-Peñarrocha, et al. "Benefits of Craniosacral Therapy in Patients with Chronic Low Back Pain: A Randomized Controlled Trial." *Journal of Alternative and Complementary Medicine* 22, no. 8 (August 2016): 650–657.

4. Bialoszewski, Dariusz, Marcin Bebelski, Monika Lewandowska, and Anna Slupik. "Utility of Craniosacral Therapy in Treatment of Patients with Non-Specific Low Back Pain. Preliminary Report." *Ortopedia Traumatologia Rehabilitacja* 16, no. 6 (November–December 2014): 605–615.

5. Haller, Heidemarie, Romy Lauche, Holger Cramer, et al. "Craniosacral Therapy for the Treatment of Chronic Neck Pain: A Randomized Sham-Controlled Trial." *Clinical Journal of Pain* 32, no. 5 (2016): 441–449.

6. Arnadottir, T. S., and A. K. Sigurdardottir. "Is Craniosacral Therapy Effective for Migraine? Tested with HIT-6 Questionnaire." *Complementary therapies in Clinical Practice* 19, no. 1 (February 2013): 11–14.

7. Rao, Keerthi, and Subhash Khatri. "Effectiveness of Craniosacral Therapy in Cervicogenic Headache." *MOJ Yoga & Physical Therapy* 2, no. 4 (2017): 121–124.

8. Matarán-Peñarrocha, Guillermo A., Adelaida María Castro-Sánchez, Gloria Carballo García, et al. "Influence of Craniosacral Therapy on Anxiety, Depression and Quality of Life in Patients with Fibromyalgia." *Evidence-Based Complementary and Alternative Medicine* 2011 (2011): Article ID 178769.

9. Elden, Helen, Hans-Christian Östgaard, Anna Glantz, et al. "Effects of Craniosacral Therapy as Adjunct to Standard Treatment for Pelvic Girdle Pain in Pregnant Women: A Multicenter, Single Blind, Randomized Controlled Trial." *Acta Obstetricia et Gynecologica Scandinavica* 92, no. 7 (July 2013): 775–782.

10. Jäkel, Anne, and Philip von Hauenschild. "A Systematic Review to Evaluate the Clinical Benefits of Craniosacral Therapy." *Complementary Therapies in Medicine* 20, no. 6 (2012): 456–465.

REFERENCES AND FURTHER READINGS

Arnadottir, T. S., and A. K. Sigurdardottir. "Is Craniosacral Therapy Effective for Migraine? Tested with HIT-6 Questionnaire." *Complementary Therapies in Clinical Practice* 19, no. 1 (February 2013): 11–14.

Bialoszewski, Dariusz, Marcin Bebelski, Monika Lewandowska, and Anna Slupik. "Utility of Craniosacral Therapy in Treatment of Patients with Non-Specific Low Back Pain. Preliminary Report." *Ortopedia, Traumatologia Rehabilitacja* 16, no. 6 (November–December 2014): 605–615.

Castro-Sánchez, A. M., I. C. Lara-Palomo, G. A. Matarán-Peñarrocha, et al. "Benefits of Craniosacral Therapy in Patients with Chronic Low Back Pain: A Randomized Controlled Trial." *Journal of Alternative and Complementary Medicine* 22, no. 8 (August 2016): 650–657.

Elden, Helen, Hans-Christian Östgaard, Anna Glantz, et al. "Effects of Craniosacral Therapy as Adjunct to Standard Treatment for Pelvic Girdle Pain in Pregnant Women: A Multicenter, Single Blind, Randomized Controlled Trial." *Acta Obstetricia et Gynecologica Scandinavica* 92, no. 7 (July 2013): 775–782.

Haller, Heidemarie, Romy Lauche, Holger Cramer, et al. "Craniosacral Therapy for the Treatment of Chronic Neck Pain: A Randomized Sham-Controlled Trial." *Clinical Journal of Pain* 32, no. 5 (2016): 441–449.

Haller, Heidemarie, Romy Lauche, Tobias Sundberg, et al. "Craniosacral Therapy for Chronic Pain: A Systematic Review and Meta-Analysis of Randomized Controlled Trials." *BMC Musculoskeletal Disorders* 21, no. 1 (January 2020): 1–14.

Harrison, Rachel E., and John S. Page. "Multipractitioner Upledger CranioSacral Therapy: Descriptive Outcome Study 2007–2008." *Journal of Alternative and Complementary Medicine* 17, no. 1 (2011): 13–17.

Jäkel, Anne, and Philip von Hauenschild. "A Systematic Review to Evaluate the Clinical Benefits of Craniosacral Therapy." *Complementary Therapies in Medicine* 20, no. 6 (December 1, 2012): 456–465.

Matarán-Peñarrocha, Guillermo A., Adelaida María Castro-Sánchez, Gloria Carballo García, et al. "Influence of Craniosacral Therapy on Anxiety, Depression and Quality of Life in Patients with

Fibromyalgia." *Evidence-Based Complementary and Alternative Medicine* 2011 (2011): Article ID 178769.

Rao, Keerthi, and Subhash Khatri. "Effectiveness of Craniosacral Therapy in Cervicogenic Headache." *MOJ Yoga & Physical Therapy* 2, no. 4 (2017): 121–124.

Exercise

INTRODUCTION

When one is in pain, it is very tempting to want to stay in bed or participate in as little physical activity as possible. To say the least, it is simply counterintuitive to want to exercise. Yet, in many instances, exercise is exactly what the body needs to support the healing process. Exercise improves the pain threshold; people develop a higher tolerance for their pain. Continuing to exercise prevents the weakening of muscles and the deterioration of joints. Exercise increases the flow of oxygen to the brain, which plays a role in modulating the pain response. Staying inactive may only contribute to a downward spiral of increasing pain and an ever-growing list of additional pain-related problems.

Cardiovascular exercises are known to reduce pain, especially low back pain and joint pain. For example, people dealing with the ongoing pain of osteoarthritis may obtain relief from exercise, such as walking or swimming. Walking is a low-impact activity that increases blood flow and reduces stiffness and pain in muscles and joints. Swimming or water exercises relax muscles, and the buoyancy of the water is useful for people with musculoskeletal or joint pain. Exercising in water enables people to exercise without putting any stress on muscles and joints, and it is particularly useful for people with mobility issues.

Stretching exercises are also valuable for people dealing with pain. Stretching loosens stiff muscles and joint tissues, permitting greater freedom of movement, and supports better balance and dexterity.

ADMINISTRATION AND REGULATION

In many instances, before beginning an exercise routine, it may be a good idea to check with a health-care provider, especially if you have any preexisting conditions, such as high blood pressure, heart disease, diabetes, kidney disease, recent treatment for cancer, or a history of injury, back pain, or hip, knee, or shoulder problems. Some people begin an exercise program with a visit to a physical or occupational therapist, fitness specialist, or personal trainer. Some people will only exercise with a personal/athletic trainer. These professionals may help devise programs to meet individual's specific needs and requirements. For those who like to swim or participate in water exercises, your local YMCA or community center may have a pool. People who prefer stretching in groups should consider yoga or Tai Chi classes. These disciplines include slow motions and poses that improve flexibility and strength. In any case, it is best to begin any exercise program slowly and gradually increase the amount and degree of exercising. Though there are people who can barely exercise once or twice a week, others exercise daily. Aim for exercising at least 30 to 60 minutes, three or four times per week. Five, six, or seven times a week is even better.

Although people may exercise within their home or neighborhood, many people decide to join a gym. All gyms must adhere to the regulations of their city or town and the state in which they operate. Of course, these will vary from community to community and from state to state. Before signing a gym contract, be sure you are comfortable with the rules, regulations, and requirements, and, of course, the cost. Costs vary widely from $10 or $20 dollars per month (plus extras) to several hundred or even higher. If cost is an issue, be sure to check your local YMCA or community center. There is a good chance they also offer classes.

BENEFITS AND RISKS

For those dealing with pain, the goal of exercise is to reduce pain while also supporting health. Exercise may decrease inflammation, increase mobility, and reduce overall levels of pain. People who exercise regularly may be able to postpone or avoid surgery for a pain-related problem, such as osteoarthritis or an old injury. They may be able to reduce or discontinue their intake of pain medication.

However, exercise is not always useful for pain. Sometimes, especially when exercising improperly, pain may worsen. Also, injuries may occur during exercise and many other aspects of life. Sometimes, a medical provider will advise against exercise. For example, exercise will only increase the intense pain associated with a stress fracture. People dealing with a stress fracture will be told to refrain from exercise for six to eight weeks.

Participating in certain group exercise programs, such as a basketball or volleyball team, should probably be avoided. Basketball and volleyball involve jumping, landing, and moving quickly in different directions. The games place lots of pressure on the joints. In fact, any sport that places too much stress on joints should be avoided, especially in those who have already been injured.

RESEARCH FINDINGS

Therapeutic Exercise Is Beneficial to Women Suffering from Primary Dysmenorrhea or Menstrual Pain

In a systematic review and meta-analysis published in 2019 in the journal *Physical Therapy*, researchers from Spain evaluated the use of therapeutic exercises for the treatment of menstrual pain. The researchers located 16 randomized, controlled trials that met their criteria for a systematic review; of these, 11 met their criteria for a meta-analysis. The trials, which were all published in English or Spanish before January 31, 2018, included women between the ages of 16 and 25 years. Though there was a great deal of heterogeneity in the types of exercise studied, the researchers nevertheless learned that therapeutic exercise had a significantly greater effect on intensity levels of menstrual pain. However, two studies found no differences between the groups. Five of the eight trials that measured the duration of pain found that exercise significantly reduced the duration of pain. Still, the most effective exercise programs were stretching and isometric exercises for 8 weeks for pain intensity and duration, yoga for 12 weeks for pain intensity and quality of life, and aerobic exercises for 12 weeks for quality of life. The researchers concluded that "therapeutic exercise for 8 to 12 weeks is a useful therapeutic option for young women with primary dysmenorrhea because it produces a decrease in pain intensity and, to a lesser extent, a decrease in pain duration."[1]

Tai Chi Seems to Be Useful for Some Types of Chronic Pain

In a systematic review and meta-analysis published in 2016 in the journal *Scientific Reports*, researchers from China wanted to learn if Tai Chi would help people with chronic pain from problems such as low back pain, osteoarthritis, osteoporosis, and fibromyalgia. Their cohort consisted of 18 randomized, controlled trials; all of the participants had chronic pain conditions that lasted for at least six months. The trials, which were written in English or Chinese, assessed the immediate effects of Tai Chi as well as the follow-up and long-term effects. They included a total of 1,260 subjects with a mean age of 61.43 years. The duration of the trials ranged from 6 to 28 weeks; follow-up times ranged from 6 to 36 weeks. The trials were conducted in the United States, Australia, China, and Korea between 2000 and 2015. The researchers learned that Tai Chi achieved better pain control than the control interventions, and it seemed especially useful for osteoarthritis pain, low back pain, and osteoporosis pain. It appears to take about 6 weeks of Tai Chi before the benefits are fully evident. A longer duration of exercise may achieve better results. However, "there was insufficient evidence to support or refute the value of Tai Chi compared with other active therapies for chronic pain conditions."[2]

Aerobic Exercise Appears to Increase the Tolerance for Pain

In a trial published in 2016 in the journal *Medicine & Science in Sports & Exercise*, researchers from Australia examined the effect of aerobic exercise on pain sensitivity in healthy people. The initial cohort consisted of 5 males and 22 females with no history of chronic pain or chronic disease. All of the subjects participated in either a six-week structured aerobic exercise program or six weeks of their usual physical activity. It is important to note that the subjects were not randomly assigned to each group. Rather, they selected their activity. The exercise program consisted of cycling three times per week for 30 minutes. There was an initial assessment, 18 exercise sessions, and a final assessment. The control subjects only attended the first and final sessions. During the trial, the subjects completed several questionnaires. The final analyses included 24 subjects. The researchers determined that the moderate to vigorous exercise increased the pain tolerance of their healthy subjects. The researchers commented that "this is the first study to clearly demonstrate an effect of chronic exercise on pain sensitivity in healthy, nonathletic adults."[3]

Retro Walking May Be Better Than Forward Walking for People with Knee Osteoarthritis

In a three-arm, single-blind, randomized, controlled trial published in 2019 in the journal *BMC Musculoskeletal Disorders*, researchers from Saudi Arabia, China, and India compared the effect of a retro walking program and a forward walking program to a control in people with knee osteoarthritis. (Retro walking is walking backward on the ground or a treadmill.) The cohort consisted of 68 subjects (38 female) with a mean age of 55.6 years; all of the subjects had physician-diagnosed knee osteoarthritis. For six weeks, the subjects in the retro (n = 23) and forward (n = 23) walking groups completed 10 minutes of supervised walking three days per week, and they were told to increase their walking time up to 30 minutes. During warm-up and cool-down sessions, the subjects were instructed to perform ankle toe movements, heel-raise exercises, and hamstring and gastrocnemius-soleus stretches (stretching the broad, flat muscle in the calf). The subjects in all three groups (the control group had 22 subjects) participated in a routine physiotherapy program, which consisted of a combination of closed and open kinematic chain exercises including straight leg raising, isometric quadriceps, isometric hip adduction, terminal knee extension, semi-squat, and leg press. All outcomes were measured by a physical therapist who has been in clinical practice for more than 10 years. The researchers learned that the subjects in the retro walking group had effective reductions in pain and improvements in function, quadriceps muscle strength, and performance. And, these reductions were greater than those seen in the forward walking group and control group. The researchers concluded that retro walking is more advantageous that forward walking. "After some training, people can easily be able to do the retro-walking in the public parks."[14]

Therapeutic Exercise Seems to Help People Dealing with Fibromyalgia

In a systematic review and meta-analysis published in 2017 in the journal *Biomedical Research International*, researchers from Spain investigated the ability of therapeutic exercise to help people suffering from fibromyalgia. The researchers included randomized, controlled trials that used aerobic, strengthening, or stretching exercises, or a combination of these. Sixteen studies were included in the systematic review, and 14 were included in the meta-analysis. The trials were conducted in the United States, the United Kingdom, Norway, Brazil, Spain, Sweden, and Turkey, and they tended to be small and heterogeneous. The researchers learned that exercise was useful for the symptoms associated with fibromyalgia, but they were unable to determine definitively which exercises were the most effective. It appeared that aerobic exercise and muscle strengthening were the best for reducing pain and the severity of the disease. The researchers concluded that it would be interesting to "conduct primary research into the type of exercise likely to yield the highest rate of adherence to an exercise treatment regime using a larger sample."[5]

Exercise Helps Children and Adolescents with Juvenile Idiopathic Arthritis

In a systematic review and meta-analysis published in 2018 in the journal *Archives of Physical Medicine and Rehabilitation*, researchers from Alberta, Canada, examined the efficacy of exercise for children and adolescents with juvenile idiopathic arthritis, the most common chronic childhood rheumatic disease. The researchers examined nine randomized, controlled trials and one longitudinal cohort study. All of the randomized, controlled trials were considered to be of moderate quality. The exercise interventions in the randomized, controlled trials included aquatic, strengthening, proprioceptive, aerobic, and Pilates exercises. The duration of the exercise programs ranged from 10 to 48 weeks, with a median of 12 weeks. Exercise exposures involved 20 to 48 sessions with partial or complete therapist supervision. However, there was substantial heterogeneity in study outcomes and limited statistical reporting across studies. Also, there was a consistent lack of reporting on adverse events. The researchers learned that an exercise program appeared to have several benefits for children and teens with juvenile idiopathic arthritis, including improving pain and body strength. They concluded that the "exercise programs emphasizing strength, flexibility, and balance using supervised or partially supervised training sessions were commonly associated with improvements in pediatric activity, body function and structure and QOL [quality of life]." Conversely, high-impact exercise tended to increase pain and was not recommended for these children and teens.[6]

Children Who Play String Instruments May Benefit from Pilates and Therapeutic Exercise for Back Pain and Postural Alignment

In a randomized, controlled pilot trial with two parallel interventions, researchers from Spain wanted to learn if children who played string instruments would benefit from Pilates and therapeutic exercise. They explained that playing some string instruments may cause back pain and alterations of the spine. The cohort consisted of 25 children between the ages of 10 and 14 years who were enrolled in one of two music schools. They played or were learning to play violin, viola, cello, or double bass. One group of children performed Pilates and therapeutic exercise (eight females and five males), and the other group only performed therapeutic exercises (nine females and three males). The sessions were held for 50 minutes, once per week, for four weeks. The classes were taught by a physical therapist, and periodic pain assessments were conducted. For example, the children were asked if their backs hurt before, during, and after playing their instruments. If they did experience pain, they were asked to rate their pain between 0 and 10. The researchers learned that the only children who experienced pain relief were in the Pilates/therapeutic exercise group. The researchers concluded that "the application of a low dose of Pilates method combined with therapeutic exercise could be a beneficial intervention in the reduction of pain before and after practice in children who play string instruments."[7]

Motor Control Exercise Does Not Appear to Be More Effective Than Other Exercises for People with Low Back Pain

In a systematic review published in 2016 in the journal *Spine*, researchers from Australia, Brazil, the Netherlands, and Canada wanted to learn if motor control exercise would help people with nonspecific low back pain. (Used to manage nonspecific low back pain, this type of exercise focuses on the activation of the deep spine muscles. Patients are taught how to isolate the deep spinal muscles while maintaining normal respiration.) The cohort consisted of 32 randomized, controlled trials with 2,628 subjects. Twenty-nine trials evaluated patients with chronic low back pain, and three trials had patients with acute low back pain. The trials compared motor control exercise to placebos, no treatment, another active treatment, or motor control exercise as a supplement to another treatment. Most of the trials had a low risk of bias, and they included primarily middle-aged subjects recruited from primary or tertiary care. The researchers found no clinically important differences for any outcomes between motor control exercise and any other type of exercise for both acute and chronic low back pain. As a result, the researchers concluded that "the choice of exercise for chronic LBP [low back pain] should depend on patient or therapist preferences, therapist training, costs, and safety."[8]

Different Types of Exercising, Even Free Physical Activity, May Help Patellofemoral Pain

In a single-blind, randomized, controlled trial published in 2019 in *The American Journal of Sports Medicine*, researchers from Norway compared three treatments for patellofemoral pain (PFP)—hip-focused exercise, knee-focused exercise, and free physical exercise. (Patellofemoral pain syndrome occurs when the nerves sense pain in the soft tissues and bone around the kneecap. It is most often seen in women and young adults.) The cohort consisted of 112 subjects between the ages of 16 and 40 years, with a mean age of 27.6 years. All of the subjects had symptoms of PFP for at least three months. In addition to patient education, for 6 weeks, 39 subjects received isolated hip-focused exercise, 37 received traditional knee-focused exercise, and 36 participated in free physical activity (control). Each week, there were three sessions. Assessments were conducted at baseline, six weeks, and three months. The researchers learned that after three months, there were no significant pain differences between the subjects in the three groups. And, they concluded that "guided exercises improved muscle strength but did not translate to additional gains in other outcomes over the control group."[9]

An Internet-Based Exercise Intervention May Improve the Pain and Other Symptoms Experienced by Breast Cancer Survivors

In a two-arm, assessor-blind, parallel, randomized, controlled trial published in 2016 in the journal *Cancer*, researchers from Spain evaluated the ability of an internet-based exercise intervention to help breast cancer survivors. Breast cancer survivors with diagnoses ranging from stage 1 to stage 3A were placed either in an intervention group ($n = 40$) or a control group ($n = 41$). After completing baseline assessments, the subjects in the intervention group received in-person instructions on how to assess and use their individually designed exercise programs. The schedule consisted of three sessions per week, on nonconsecutive days, that lasted for about 90 minutes. Each session included a warm-up, resistance and aerobic exercise training, and a cool-down. According to the researchers, there was high acceptance and adherence to the intervention. Assessments were conducted at baseline, at eight weeks, when the program ended, and at six months. In addition to pain, assessments were conducted on quality of life, muscle strength, and fatigue. The researchers learned that the subjects in the intervention group had improvements in pain and the other factors studied, and these findings were maintained at the six-month follow-up. The researchers commented that non-face-to-face programs may "be an effective alternative to traditional cancer rehabilitation."[10]

Some Trials of the Use of Exercise to Help People with Knee or Hip Osteoarthritis or Hip and Knee Osteoarthritis Have Inherent Limitations

In a systematic review published in 2018 in the *Cochrane Database of Systematic Reviews*, researchers from the United Kingdom evaluated randomized, controlled trials the compared land or water-based exercise programs to control groups consisting of no treatment or nonexercise interventions. The trials evaluated levels of pain or function and at least one psychosocial outcome such as depression or anxiety. Twenty-one trials with 2,372 subjects met the inclusion criteria. The subjects were all 45 years and older with a clinical diagnosis of osteoarthritis or self-reported chronic hip or knee pain for more than six months. However, there were wide variations in many aspects of the exercise programs, such as the frequency and duration and mode of delivery, and there were differences in the symptoms and duration of symptoms experienced by the subjects. The outcomes measured, the methodological quality, and reporting varied. Further, the trials failed to provide information on adverse events, and for 20 of the trials there was a high risk of bias. Still, the researchers concluded that participating in an exercise program "may slightly improve physical function, depression and pain." Yet, "without adequate information and advice from healthcare professionals, people do not know what they should and should not do, and, as a consequence, avoid activity for fear of causing harm."[11]

NOTES

1. Carroquino-Garcia, Paloma, José Jesús Jiménez-Rejano, Esther Medrano-Sanchez, et al. "Therapeutic Exercise in the Treatment of Primary Dysmenorrhea: A Systematic Review and Meta-Analysis." *Physical Therapy* 99, no. 10 (October 28, 2019): 1371–1380.

2. Kong, Ling Jun, Romy Lauche, Petra Klose, et al. "Tai Chi for Chronic Pain Conditions: A Systematic Review and Meta-Analysis of Randomized Controlled Trials." *Scientific Reports* 6 (2016): 25325.

3. Jones, Matthew D., John Booth, Janet L. Taylor, and Benjamin K. Barry. "Aerobic Training Increases Pain Tolerance in Healthy Individuals." *Medicine & Science in Sports & Exercise* 46, no. 8 (August 2014): 1640–1647.

4. Alghadir, Ahmad H., Shahnawaz Anwer, Bibhuti Sarkar, et al. "Effect of 6-Week Retro or Forward Walking Program on Pain, Functional Disability, Quadriceps Muscle Strength, and Performance in Individuals with Knee Osteoarthritis: A Randomized Controlled Trial." *BMC Musculoskeletal Disorders* 20 (2019): 159.

5. Sosa-Reina, M. Dolores, Susana Nunez-Nagy, Tomás Gallego-Izquierdo, et al. "Effectiveness of Therapeutic Exercise in Fibromyalgia Syndrome: A Systematic Review and Meta-Analysis of Randomized Clinical Trials." *Biomedical Research International* 2017 (2017): 2356346.

6. Kuntze, Gregor, Colleen Nesbitt, Jackie L. Whittaker, et al. "Exercise Therapy in Juvenile Idiopathic Arthritis: Systematic Review and Meta-Analysis." *Archives of Physical Medicine and Rehabilitation* 99, no. 1 (January 2018): 178–193.

7. Poncela-Skupien, Carolina, Elena Pinero-Pinto, Carmen Martinez-Cepa, et al. "How Does the Execution of the Pilates Method and Therapeutic Exercise Influence Back Pain and Postural Alignment in Children Who Play String Instruments? A Randomized Controlled Pilot Study." *International Journal of Environmental Research and Public Health* 17, no. 20 (October 13, 2020): 7436.

8. Saragiotto, Bruno T., Christopher G. Maher, Tiâ P. Yamato, et al. "Motor Control Exercise for Nonspecific Low Back Pain: A Cochrane Review." *Spine* 41, no. 16 (August 15, 2016): 1284–1295.

9. Hott, Alexandra, Jens Ivar Brox, Are Hugo Pripp, et al. "Effectiveness of Isolated Hip Exercise, Knee Exercise, or Free Physical Activity for Patellofemoral Pain: A Randomized Controlled Trial." *The American Journal of Sports Medicine* 47, no. 6 (May 2019): 1312–1322.

10. Galiano-Castillo, Noelia, Irene Cantarero-Villanueva, Carolina Fernández-Lao, et al. "Telehealth System: A Randomized Controlled Trial Evaluating the Impact of an Internet-Based Exercise Intervention on Quality of Life, Pain, Muscle Strength, and Fatigue in Breast Cancer Survivors." *Cancer* 122, no. 20 (October 15, 2016): 3166–3174.

11. Hurley, Michael, Kelly Dickson, Rachel Hallett, et al. "Exercise Interventions and Patient Beliefs for People with Hip, Knee or Hip and Knee Osteoarthritis: A Mixed Methods Review." *Cochrane Database of Systematic Reviews* 4, no. 4 (April 17, 2018): CD010842.

REFERENCES AND FURTHER READINGS

Alghadir, Ahmad H., Shahnawaz Anwer, Bibhuti Sarkar, et al. "Effect of 6-Week Retro or Forward Walking Program on Pain, Functional Disability, Quadriceps Muscle Strength, and Performance in Individuals with Knee Osteoarthritis: A Randomized Controlled Trial (Retro-Walking Trial)." *BMC Musculoskeletal Disorders* 20 (2019): 159.

Carroquino-Garcia, Paloma, José Jesús Jiménez-Rejano, Esther Medrano-Sanchez, et al. "Therapeutic Exercise in the treatment of Primary Dysmenorrhea: A Systematic Review and Meta-Analysis." *Physical Therapy* 99, no. 10 (October 28, 2019): 1371–1380.

Galiano-Castillo, Noelia, Irene Cantarero-Villanueva, Carolina Fernández-Lao, et al. "Telehealth System: A Randomized Controlled Trial Evaluating the Impact of an Internet-Based Exercise Intervention on Quality of Life, Pain, Muscle Strength, and Fatigue in Breast Cancer Survivors." *Cancer* 122, no. 20 (October 15, 2016): 3166–3174.

Hott, Alexandra, Jens Ivar Brox, Are Hugo Pripp, et al. "Effectiveness of Isolated Hip Exercise, Knee Exercise, or Free Physical Activity for Patellofemoral Pain: A Randomized Controlled Trial." *The American Journal of Sports Medicine* 47, no. 6 (May 2019): 1312–1322.

Hurley, Michael, Kelly Dickson, Rachel Hallett, et al. "Exercise Interventions and Patient Beliefs for People with Hip, Knee or Hip and Knee Osteoarthritis: A Mixed Methods Review." *Cochrane Database of Systematic Reviews* 4, no. 4 (April 17, 2018): CD010842.

Jones, Matthew D., John Booth, Janet L. Taylor, and Benjamin K. Barry. "Aerobic Training Increases Pain Tolerance in Healthy Individuals." *Medicine & Science in Sports & Exercise* 46, no. 8 (August 2014): 1640–1647.

Kong, Ling Jun, Romy Lauche, Petra Klose, et al. "Tai Chi for Chronic Pain Conditions: A Systematic Review and Meta-Analysis of Randomized Controlled Studies." *Scientific Reports* 6 (2016): 25325.

Kuntze, Gregor, Colleen Nesbitt, Jackie L. Whittaker, et al. "Exercise Therapy in Juvenile Idiopathic Arthritis: A Systematic Review and

Meta-Analysis." *Archives of Physical Medicine and Rehabilitation* 99, no. 1 (January 2018): 178–193.

Poncela-Skupien, Carolina, Elena Pinero-Pinto, Carmen Martinez-Cepa, et al. "How Does the Execution of the Pilates Method and a Therapeutic Exercise Influence Back Pain and Postural Alignment in Children Who Play String Instruments? A Randomized Controlled Pilot Study." *International Journal of Environmental Research and Public Health* 17, no. 20 (October 13, 2020): 7436.

Saragiotto, Bruno T., Christopher G. Maher, Tiê P. Yamato, et al. "Motor Control Exercise for Nonspecific Low Back Pain: A Cochrane Review." *Spine* 41, no. 16 (August 15, 2016): 1284–1295.

Sosa-Reina, M. Dolores, Susana Nunez-Nagy, Tomás Gallego-Izquierdo, et al. "Effectiveness of Therapeutic Exercise in Fibromyalgia Syndrome: A Systematic Review and Meta-Analysis of randomized Clinical Trials." *Biomedical Research International* 2017 (2017): 2356346.

Herbal Supplements

INTRODUCTION

There are a host of different herbs that are supposedly useful for pain. Every day, countless numbers of people who are dealing with pain purchase various herbs to treat their acute or chronic malady or maladies.

But what exactly is a medicinal herb? A medicinal herb is a plant or a part of a plant that is used for its therapeutic value. Herbal supplements are prepared from living or dried plants and may contain a wide variety of interrelated compounds. Herbal medicine is the practice of using herbs to promote health and prevent and treat illness. Until modern times, herbal remedies were the primary form of medicine.

In all probability, people are less likely to use herbal supplements when faced with acute pain. Depending on the type and degree of pain, they may use short-term opioids or over-the-counter pain relievers, such as ibuprofen or acetaminophen. It is when a person is faced with chronic pain that he or she may begin to research herbal alternatives. And, although there is a good deal of marketing of the many and varied benefits of herbal supplements, there is not a great deal of solid research on their use for pain or how many people turn to this alternative. Nevertheless, in view of the millions of people who live with chronic or debilitating pain, it is a topic that needs to be addressed.

There are many herbal supplements that claim to be useful for pain. These include Boswellia, capsaicin, peppermint oil, and ginger, which are discussed in this entry, as well as bromelain, cloves, eucalyptus, lavender, rosemary, and white willow bark. There is not always good research to back the claims made by those who manufacture and market these products.

ADMINISTRATION AND REGULATION

As with all types of supplements, it is very important to follow the administration instructions on the label. If the daily recommended dosage is one capsule, then that is the amount that should be taken. On the other hand, if the daily dosage is four capsules, then it is okay to work up to that amount over a period of time. Though some herbal supplements are quick acting, many are slower, especially when treating a long-term problem, such as chronic pain.

While herbal supplements are regulated by the Food and Drug Administration (FDA), they do not receive nearly the same scrutiny as food and drugs. They fall under the category of dietary supplements. Thus, it is not necessary for manufacturers to seek FDA approval before selling herbal supplements. If they have supporting research, companies are able to make nonspecific claims for their herbal products. But, the companies need to include a disclaimer that the FDA has not evaluated the claim. Manufacturers must follow good manufacturing practices. If the FDA determines that a product is unsafe, it is able to take action against the manufacturer or distributor or both; it may issue a warning or insist that the product be removed from the market. However, there is no guarantee that all herbal products are safe and free from contaminants.

The FDA does require that herbal supplements have the following information on their labels: the name of the herbal supplement, the name and address of the manufacturer or distributor, a complete list of ingredients either in the Supplement Facts panel or listed beneath it, and serving size, amount, and active ingredients.

There is no reliable way to know how many people in the United States turn to herbal supplements for pain relief. Still, one may safely speculate that it is in the millions. Herbal supplements tend to be less expensive than traditional medications, though that is not always the case. Some herbal supplements are expensive. To save money, it is a good idea to compare prices online.

BENEFITS AND RISKS

People tend to use herbal supplements for chronic pain to avoid some of the myriad of problems associated with opioids or even the side effects of nonsteroidal anti-inflammation drugs (gastrointestinal upset) or acetaminophen (liver concerns, especially in higher doses). In all probability, these people are convinced that herbal supplements are a less expensive and safer alternative. And in many instances, that is absolutely true. When used appropriately, the vast majority of herbal supplements are safe and have few or no adverse side effects. Serious side effects tend to be rare.

But, herbal supplements may have risks. They may interact with conventional prescription or over-the-counter medicines or may trigger a stronger-than-expected or allergic reaction. On some rare occasions, this may be life-threatening. Herbal supplements may interfere with medications used during surgical procedures, such as anesthetics, and cause dangerous complications. That is why medical providers recommend that people stop using herbal supplements before a scheduled procedure or surgery. Other side effects associated with herbal supplements include nausea, dizziness, headache, and upset stomach. If the herbal supplements are strong enough to relieve pain, they may be strong enough to cause problems. In addition, there is at least the potential for contamination, adulteration, and toxicity. Further, herbs may contain multiple compounds, many of which may not be identified. It is also quite apparent that some herbal supplements are of lower quality than others. Whenever possible, select herbal supplements that have been tested by independent sources. The FDA maintains lists of supplements that are under regulatory review or that have been reported to cause adverse effects.

RESEARCH FINDINGS

Boswellia

Boswellia Appears to Be Useful for Knee Osteoarthritis

In a double-blind, placebo-controlled, clinical trial published in 2019 in the journal *Phytotherapy Research*, researchers from Utah and New Jersey (USA) and India evaluated the safety and efficacy of Boswellin® for knee osteoarthritis. The initial cohort consisted of 17 male and 31 female subjects with newly diagnosed mild to moderate knee osteoarthritis. They had a mean age of 58.7 years. For 120 days, the subjects took either two tablets per day of Boswellin (169.33 mg *Boswellia serrate* extract) or two tablets per day of a placebo that was identical in appearance. To ensure compliance, study personnel conducted regular home visits. The severity of osteoarthritis was assessed via questionnaire, radiography, and physical examination at baseline and at the end of the trial. Other assessments, such as vital signs, were measured periodically. The subjects recorded their daily medications and adverse effects in a diary. Forty-two subjects in the treatment group and 40 in the placebo group completed the trial. The researchers learned that when compared to the placebo, the subjects taking the herbal tablets had reductions in pain and stiffness, which resulted in significant improvements in physical function. At the same time, there were no reports of serious adverse events. The researchers concluded that Boswellin "exerted anti-inflammatory/anti-arthritic activity efficaciously in reducing joint pain and improving the physical functional ability."[1]

In a systematic review and meta-analysis published in 2018 in the journal *Seminars in Arthritis and Rheumatism*, researchers from Boston, Massachusetts (USA), examined the efficacy of Boswellia and curcumin for knee osteoarthritis. They located 11 randomized controlled trials that met their criteria. All of the trials compared Boswellia or curcumin formulations administered alone or in combination against either a matching placebo or nonsteroidal anti-inflammation drugs (NSAIDs). Unfortunately, the quality of the studies tended to be low, and 79 percent included fewer than 100 participants. Still, the researchers learned that Boswellia and curcumin are both better than placebos at relieving symptoms of knee osteoarthritis, and they have little risk of creating safety concerns. The researchers concluded that both herbal supplements could be valuable additions to the products available for the treatment of knee osteoarthritis. However, "the current body of evidence is not adequate in size and quality to make any meaningful clinical practice recommendations."[2]

Boswellia Has Pain-Relieving Properties

In a randomized, double-blind, placebo-controlled, crossover trial published in 2014 in the *Indian Journal of Pharmacology*, researchers from India tested the pain-relieving properties of Boswellia in healthy volunteers using an experimental mechanical pain model. The cohort consisted of 12 healthy male subjects between the ages of 18 and 45 years. They took either a single oral dose of two 125-mg capsules of *Boswellia serrate* or two identical placebo capsules. After a 2-week washout period, they took the alternative supplement. All of the subjects who had taken *Boswellia serrate* took the placebo, and all who had taken the placebo took the *Boswellia serrate*. Using a validated mechanical pain model by Randall Selitto (Ugo basile analgesymeter), mechanical pain was forced on the nail bed of the nondominant hand index finger. Assessments were conducted at baseline and at 1 hour, 2 hours, and 3 hours after test drug or placebo administration. The researchers determined that, when compared to the placebo, the mean pain threshold force and time significantly increased at 2 and 3 hours of herbal administration. And, when compared to baseline, Boswellia significantly increased the mean pain threshold force three hours after taking the herb. The researchers concluded that "*Boswellia serrate* significantly increased pain threshold force and time and pain tolerance force and time when compared to baseline and placebo with good safety and tolerability."[3]

When Combined with Turmeric, Boswellia Seems to Help People after Arthroscopic Supraspinatus Tendon Repair Surgery

In a prospective, randomized, trial published in 2015 in the journal *Musculoskeletal Surgery*, researchers from Italy investigated the ability of a combination of Boswellia and turmeric to help people recover from pain following arthroscopic supraspinatus (SSP) tendon repair (surgical repair of rotator cuff tears). The cohort consisted of 104 people who had surgical SSP repair from May 1 to December 31, 2013. Three weeks before surgery, the subjects were placed in a group to take the combination herb (Tendisulfur®) or a group to take placebos. They remained on the herbs or placebos for two months. The subjects were also prescribed conventional analgesic therapy with tramadol or paracetamol. The final analysis included 100 subjects, with 50 in each group. The subjects were assessed immediately before the operation and at weeks 1, 2, 4, 6, 8, 12, and 24. The researchers found that the subjects in the treatment group had significant reductions in overall pain scores at all time points, and the night pain scores had a similar trend. But, the subjects in the placebo group experienced significantly lower pain after the first two time points. Still, the researchers underscored the importance of early postoperative pain relief, and that relief during that early postoperative period was better with the herbal supplements.[4]

Capsaicin

Capsaicin Appears to Help People with Pain from Diabetic Peripheral Neuropathy

In a systematic review and meta-analysis published in 2017 in the journal *Clinical Therapeutics*, researchers from the Netherlands compared the efficacy of an 8 percent capsaicin patch to oral medications for diabetic peripheral neuropathy. Searches were limited to studies published in English after 1950. The researchers located 25 randomized controlled trials that met their criteria, such as having a study duration of four weeks or longer. The oral agents evaluated in the trials were pregabalin, duloxetine, gabapentin, and amitriptyline. Most of the trials had placebos and a parallel design, and a majority were conducted in North America, with the remainder conducted in Asia and Europe. Trial duration ranged from 4 to 15 weeks, and the number of subjects ranged from 25 to 804. Mean ages ranged from 48 to 76 years, and mean baseline pain scores—based on an 11-point rating scale—ranged from 5.5 to 7.3. The researchers learned that the capsaicin 8 percent patch "exhibited a numerical advantage" to pregabalin and gabapentin and had "similar efficacy" to duloxetine. There was insufficient evidence to compare the patch to amitriptyline. Moreover, the oral medications were much more likely to have side effects, such as excessive sleepiness, dizziness, and diarrhea. The researchers concluded that "localized treatment with the capsaicin 8% patch had similar efficacy but offered tolerability benefits in terms of systemic adverse events."[5]

Capsaicin May Be as Useful for Pain Relief as Topical Nonsteroidal Anti-Inflammatory Drugs

In a systematic review and meta-analysis published in 2018 in the journal *Osteoarthritis and Cartilage*, researchers from the United Kingdom compared the efficacy of topical capsaicin to topical NSAIDs for the relief of pain from osteoarthritis. The researchers included 28 trials with a total of 7,372 subjects; 3,473 subjects took placebos, 3,693 subjects used topical NSAIDs, and 206 subjects used topical capsaicin. The meta-analysis included 23 studies on NSAIDs and 5 on capsaicin. All of the trials were described as double-blind, though they may not have actually been structured in that way, and all but one had a parallel design. Many of the trials had considerable risk of bias. No trials directly compared capsaicin to topical NSAIDs; the two treatments were compared to placebos. The researchers determined that capsaicin and topical NSAIDs were both superior to placebo for pain relief. However, capsaicin was only statistically superior to placebo, when used at "licensed doses." No significant pain relief differences were found between the topical capsaicin and topical NSAIDs. The researchers emphasized that "larger and better conducted RCTs [randomized controlled trials], particularly for capsaicin, are required to confirm this."[6]

High Concentrations of Topical Capsaicin May Offer Some Help for Chronic Neuropathic Pain in Adults

In a systematic review published in 2017 in the *Cochrane Database of Systematic Reviews*, researchers based in the United Kingdom evaluated the ability of high concentrations (8%) of topical capsaicin to help people with chronic neuropathic pain. The researchers included eight randomized, double-blind, controlled studies that had a duration of at least six weeks; the studies had a total of 2,488 subjects. The studies were thought to have good methodological quality, and only one study was considered to be at high risk of bias. Two studies used a placebo control, and six used 0.04 percent topical capsaicin as the placebo. Efficacy outcomes were inconsistently reported. The researchers learned that, when compared to placebos, the high concentration capsaicin offered subjects with postherpetic neuropathic pain moderate to substantial levels of pain relief. They experienced a 30 to 50 percent reduction in pain. Still, because the quality of the evidence was "moderate or very low," the results should be interpreted with caution. The most common adverse events were erythema (superficial reddening) and pain over the application sites. However, these reactions tended to be minimal and transitory. The researchers added that the subjects who did obtain high levels of pain relief tended to have "additional improvements in sleep, fatigue, depression, and quality of life."[7]

Peppermint Oil

Enteric-Coated Peppermint Oil May or May Not Be Useful for the Symptoms Associated with Irritable Bowel Syndrome, Including Pain

In a systematic review and meta-analysis published in 2019 in the journal *BMC Complementary and Alternative Medicine*, researchers from several locations, but based in Baltimore, Maryland (USA), evaluated the ability of peppermint oil to help people deal with the symptoms of irritable bowel syndrome, including pain. The researchers located 12 randomized, controlled trials with 835 subjects that met their criteria. The trials were published between 1979 and 2016 and included subjects from Asia, Europe, and North America. Studies ranged from 18 to 178 subjects and were usually located in teaching hospitals. Most studies were double-blind, parallel-group, randomized, controlled trials with follow-up durations ranging from 3 to 12 weeks. Three studies had crossover designs. The researchers determined that treatment with peppermint oil significantly improved abdominal pain and global symptoms of irritable bowel syndrome. At the same time, peppermint oil appeared to have "a good safety profile." The researchers concluded that "enteric-coated peppermint oil is a safe and effective therapy for the relief of abdominal pain and global symptoms in adults with IBS."[8]

In a systematic review and meta-analysis published in 2014 in the *Journal of Clinical Gastroenterology*, researchers from La Jolla, California (USA), similarly assessed the efficacy and safety of enteric-coated peppermint oil capsules for treating the symptoms associated with irritable bowel syndrome, such as abdominal pain. The researchers included 9 randomized controlled trials with a total of 726 subjects and a study duration of at least two weeks. Seven studies were double-blind, placebo-controlled parallel-group trials in adult patients with active irritable bowel syndrome. One study was a double-blind, placebo-controlled, parallel-group trial in pediatric patients with active irritable bowel syndrome. The remaining study was a double-blind, placebo-controlled crossover trial that provided outcome results before the first crossover. The studies used various doses of peppermint oil, and they tended to be of higher methodological quality. Few adverse effects were reported. The researchers noted that they found "moderate-quality evidence" that peppermint oil is a safe and effective short-term therapy for active irritable bowel syndrome. They concluded that "future studies should be conducted to assess the long-term efficacy and safety of peppermint oil treatment and to determine whether peppermint oil is equivalent or superior to antispasmodic and antidepressant drugs."[9]

In a randomized, double-blind trial published in 2020 in the journal *Gastroenterology*, researchers based in the Netherlands also explored the efficacy and safety of enteric-coated peppermint oil for the symptoms associated with irritable bowel syndrome. The initial cohort consisted of 189 subjects (mean overall age of 34 years) with irritable bowel syndrome at four hospitals in the Netherlands; for eight weeks, they were randomly assigned to take small intestinal-release peppermint oil, or ileocolonic-release peppermint oil, or a placebo. Study visits were conducted at the start of pretreatment, at randomization, and at the end of treatment. In addition, there were telephone assessments at the beginning of weeks two, four, and six. Subjects answered daily questions, including inquiries on levels of pain. One hundred and seventy-eight subjects completed the trial, and there were follow-ups six months after the trial ended. Overall compliance of all three groups was very high. Interestingly, there were no significant differences in levels of pain relief and overall symptom relief between the groups. Yet when compared to the placebo, the small intestinal-release peppermint oil did reduce secondary outcomes of abdominal pain, discomfort, and IBS severity. Though mild, adverse events occurred more often in the peppermint groups. The researchers commented that their findings "do not support further development of ileocolonic–release peppermint oil for the treatment of IBS."[10]

Ginger

Ginger Seems Useful for the Symptoms of Primary Dysmenorrhea

In a systematic review and meta-analysis published in 2015 in the journal *Pain Medicine*, researchers from Korea and Rockwell, North Carolina (USA), evaluated randomized, controlled trials on the use of ginger to treat primary dysmenorrhea, defined as pain during at least 50 percent of the menstrual cycle or on the first three days and a pain score of 3 to 4 based on a 10 visual analog scale. The researchers located seven trials that met their criteria and had a low to moderate risk of bias. The ages of the subjects varied, but they were within the range of 13 to 30 years; most of the subjects were teens. The studies included between 22 and 150 subjects. Each trial consisted of two cycles. In four of the trials, subjects in the experimental group took between 750 and 2,000 mg ginger powder capsules per day for the first three days of the menstrual cycle; those in the control groups took placebos. In three trials, analgesic medications or exercise were used as positive controls. The severity of pain was assessed before and after the intervention. The researchers learned that ginger offered a "highly significant" degree of relief from primary dysmenorrhea in the studies in which analgesics were used as a positive control. Ginger powder was as effective as analgesic drug treatment. Furthermore, all of the studies found ginger to be an effective treatment for dysmenorrhea pain. As there was no clear difference in efficacy between the doses, the researchers suggested that it is probably best to begin with the lowest dose. The researchers concluded that "the strength of the study was the consistency of benefit among all of the studies and a very highly statistically significant effect of ginger for treating pain."[11]

In a randomized, crossover, clinical trial published in 2018 in the *Taiwanese Journal of Obstetrics & Gynecology*, researchers from Iran compared the effect of ginger and Novafen, a medicine containing acetaminophen, ibuprofen, and caffeine, for menstrual pain. The cohort consisted of 168 female Babol University of Medical Sciences students between the ages of 18 and 26 years; all of the students, who had an average age of 21.83 years, had primary menstrual pain. The students were divided into two groups. During the first month of the trial, the students in the first group took Novafen during the first two days of their menstrual cycle; they took four 200-mg capsules per day. The students in the second group took ginger during the first two days of their menstrual cycle; they took four 200-mg ginger capsules per day. During the second month of the trial, the students took the opposite medication/supplementation. The researchers learned that both treatments effectively reduced menstrual pain. Though the reduction in the ginger group was slightly higher than the Novafen group, the difference was not statistically significant. The researchers concluded that "treatment with natural herbal medicine, non-synthetic drug, to reduce primary dysmenorrhea is recommended."[12]

Ginger May or May Not Be Useful for Knee Osteoarthritis

In a systematic review and meta-analysis published in 2020 in the journal *Pain Physician*, researchers from Chile wanted to determine if ginger would improve the pain and functioning associated with knee osteoarthritis. The researchers located seven clinical trials that met their criteria. These studies included 371 subjects; the age range of the subjects was between 52.7 and 65.2 years, with an average of 55.6 years. The majority of the trials had a medium to high risk of bias; only about one-fourth had a low risk of bias. The evidence tended to be heterogeneous and of poor methodological quality. The researchers observed that they had "insufficient evidence to support the use of ginger compared with placebo for the pain relief and function improvement in patients with knee OA [osteoarthritis]."[13]

NOTES

1. Majeed, Muhammed, Shaheen Majeed, Narayanan K. Narayanan, and Kalyanam Nagabhushanam. "A Pilot, Randomized, Double-Blind, Placebo-Controlled Trial to Assess the Safety and Efficacy of a Novel *Boswellia serrate* Extract in the Management of Osteoarthritis of the Knee." *Phytotherapy Research* 33 (2019): 1457–1468.

2. Bannuru, Raveendhara, Mikala C. Osani, Fatimah Al-Eid, and Chenchen Wang. "Efficacy of Curcumin and Boswellia for Knee Osteoarthritis: Systematic Review and Meta-Analysis." *Seminars in Arthritis and Rheumatism* 48 (2018): 416–429.

3. Prabhavathi, K., U. Shobha Jagdish Chandra, Radhika Soanker, and P. Usha Rani. "A Randomized, Double Blind, Placebo Controlled Cross Over Study to Evaluate the Analgesic Activity of *Boswellia serrate* in Healthy Volunteers Using Mechanical Pain Model." *Indian Journal of Pharmacology* 46, no. 5 (September-October 2014): 475–479.

4. Merolla, G., F. Dellabiancia, A. Ingardia, et al. "Co-Analgesic Therapy for Arthroscopic Spraspinatus Tendon Repair Using a Dietary Supplement Containing *Boswellia serrate* and *Curcuma longa*: A Prospective Randomized Placebo-Controlled Study." *Musculoskeletal Surgery* 99, Supplement 1 (2015): S43–S52.

5. Van Nooten, Floortje, Maarten Treur, Krystallia Pantiri, et al. "Capsaicin 8% Patch Versus Oral Neuropathic Pain Medications for the Treatment of Painful Diabetic Peripheral Neuropathy: A Systematic Literature Review and Network Meta-Analysis." *Clinical Therapeutics* 39, no. 4 (April 2017): 787–803.e18.

6. Persson, M. S. M., J. Stocks, D. A. Walsh, et al. "The Relative Efficacy of Topical Non-Steroidal Anti-Inflammatory Drugs and Capsaicin in Osteoarthritis: A Network Meta-Analysis of Randomized Controlled Trials." *Osteoarthritis and Cartilage* 26 (2018): 1575–1582.

7. Derry, Sheena, Andrew S. C. Rice, Peter Cole, et al. "Topical Capsaicin (High Concentrations) for Chronic Neuropathic Pain in Adults." *Cochrane Database of Systematic Reviews* 1, no. 1 (January 13, 2017): CD007393.

8. Alammar, N., L. Wang, B. Saberi, et al. "The Impact of Peppermint Oil on the Irritable Bowel Syndrome: A Meta-Analysis of the Pooled Clinical Data." *BMC Complementary and Alternative Medicine* 19 (2019): 21–30.

9. Khanna, Reena, John K. MacDonald, and Barrett G. Levesque. "Peppermint Oil for the Treatment of Irritable Bowel Syndrome: A Systematic Review and Meta-Analysis." *Journal of Clinical Gastroenterology* 48, no. 6 (July 2014): 505–512.

10. Weerts, Zsa Zsa R. M., Ad A. M. Masclee, Ben J. M. Witteman, et al. "Efficacy and Safety of Peppermint Oil in a Randomized, Double-Blind Trial of Patients with Irritable Bowel Syndrome." *Gastroenterology* 158 (2020): 123–136.

11. Daily, James W., Xin Zhang, Da Sol Kim, and Sunmin Park. "Efficacy of Ginger for Alleviating the Symptoms of Primary Dysmenorrhea: A Systematic Review and Meta-Analysis of Randomized Clinical Trials." *Pain Medicine* 16, no. 12 (December 2015): 2243–2255.

12. Adib Rad, Hajar, Zahra Basirat, Fatemeh Bakouei, et al. "Effect of Ginger and Novafen on Menstrual Pain: A Cross-Over Trial." *Taiwanese Journal of Obstetrics & Gynecology* 57 (2018): 806–809.

13. Araya-Quintanilla, F., H. Gutiérrez-Espinoza, M. J. Muñoz-Yanez, et al. "Effectiveness of Ginger on Pain and Function in Knee Osteoarthritis: A PRISMA Systematic Review and Meta-Analysis." *Pain Physician* 23 (2020): E151–E161.

REFERENCES AND FURTHER READINGS

Adib Rad, Hajar, Zahra Basirat, Fatemeh Bakouei, et al. "Effect of Ginger and Novafen on Menstrual Pain: A Cross-Over Trial." *Taiwanese Journal of Obstetrics & Gynecology* 57 (2018): 806–809.

Alammar, N., L. Wang, B. Saberi, et al. "The Impact of Peppermint Oil on the Irritable Bowel Syndrome: A Meta-Analysis of the Polled Clinical Data." *BMC Complementary and Alternative Medicine* 19 (2019): 21–30.

Araya-Quintanilla, F., H. Gutiérrez-Espinoza, M. J. Muñoz-Yanez, et al. "Effectiveness of Ginger on Pain an Function inn Knee Osteoarthritis: A PRISMA Systematic Review and Meta-Analysis." *Pain Physician* 23 (2020): E151–E161.

Bannuru, Raveendhara R., Mikala C. Osani, Fatimah Al-Eid, and Chenchen Wang. "Efficacy of Curcumin and Boswellia for Knee Osteoarthritis: Systematic Review and Meta-Analysis." *Seminars in Arthritis and Rheumatism* 48 (2018): 416–429.

Daily, James W., Xin Zhang, Da Sol Kim, and Sunin Park. "Efficacy of Ginger for Alleviating the Symptoms of Primary Dysmenorrhea: A Systematic Review and Meta-Analysis of Randomized Clinical Trials." *Pain Medicine* 16, no. 12 (December 2015): 2243–2255.

Derry, Sheena, Andrew S. C. Rice, Peter Cole, et al. "Topical Capsaicin (High Concentrations) for Chronic Neuropathic Pain in Adults." *Cochrane Database of Systematic Reviews* 1, no. 1 (January 13, 2017): CD007393.

Khanna, Reena, John K. MacDonald, and Barrett G. Levesque. "Peppermint Oil for the Treatment of Irritable Bowel Syndrome: A Systematic

Review and Meta-Analysis." *Journal of Clinical Gastroenterology* 48, no. 6 (July 2014): 505–512.

Majeed, Muhammed, Shaheen Majeed, Narayanan K. Naraynan, and Kalyanam Nagabhushanam. "A Pilot, Randomized, Double-Blind, Placebo-Controlled Trial to Assess the Safety and Efficacy of a Novel *Boswellia serrate* Extract in the Management of Osteoarthritis of the Knee." *Phytotherapy Research* 33 (2019): 1457–1468.

Merolla, G., F. Dellabiancia, A. Ingardia, et al. "Co-Analgesic Therapy for Arthroscopic Supraspinatus Tendon Repair Pain Using Dietary Supplement Containing *Boswellia serrate* and *Curcuma Longa*: A Prospective Randomized Placebo-Controlled Study." *Musculoskeletal Surgery* 99, Supplement 1 (2015): S43–S52.

Persson, M. S. M., J. Stocks, D. A. Walsh, et al. "The Relative Efficacy of Topical Non-Steroidal Anti-Inflammatory Drugs and Capsaicin in Osteoarthritis: A Network Meta-Analysis of randomized Controlled Trials." *Osteoarthritis and Cartilage* 26 (2018): 1575–1582.

Prabhavathi, K., U. Shobha Jagdish Chandra, Radhika Soanker, and P. Usha Rani. "A Randomized, Double-Blind, Placebo Controlled, Cross Over Study to Evaluate the Analgesic Activity of *Boswellia serrate* in Healthy Volunteers Using Mechanical Pain Model." *Indian Journal of Pharmacology* 46, no. 5 (September–October 2014): 475–479.

Van Nooten, Floortje, Maarten Treur, Krystallia Pantiri, et al. "Capsaicin 8% Patch Versus Oral Neuropathic Pain Medications for the Treatment of Painful Diabetic Peripheral Neuropathy: A Systematic Literature Review and Network Meta-Analysis." *Clinical Therapeutics* 39, no. 4 (April 2017): 787–803.e18.

Weerts, Zsa Zsa R. M., Ad A. M. Masclee, Ben J. M. Witteman, et al. "Efficacy and Safety of Peppermint Oil in a Randomized, Double-Blind Trial of Patients with Irritable Bowel Syndrome." *Gastroenterology* 158 (2020): 123–136.

Homeopathy

INTRODUCTION

Also known as homeopathic medicine, homeopathy is a medical system that was developed more than 200 years ago in Germany. It has two primary principles. The first, known as "like cures like," contends that a medical problem may be ameliorated by a substance that produces similar symptoms in healthy people. And the second, known as the "law of minimum dose," is the belief that the lower the dose of a medication, the greater its effectiveness. Homeopathic products tend to be very diluted.

Homeopathy treatments, known as remedies, are derived from a variety of sources, including plants, minerals, or animals. They are often made into pellets, which should be placed under the tongue. However, they may be sold as ointments, gels, drops, creams, and tablets. Treatments are customized for each person; people with the same condition may be advised to take different remedies. When recommending remedies, a practitioner factors in the patient's constitution, emotional and mental make-up, how the patient responds to physical emotional, and mental influences and stress, as well as the patient's personality, temperament, genetic predispositions, and family history of particular diseases.

Though homeopathy has been embraced by some traditional and integrative healthcare providers, it remains controversial. Many question how a product that has few or no active ingredients can have any noticeable effect on the body, and it is a challenge to conduct research on products that are individualized; there are no uniform prescribing standards. There are hundreds, perhaps even thousands, of different homeopathic remedies. A few of the most commonly used treatments for pain include arnica, bryonia alba, guaiacum, hypericum, and rhus toxicodenrun. A practitioner will recommend a treatment based on a person's symptoms and the overall impact of the medical problem on that person. Practitioners, who usually work in an office setting, take a holistic approach to treating their patients.

ADMINISTRATION AND REGULATION

In an article published in 2018 in the journal *Homeopathy*, two Boston-area physicians described the use of homeopathy in the United States. According to these physicians, just over 2 percent of the adult U.S. population and 1.8 percent of the youth population use homeopathy, primarily for respiratory, otorhinolaryngology (ears, nose, and throat), and musculoskeletal complaints. But, the remedies may be used for other medical conditions including, fatigue, sleep, stress, chronic pain, and gastrointestinal, and neurological problems. Only 19 percent of those who use homeopathy remedies actually visit a provider for treatment; the vast majority self-prescribe their treatment(s). Homeopathy users are more likely to be white, female, aged 30–44 years, and live in the western part of the United States. They tend to be married, have at least a high school education, and have a lower body mass index.[1]

There are no national certification programs for homeopathic practitioners. The administration of homeopathy varies from state to state. Generally, people who are licensed health-care providers are able to practice homeopathy. As a result, some physicians, chiropractors, osteopaths, and other medical providers, who work in a wide variety of settings, train in homeopathy and prescribe remedies to their patients. In some states, nonlicensed professionals may also practice homeopathy. (The training of naturopathic doctors includes homeopathy.) Costs associated with health-care practitioners would be a function of the type of medical provider and the health insurance coverage. Some health insurance providers may refuse to cover homeopathic consultations. The remedies themselves, in their various different forms, are quite inexpensive and are readily available in "health food" type stores and online.

Under the Federal Food, Drug, and Cosmetic Act (FDCA), homeopathic products are regulated as drugs. However, the U. S. FDA Administration does not evaluate them for effectiveness or safety. The FDA allows homeopathic products that meet certain conditions to be sold without agency preapproval. For example, homeopathic products must contain active ingredients listed in the *Homeopathic Pharmacopeia of the United States*. Further, the FDA requires that the label on the product, the outer container, or the accompanying leaflet include at least one medical problem to be treated, a list of ingredients, the number of active ingredient dilutions, and directions for use.

BENEFITS AND RISKS

Homeopathic practitioners contend that the remedies are effective and inexpensive tools to treat a wide variety of medical problems. Acute and chronic problems may be addressed during the course of one session with a practitioner or, as has been noted, by individuals who conduct their own homeopathic research and select their own remedies. Homeopathy supports the body's ability to heal itself. After taking remedies, people may report improvements in overall energy, quality of sleep, digestion, and general health. Sometimes, people report the disappearance of other symptoms seemingly unrelated to the condition being treated. Furthermore, there are reports of homeopathy being useful for people having surgery. The remedies have been used both before and after surgery to speed healing.

It is possible that homeopathic products may contain potentially harmful ingredients, such as mercury or iron, that cause side effects or drug interactions. There have been reports of such problems. In addition, some people have replaced their traditional medications with homeopathic treatments and have subsequently become ill. People concerned about alcohol consumption should know that liquid homeopathic products may contain alcohol. In addition, homeopathic practitioners have reported that some patients experience a response known as "homeopathic aggravation," a temporary worsening of symptoms.

Though there are many traditionally trained medical providers who do prescribe homeopathy, it should be underscored that homeopathy and its underlying principles are not supported by mainstream allopathic medicine, and there are legitimate safety concerns. There are no FDA-approved products labeled as homeopathic. As a result, homeopathic products are sold in the United States without FDA evaluation for safety or effectiveness. There are no homeopathic products that have been approved by the FDA to treat, cure, prevent, or mitigate any diseases or conditions.

RESEARCH FINDINGS

Homeopathy Appears to Be Useful for Endometriosis-Associated Pelvic Pain

In a 24-week, randomized, double-blind, placebo-controlled, clinical trial published in 2017 in the *European Journal of Obstetrics & Gynecology and Reproductive Biology*, researchers from São Paulo, Brazil, wanted to determine if the homeopathic treatment potentized estrogen would be useful for women suffering from endometriosis-associated pelvic pain. The initial cohort consisted of 50 women between the ages of 18 and 45 years with a diagnosis of deeply infiltrating endometriosis and pelvic pain. Three different doses of potentized estrogen (12cH, 18cH, and 24cH) or a placebo were administered sequentially every eight weeks to 23 women in the intervention group and 27 women in the placebo group. The vials containing potentized estrogen and the placebo were identical in appearance. Pain measurements were taken at baseline and every eight weeks throughout the trial; quality of life, depression, and anxiety assessments were also conducted. Seventeen women in the intervention group and 24 women in the placebo group completed the trial. The researchers learned that the potentized estrogen was "significantly superior" than the placebo in reducing endometriosis-associated pelvic pain. The women taking the placebo did not experience any significant improvement in pain. In addition, the women in the intervention group had improvements in bodily pain, vitality, mental health, and depression. Because of its safety and low cost, the researchers commented that "homeopathy might be added to routine conventional treatment of endometriosis as a complementary therapeutic resource." There was therapeutic efficacy, "regardless of the potency used."[2]

Homeopathic Treatments May Be Useful for Women Dealing with Joint Pain and Stiffness Linked to Aromatase Inhibitor Treatment for Early Breast Cancer

In a prospective, unrandomized, observational, pilot trial published in 2016 in the journal *Homeopathy*, researchers from France noted that women with early hormone receptor–positive breast cancer may be treated with a class of medications known as aromatase inhibitors. Unfortunately, this medication often causes joint pain and stiffness. In some cases, because of these chronically painful side effects, women discontinue their medication. The researchers wanted to learn if the homeopathic treatments, *Ruta graveolens* 5cH and *Rhus toxicodendron* 9cH, would be useful for these side effects. The researchers recruited 40 patients with a mean age of 64.9 years; all of the women were taking aromatase inhibitors. The 20 women in one group received homeopathy and standard treatment for three months; the 20 women in the other group received only standard therapy. The researchers found a significant difference in the pain scores between the baseline levels and the levels after three months. The pain scores of the women in the intervention group decreased significantly. Nine women in the standard therapy group and one in the combination group increased their consumption of pain medication. The women in the standard group had more pain-related sleep problems, and they required more time for their morning stiffness to dissipate. The researchers emphasized the need for a larger study to confirm their results.[3]

When Combined with Physiotherapy, Homeopathy Appears to Be Useful for Chronic Low Back Pain from Osteoarthritis

In a six-week randomized, double-blind, placebo-controlled, pilot trial published in 2016 in the journal *Alternate Therapies in Health & Medicine*, researchers from South Africa evaluated the ability of a combination of physiotherapy and a homeopathic complex to help people suffering from chronic low back pain from osteoarthritis. The cohort consisted of 30 men and women, between the ages of 45 and 75 years, who were receiving physiotherapy treatment for osteoarthritis of the lumbar spine at a private physiotherapy practice in Gauteng, South Africa. Fifteen subjects were placed in an intervention group, and 15 were in a placebo group. Every two weeks, the subjects in both groups received massages, thermal therapy, and joint mobilization. In addition, the subjects in the intervention group took a homeopathic complex that contained 6cH each of *Arnica Montana*, *Bryonia alba*, *Causticum*, *Kalmia latifolia*, *Rhus toxicodendron, and Calcarea fluorica.* The other subjects took a placebo. The researchers found that the subjects in the intervention group significantly outperformed the control group with regard to pain, daily functioning, and range of motion. However, there was no significant difference between the two groups in the need for conventional pain medication. While acknowledging that the sample size of their trial was too small to be conclusive, the researchers noted that the combination of physiotherapy and the homeopathic complex "can significantly improve the symptoms associated with CLBP [chronic low back pain] due to OA [osteoarthritis]."[4]

Homeopathy Seems to Help Children with Migraines

In an observational, prospective, open, nonrandomized, noncomparative, multicenter trial published in 2013 in *The Journal of Alternative and Complementary Medicine*, researchers based in France wanted to learn if homeopathic treatments would help children who suffer from migraines. The cohort consisted of 59 physicians (general practitioners and pediatricians) from 12 different countries, who had training in homeopathic medicine, and 168 children between the ages of 5 and 15 years, who suffered from migraines. The mean age of the children was 11 years, and 60 percent were female. The physicians individualized the homeopathic treatments for each patient. The mean duration of follow-up was 104 days. The researchers learned that after three months of homeopathic treatments the children had a two-thirds statistically significant reduction in the incidence of migraines. Moreover, the intensity of the migraines significantly lessened. At baseline, over two-thirds of the children complained of severe/intolerable headaches; after three months, that figure was down to 19.1 percent. And, the migraines were significantly shorter. The percentage of children having a migraine that lasted more than six hours decreased from 36.5 percent to 13.5 percent. The researchers concluded that their findings "suggest that homeopathic medicines may decrease the frequency, intensity, and duration of migraine attacks, and may significantly reduce absenteeism from school."[5]

Homeopathy May Be Helpful in the Treatment of Fibromyalgia

In a literature review and meta-analysis published in 2014 in the journal *Complementary Therapies in Medicine*, researchers from Germany examined the use of homeopathic medicine to treat fibromyalgia between October 2012 and February 2013. Including subjects of all ages, the researchers found ten case reports, three observational studies, and one nonrandomized and four randomized controlled trials that met their criteria. (As no standardized mean differences could be calculated, the case reports were excluded from the meta-analysis.) According to the researchers, while the studies included in the meta-analysis tended to have "low methodology quality," they were "sufficiently homogenous in terms of conditions treated, interventions and outcomes." Also, there was solid evidence that people with fibromyalgia may well benefit from homeopathic treatment, and homeopathy may be a complementary treatment for that painful, disabling disorder. There is "a sufficient basis for discussing the possible benefits of homeopathy for patients suffering from fibromyalgia syndrome."[6]

Homeopathy May or May Not Help People with the Pain of Knee Osteoarthritis

In a prospective, observational trial published in 2016 in the *Indian Journal of Research in Homeopathy*, researchers from India wanted to learn if homeopathy could help people dealing with the problems associated with knee osteoarthritis, such as pain, stiffness, and disease progression. The cohort consisted of 131 subjects (107 females and 24 males) with osteoarthritis of the knee, diagnosed by orthopedic surgeons during a clinical examination at the outpatient department of a medical college and hospital. Each subject was prescribed a single homeopathic medicine at a time in one to three doses and was assessed for pain, morning stiffness, and the impact on activities of daily living. Subjects were treated for a minimum of 12 months; the mean period of treatment was 27 months. The researchers learned that the homeopathic treatments reduced pain and stiffness. The researchers commented that "this long-term adherence to a therapy with substantial relief in pain and improvements in ADL [activity of daily living] signifies the clinical effect of homeopathic medicines." However, because the subjects continued to take their normal pain medications, the trial failed to determine if the improvements were only from the homeopathic remedies. Further research is needed.[7]

In a prospective, parallel-arm, double-blind, randomized, placebo-controlled pilot trial published in 2015 in the *Journal of Evidence-Based Complementary & Alternative Medicine*, researchers from India evaluated the ability of homeopathy to help people with pain from knee osteoarthritis. The cohort consisted of 60 subjects with acute painful episodes of knee osteoarthritis; the trial was conducted from January to October 2014. Thirty subjects were placed in an intervention group, which received individualized treatments over two weeks, and 30 were in a placebo group. Changes in symptoms, such as pain, stiffness, and loss of function, were noted. Fifty-four subjects completed the trial; the drop-out rate was 10 percent. The researchers found that significant reductions were achieved in all the outcomes across the two groups. The homeopathy treatments did not appear to be better than the placebo treatment for the pain and other problems associated with knee osteoarthritis. "Although evidences seemed to be inadequate in support of efficacy of individualized homeopathy over placebo in acute painful episodes of knee osteoarthritis, larger randomized controlled trials in a multicenter design seem quite feasible in [the] near future."[8]

Homeopathy May Help Women Suffering from Post-Caesarian Backaches

In a three-month open, observational, noncontrolled clinical trial published in 2019 in the *Indian Journal of Research in Homeopathy*, researchers from India investigated the ability of homeopathic remedies to help women deal with backaches following delivery of a baby by caesarian section. The initial cohort consisted of 50 women who suffered from backaches after delivering babies by caesarian section. "Experienced homeopathic physicians" prescribed different homeopathic remedies. Assessments were made at baseline and during treatment. Forty-five women completed the trial, and no adverse effects were reported. The researchers found that the women experienced statistically significant reductions in pain. Still, the researchers underscored the need for more research on this potential treatment. This research should be randomized "with enhanced methodological rigour."[9]

Homeopathy May or May Not Be Useful for Women Suffering from Primary Dysmenorrhea or Menstrual Pain

In a double-blind, placebo-controlled, randomized trial, with two parallel arms, published in 2016 in the *Iranian Red Crescent Medical Journal*, researchers from Iran wanted to determine if homeopathy would be useful for the pain and discomfort associated with menstrual periods, a condition known as dysmenorrhea.

The initial cohort consisted of 60 students who resided in three dormitories of the Tabriz University of Medical Sciences in Tabriz, Iran. All of the women had moderate or severe menstrual pain. Assessments were made during two cycles before and two cycles after the intervention. The women were given diaries in which they recorded menstrual pain intensity and the number of analgesic pills they took, during the two days before and the three days after the start of menstrual bleeding. Six participants were excluded because of noncompliance with the diary completion. As a result, 54 women were referred to a homeopath for consultation and were given homeopathic treatment or a placebo. Twenty-seven women received a homeopathic remedy, and 27 women received a placebo. One intervention woman and six placebo women were lost to follow-up. Hence, 47 women completed the entire trial. The researchers failed to observe any significant differences in menstrual pain intensity and the need for analgesics between the groups. The results were the same for the intervention and placebo, However, when compared to the preintervention status, the homeopathic treatment "showed a significant decrease in pain intensity and improvement in quality of life after homeopathic treatment." After taking the homeopathic medication, the subjects experienced significant pain relief. No side effects were reported by any of the subjects.[10]

The Homeopathic Remedy Arnica Montana May Be Useful for Women Undergoing Total Mastectomy, but It Does Not Appear to Affect Pain

In a randomized, double-blind, placebo-controlled trial published in 2017 in the *Journal of Intercultural Ethnopharmacology*, researchers from Italy wanted to learn if the homeopathic remedy Arnica montana would benefit women who undergo a total mastectomy for breast cancer. Specifically, would it reduce blood loss and seroma production? The trial was carried out in a single university hospital from 2012 to 2014. The initial cohort consisted of 53 women who had unilateral total mastectomies with or without reconstruction. The women received either five sublingual drops of Arnica montana 1000K three times a day (n = 26) or a placebo (n = 27) with the same administration, from one day before the surgery to the fourth day after the surgery. The same operating team operated on all the women, though the members of the surgical team were not aware who took the remedy and who took the placebo. Three of the women in the treatment group were excluded, as were seven in the placebo group. The researchers learned that the women in the treatment group had lower mean volume of collected blood and serum. However, there were no statistically significant differences in the perception of pain between the two groups. Also, "the presence of bruising and hematomas or breast swelling did not differ significantly by treatment group."[11]

Topical Arnica May Have Little Effect on Performance, Pain, and Muscle Damage after Intense Exercise

In a double-blind, randomized, placebo-controlled trial published in 2014 in the *European Journal of Sport Science*, researchers from Australia wanted to determine if topical arnica would be useful in reducing pain, indicators of inflammation, and muscle damage in well-trained males. The cohort consisted of 20 well-trained males from a variety of sports with a mean age of 25.3 years. At baseline, all of the men were free from injuries or conditions associated with inflammation. They were given either a 50-gram arnica gel tube or a placebo; both types had the same color, smell, and texture. For five days, the men applied the gels to their quadriceps and gastrocnemius muscles immediately after a downhill run and then reapplied to the same regions every four hours. Each subject recorded the date and time of applications on a compliance checklist. No adverse effects were reported. The researchers learned that the topical arnica had "minimal" effect on performance and blood markers. However, the arnica "may have influenced the participants' perception of pain in their lower limbs" three days after exercising. The researchers concluded that further research is needed to learn more about the *timing* of topical arnica application.[12]

Homeopathic Remedies May or May Not Be Useful for Irritable Bowel Syndrome, a Potentially Painful and Debilitating Condition

In a review published in 2019 in the *Cochrane Database of Systematic Reviews*, researchers from the United Kingdom evaluated the ability of clinical homeopathy and individualized homeopathy to ameliorate the symptoms associated with irritable bowel syndrome. (Clinical homeopathy occurs when a specific remedy is prescribed for a specific condition. Individualized homeopathy is when a remedy is prescribed based on a person's symptoms and after a detailed consultation.) The cohort consisted of four randomized, controlled trials with 307 participants. Two of the trials compared clinical homeopathy to placebo for irritable bowel syndrome with constipation, and one trial compared individualized homeopathy to the usual care for the treatment of irritable bowel syndrome in female patients. The fourth trial had three arms and compared homeopathic treatment to supportive listening or usual care. Though the risk of bias was unclear in the first three studies, the risk of bias in the fourth study was low. Still, the researchers were unable to find definitive results. "No firm conclusions regarding the effectiveness and safety of homeopathy for the treatment of IBS [irritable bowel syndrome] can be drawn."[13]

Adverse Effects of Homeopathy Appear to Be Somewhat Common

In a systematic review and meta-analysis published in 2016 in the journal *Complementary Therapies in Medicine*, researchers from Norway and China wanted to learn more about adverse reactions that may occur from homeopathic medicine. The cohort consisted of 41 randomized, controlled trials with 6,055 participants. A subtotal of 39 studies, with 5,902 participants, were included in the meta-analysis. The methodology in the majority of the trials was high quality. Twenty-eight trials (68%) reported adverse effects, and five trials (12%) reported homeopathic aggravations. Thus, 491 participants experienced 690 adverse events, 426 in the treatments groups and 264 in the control groups. The adverse events were mostly categorized as gastrointestinal disorders, headache/dizziness, or dermatitis. One hundred seven participants experienced a total of 158 homeopathic aggravations, 91 in the treatment groups and 67 in the control groups. The researchers concluded that adverse effects and homeopathic aggravations are "commonly reported in trials." Moreover, the meta-analysis found "that the proportion of patients experiencing adverse effects to be similar for patients randomized to homeopathic treatment compared to patients randomized to placebo and conventional medicine."[14]

NOTES

1. Dossett, Michelle L., and Gloria Y. Yeh. "Homeopathy Use in the USA and Implications for Public Health: A Review." *Homeopathy* 107, no. 1 (February 2018): 3–9.

2. Teixeira, M. Z., S. Podgaec, and E. C. Baracat. "Potentized Estrogen in Homeopathic Treatment of Endometriosis-Associated Pelvic Pain: A 24-Week, Randomized, Double-Blind, Placebo-Controlled Study." *European Journal of Obstetrics & Gynecology and Reproductive Biology* 211 (April 2017): 48–55.

3. Karp, J. C., C. Sanchez, P. Guilbert, et al. "Treatment with *Ruta graveolens* 5cH and *Rhus toxicodendron* 9cH May Reduce Joint Pain and Stiffness Linked to Aromatase Inhibitors in Women with Early Breast Cancer: Results of a Pilot Observational Study." *Homeopathy* 105, no. 4 (2016): 299–308.

4. Morris, Mary, Janice Pellow, Elizabeth M. Solomon, and Tebogo Tsele-Tebakang. "Physiotherapy and a Homeopathic Complex for Chronic Low-Back Pain Due to Osteoarthritis: A Randomized, Controlled Pilot Study." *Alternative Therapies in Health & Medicine* 22, no. 1 (February 2016): 48–56.

5. Danno, Karine, Aurélie Colas, Jean-Louis Masson, and Marie-France Bordet. "Homeopathic Treatment of Migraine in Children: Results of a Prospective, Multicenter, Observational Study." *Journal of Alternative and Complementary Medicine* 19, no. 2 (2013): 119–123.

6. Boehm, K., C. Raak, H. Cramer, et al. "Homeopathy in the Treatment of Fibromyalgia—A Comprehensive Literature-Review and Meta-Analysis." *Complementary Therapies in Medicine* 22, no. 4 (August 2014): 731–742.

7. Motiwala, F. F., Tapas Kundu, Kamlesh Bagmar, et al. "Effect of Homeopathic Treatment on Activity of Daily Living (ADL) in Knee Osteoarthritis: A Progressive Observational Study." *Indian Journal of Research in Homeopathy* 10 (2016): 182–187.

8. Koley, M., S. Saha, and S. Ghosh. "A Double-Blind Randomized Placebo-Controlled Feasibility Study Evaluating Individualized Homeopathy in Managing Pain of Knee Osteoarthritis." *Journal of Evidence-Based Complementary & Alternative Medicine* 20, no. 3 (July 2015): 186–191.

9. Nath, A., M. De, S. Singh, et al. "The Role of Homeopathic Treatment in Women Suffering from Post-Caesarean Backache: An Observational Clinical Trial." *Indian Journal of Research in Homeopathy* 13, no. 2 (2019): 81–90.

10. Mohammad-Alizadeh-Charandabi, Sakineh, Mohammad Hossein Biglu, and Khatereh Yousefi Rad. "Effect of Homeopathy on Pain Intensity and Quality of Life of Students with Primary Dysmenorrhea: A Randomized Controlled Trial." *Iranian Red Crescent Medical Journal* 18, no. 9 (September 2016): e30902.

11. Sorrentino, Luca, Salvatore Piraneo, Eliana Riggio, et al. "Is There a Role for Homeopathy in Breast Cancer Surgery? A First Randomized Clinical Trial on Treatment with *Arnica Montana* to Reduce Post-Operative Seroma and Bleeding in Patients Undergoing Total Mastectomy." *Journal of Intercultural Ethnopharmacology* 6, no. 1 (January–March 2017): 1–8.

12. Pumpa, Kate L., Kieran E. Fallon, Alan Bensoussan, et al. "The Effects of Topical Arnica on Performance, Pain and Muscle Damage after Intense Eccentric Exercise." *European Journal of Sport Science* 14, no. 3 (2014): 294–300.

13. Peckham, E. J., K. Cooper, E. R. Roberts, et al. "Homeopathy for Treatment of Irritable Bowel Syndrome." *Cochrane Database of Systematic Reviews* 9 (September 4, 2019): CD009710.

14. Stub, T., F. Musial, A. A. Kristoffersen, et al. "Adverse Effects of Homeopathy, What Do We Know? A Systematic Review and Meta-Analysis of Randomized Controlled Trials." *Complementary Therapies in Medicine* 26 (June 2016): 146–163.

REFERENCES AND FURTHER READINGS

Boehm, K., C. Raak, H. Cramer, et al. "Homeopathy in the Treatment of Fibromyalgia—A Comprehensive Literature-Review and Meta-Analysis." *Complementary Therapies in Medicine* 22, no. 4 (August 2014): 731–742.

Danno, Karine, Aurélie Colas, Jean-Louis Masson, and Marie-France Bordet. "Homeopathic Treatment of Migraine in Children: Results of a Prospective, Multicenter, Observational Study." *Journal of Alternative and Complementary Medicine* 19, no. 2 (2013): 119–123.

Dossett, Michelle L., and Gloria Y. Yeh. "Homeopathy Use in the USA and Implications for Public Health." *Homeopathy* 107, no. 1 (February 2018): 3–9.

Karp, J. C., C. Sanchez, P. Guilbert, et al. "Treatment with *Ruta graveolens* 5cH and *Rhus toxicodendron* 9cH May Reduce Joint Pain and Stiffness Linked to Aromatase Inhibitors in Women with Early Breast Cancer: Results of a Pilot Observational Study." *Homeopathy* 105, no. 4 (November 2016): 299–308.

Koley, Munmun, Subhranil Saha, and Shubhamoy Ghosh. "A Double-Blind Randomized Placebo-Controlled Feasibility Study Evaluating Individualized Homeopathy in Managing Pain of Knee Osteoarthritis." *Journal of Evidence-Based Complementary & Alternative Medicine* 20, no. 3 (2015): 186–191.

Mohammad-Alizadeh-Charandabi, Sakineh, Mohammad Hossein Biglu, and Khatereh Yousefi Rad. "Effect of Homeopathy on Pain Intensity and Quality of Life of Students with Primary Dysmenorrhea: A Randomized Controlled Trial." *Iranian Red Crescent Medical Journal* 18, no. 9 (September 2016): e30902.

Morris, Mary, Janice Pellow, Elizabeth M. Solomon, and Tebogo Tsele-Tebaksng. "Physiotherapy and a Homeopathic Complex for Chronic Low-Back Pain Due to Osteoarthritis: A Randomized, Controlled

Pilot Study." *Alternative Therapies in Health & Medicine* 22, no. 1 (February 2016): 48–56.

Motiwala, F. F., Tapas Kundu, Kamlesh Bagmar, et al. "Effect of Homeopathic Treatment on Activity of Daily Living (ADL) in Knee Osteoarthritis: A Prospective Observational Study." *Indian Journal of Research in Homeopathy* 10 (2016): 182–187.

Nath, A., M. De, S. Singh, et al. "The Role of Homeopathic Treatment in Women Suffering from Post-Caesarean Backache: A Open Observational Clinical Trial." *Indian Journal of Research in Homeopathy* 13, no. 2 (2019): 81–90.

Peckham, E. J., K. Cooper, E. R. Roberts, et al. "Homeopathy for Treatment of Irritable Bowel Syndrome." *Cochrane Database of Systematic Reviews* 9 (September 4, 2019): CD008710.

Pumpa, Kate L., Kieran E. Fallon, Alan Bensoussan, et al. "The Effects of Topical Arnica on Performance, Pain, and Muscle Damage After Intense Eccentric Exercise." *European Journal of Sport Science* 14, no. 3 (2014): 294–300.

Sorrentino, Luca, Salvatore Piraneo, Eliana Riggio, et al. "Is There a Role for Homeopathy in Breast Cancer Surgery? A First Randomized Clinical Trial on Treatment with *Arnica Montana* to Reduce Post-Operative Seroma and Bleeding in Patients Undergoing Total Mastectomy." *Journal of Intercultural Ethnopharmacology* 6, no. 1 (January–March 2017): 1–8.

Stub, T., F. Musial, A. A. Kristoffersen, et al. "Adverse Effects of Homeopathy, What Do We Know? A Systematic Review and Meta-Analysis of Randomized Controlled Trials." *Complementary Therapies in Medicine* 26 (June 2016): 146–163.

Teixeira, M. Z., S. Podgaec, and E. C. Baracat. "Potentized Estrogen in Homeopathic Treatment of Endometriosis-Associated Pelvic Pain: A 24-Week, Randomized, Double-Blind, Placebo-Controlled Study." *European Journal of Obstetrics & Gynecology and Reproductive Biology* 211 (April 2017): 48–55.

Hydrotherapy

INTRODUCTION

Also known as aquatic therapy, water therapy, and hydropathy, hydrotherapy is a complementary therapy that uses hot, warm, or cold water in a variety of different external and internal forms for health purposes. The water pressure and flow will vary depending upon the treatment, and the water may be in any form, including ice and steam.

There are several types of hydrotherapy. These include aquatic exercise, which is low impact exercise usually in a warm pool with specialized equipment. (While it is useful to know how to swim, one is able to participate in aquatic exercise without knowing this skill. Always be certain that there is at least one professional or paraprofessional with you.) It enables people to raise their heart rate and work their muscles without straining their joints. Aquatic exercise is particularly useful for elders, who are at a higher risk of falling, and people with arthritis or fibromyalgia. Warm water baths are another form of hydrotherapy. To enhance the bath, salts, essential oils, or minerals may be added. Balneotherapy is the term used for soaking in mineral-rich water or natural mineral hot springs. Warm or cold sitz baths may be used to relieve hemorrhoids or cramps. Warm or cold wraps and compresses may offer targeted relief to almost any part of the body. And, colonic therapy, which is controversial, is the practice of rinsing feces from the colon.

The use of water for therapeutic purposes probably dates back to the origins of mankind. It was widely used in ancient cultures, such as India, Egypt, and China. Father Sebastian Kneipp, a 19th-century Bavarian monk, is considered the founder of modern hydrotherapy. His use of alternating hot and cold water, known as contrast hydrotherapy, is still practiced today. Around the same time, Vincent Preissnitz founded the first hydrotherapy clinic in Gräfenberg, Germany, as part of the "naturalism movement."

Treatment included eating coarse foods and drinking huge amounts of water. Shortly thereafter, hydrotherapy came to the United States.

It is impossible to know how often people turn to hydrotherapy for the relief of pain. In all probability, it is used fairly often.

ADMINISTRATION AND REGULATION

Some hydrotherapy treatments are simple and relatively easy to do. For example, one can sit or lie down in a warm bath at home. Other practices, such as spending time in a sauna, involved specific locations and/or special equipment. Additional sites where hydrotherapy equipment may be found include hospitals, rehabilitation centers and nursing facilities, physical and occupational therapy offices, spas, swimming pools, community centers, and private clubs. Some facilities may offer group sessions for people with similar medical problems. The actual administration policies and costs will vary from location to location; some treatments may even be covered by insurance. It is best to learn as much as you can before visiting a facility or provider. If that is not possible, ask questions during an initial visit. Some facilities, such as community centers and private clubs, may offer trial memberships.

Regulations will vary according to the type of facility and the state and city/town in which it is located. In addition, most likely, there are state and local health regulations and requirements for licensure. And, there is a good chance that the people who work in the various forms of hydrotherapy require some form of licensure. On the other hand, the Centers for Disease Control and Prevention has issued recommendations for hydrotherapy tanks. Thus, it suggests that these tanks be drained and cleaned with an EPA-registered product after each person's use. And, the CDC advises against permitting people with open wounds and fecal incontinence to use the tanks.

BENEFITS AND RISKS

Hydrotherapy is useful for many different types of pain. For example, people dealing with various types of arthritis, such as osteoarthritis, psoriatic arthritis, and rheumatoid arthritis, might receive a good deal of pain relief from therapy in warm water. The warm temperature allows the muscles to relax and eases joint pain and increases the range of motion. Pushing arms and legs against the water, supports muscle strength and overall fitness. Similar relief may be obtained by people dealing with chronic back pain or recovering from knee replacement surgery.

Hydrotherapy needs to be avoided or used with caution in people with certain medical conditions. These include cardiovascular disease, high blood pressure, colds, flus, and other respiratory infections, fever, incontinence, chlorine allergy, breathing problems, kidney disease, thrombosis, skin infections, cancer, uncontrolled diabetes, asthma, epilepsy, and pregnancy. Immersion, especially for extended periods, may well be dangerous for some people. People with specific medical concerns should check with their medical provider before beginning a course of hydrotherapy. And, it is important to remember that while hydrotherapy may well be able to relieve pain, it is never a cure. Hydrotherapy should not be used as a substitute for standard medical care.

RESEARCH FINDINGS

Aquatic Exercise Helps the Pain Associated with Knee Osteoarthritis

In a systematic review and meta-analysis published in 2015 in the journal *Zeitschrift für Rheumatogie*, researchers based in China examined the use of aquatic exercise for knee osteoarthritis. The researchers located six randomized controlled trials with 398 subjects that met their criteria. The trials originated in the United States, Denmark, Taiwan, Brazil, Thailand, and Korea. Patients were recruited from outpatient clinics or community centers. On average, the subjects were in their 60s and 70s, and the majority were female. Two trials reported adverse events. Aquatic exercise included stretching, fast walking, strengthening, and/or aerobic training. The trials lasted for 6 to 18 weeks, with sessions offered two or three times per week. Control interventions included land-based exercise, treatment as usual, or home-based exercise. Because the subjects were aware of their types of treatments, blinding of subjects was impossible. As a result, all of the trials had a high risk of bias. Yet, they all had a low risk of reporting and attrition bias. "The awareness of being treated may provide a bias when compared to a control group not exposed to treatment." Still, when compared to nonexercise, the researchers found that aquatic exercise was beneficial, at least for a short period of time. Nevertheless, "studies in this area are still too few to provide further recommendations on how to apply this therapy."[1]

Aquatic Exercise and Pain Neurophysiology Education Are Better for Chronic Low Back Pain Than Aquatic Exercise Alone

In a parallel, single-blinded, randomized, controlled clinical trial published in 2015 in the journal *Clinical Rehabilitation*, researchers from Portugal wanted to determine if aquatic exercise and pain neurophysiology education were better for chronic low back pain than aquatic exercise alone. The initial cohort consisted of 62 people who were literate in Portuguese and between the ages of 18 and 65 years. Thirty subjects received both aquatic exercise and pain neurophysiology education, and 32 only participated in aquatic exercise. Aquatic exercise was held twice weekly for six weeks; there were two pain neurophysiology sessions. The subjects were assessed at baseline, six weeks after beginning the aquatic exercise program, and at a three-month follow-up. Fifty-five subjects completed the entire study. The researchers learned that the subjects in the combined program had better reductions in pain intensity, but the reductions were not statistically significant until the three-month follow-up. The researchers suggested that the education piece may help "change maladaptive pain cognitions, illness perceptions or coping strategies." Also, they concluded that "pain neurophysiology education is a clinically effective addition to aquatic exercise."[2]

Aquatic Exercise Appears to Help Obese Women with Low Back Pain

In a randomized, controlled clinical trial published in 2019 in the *Journal of Exercise Rehabilitation*, researchers from Malaysia wanted to learn if aquatic exercise would help women with obesity and low back pain. The cohort consisted of 39 women with obesity and nonspecific low back pain for more than six months; the women had yet to participate in any intervention procedures. Nineteen women were placed in an aquatic exercise groups, and 20 were in a control group; the women in both groups had similar demographic characteristics. The women in the aquatic group participated in a 12-week program held at an outdoor pool at Sultan Idris Education University. There were two weekly 60-minute aquatic exercise sessions conducted in shallow water by an aquatic exercise therapist. The subjects completed a questionnaire one day before the aquatic exercise program began and one day after the last session. On average, 92 percent of the aquatic exercise group attended the sessions. In the control group, 15 percent of the subjects had physiotherapy exercise instructions, which were completed irregularly at home. The researchers learned that the women in the aquatic exercise group experienced reductions in pain intensity. "A 12-week progressive aquatic exercise program can be more beneficial as a significant strategy to reduce pain intensity." The researchers concluded that additional studies are needed to determine the long-term effectiveness of aquatic exercises for low back pain.[3]

Physical Therapy Combined with Balneotherapy Is More Effective for Chronic Low Back Pain Than Physical Therapy Alone

In a prospective, controlled, single-blind study published in 2020 in the journal *Complementary Therapies in Medicine*, researchers from Turkey compared the short-term usefulness of physical therapy combined with balneotherapy with physical therapy alone for chronic low back pain. The initial cohort consisted of 270 subjects with chronic low back pain. They were randomly placed in a group to receive the combined therapy (n = 135) or a group to receive only physical therapy (n = 135). The three-week study included a total of 15 sessions. Assessments were conducted at baseline and the end of the study. One hundred twenty-nine subjects in the combined group and 133 subjects in the physical therapy group completed the entire study. While the subjects in both groups experienced improvements in pain, the subjects in the combined therapy group had "more pronounced improvement." Balneotherapy "may have positive contributions to reducing pain, functionality of patients, quality of life, fatigue and disability status."[4]

Aquatic Therapy Appears to Help Some People with Neck Pain

In a systematic review published in 2020 in the *International Journal of Biometeorology*, researchers from Spain investigated the use of aquatic therapy for neck pain. The researchers located 13 studies with 658 subjects that met their criteria. These included three randomized, controlled trials, two randomized studies, one single-blind, controlled study, one pilot controlled study, one pilot study, two observational retrospective studies, two prospective studies, and one not specified. The main symptoms of the subjects were neck pain, disability, cervical disc herniation, and compromised quality of life. The types of aquatic therapy varied from study to study, as did the administration of the therapy and the water temperature. Only five studies mentioned the sex of the subjects. In these, there were 42 men and 209 women. Nine of the studies concluded that aquatic therapy reduced pain, and three studies concluded that disability improved. Five studies found that functional capacity improved. However, only four of the studies could be classified as good, eight could be classified as fair, and the remaining one was weak. Nevertheless, the researchers concluded that "treatment of neck pain using different waters and techniques reduced pain and disability, and improved functional capacity, quality of life, joint mobility, balance, relaxation and mood."[5]

Aquatic Exercise May Benefit People with Parkinson's Disease

In a single-blinded, prospective, randomized, controlled trial published in 2017 in the *European Journal of Physical and Rehabilitation Medicine*, a researcher from Spain examined the ability of aquatic therapy to help people with Parkinson's disease improve pain and functioning. The cohort consisted of 30 people with Parkinson's disease from 2 Parkinson's associations in Spain. Six men and 9 women, with a mean age of 67.53 years, were assigned to receive an aquatic therapy known as aquatic Ai Chi, and seven men and eight women, with a mean age of 66.80 years, received supervised training on dry land. All of the 45-minute interventions continued for 10 weeks, with group sessions held twice weekly. The aquatic sessions were in municipal pools, and all of subjects completed the entire trial. The interventions appeared to have no adverse effects. During the trial, no medication changes were initiated. The researchers determined that more notable improvements were experienced by the subjects in the aquatic exercise group. In fact, when compared to the land therapy group, significant differences were found in baseline and one-month assessments in pain perception values. The researchers concluded that "physical exercise performed in water has positive effects" for people with Parkinson's disease. It should be considered as part of the treatment protocol by neurologists and health professionals who work in the field of neuro-rehabilitation, "as long as the necessary resources for its implementation are available."[6]

Aquatic Therapy Benefits Patients with Chronic Stroke Problems

In a study published in 2020 in the *International Journal of Environmental Research and Public Health*, the same researcher from Spain evaluated the usefulness of aquatic and land therapy for people dealing with chronic stroke problems, including perceived pain. The cohort consisted of 41 subjects with pain, depression, and quality of life issues associated with chronic stroke. They were randomly placed in an Ai Chi aquatic therapy group ($n = 13$), a land-based physiotherapy group ($n = 15$), and a combination group ($n = 13$). (Ai Chi is a water-based total body strengthening and relaxation program.) The mean age of the subjects in the three groups was the early to mid-60s. The subjects in all three groups received two 45-minute sessions of therapy each week for 12 weeks. All of the subjects completed their entire programs, and there were no adverse effects. The researcher learned that aquatic therapy improved some aspects of pain, mood, and quality of life. "Therefore, this treatment option should be considered when designing treatment protocols on behalf of neurologists and health professional working in the field of neuro-rehabilitation."[7]

Pregnant Women with Low Back Pain May Obtain a Small Benefit from Unsupervised Water Exercise

In a randomized, controlled, parallel-group trial published in 2017 in the online journal *PLoS ONE*, researchers from Denmark investigated the ability of unsupervised water exercise to help pregnant women with low back pain. The initial cohort consisted of 516 healthy pregnant women; they had a mean age of 31 years, and 86 percent had a higher education and 83 percent were exercisers. The women were assigned to participate in twice weekly water exercises for 12 weeks and standard prenatal care ($n = 258$) or standard prenatal care alone ($n = 258$). The water exercise intervention was performed between 20 and 32 gestational weeks; the exercising women were encouraged to keep a training logbook; these were distributed during an introductory session. The women had free access to several pools in Copenhagen (Denmark's capital). Data were obtained at baseline and at a follow-up; outcomes were obtained for 91 percent of the women at follow-up; 9 percent were lost to follow-up. The researchers found that the women who exercised obtained statistically significant pain relief, but the benefit was not clinically significant. Moreover, at follow-up, more women in the water exercise group, reported no low back pain. "Few women reported side effects, and only one woman withdrew from the trial as she found the exercises uncomfortable to perform."[8]

Water Immersion Seems to be Helpful During Labor and Delivery, But It May or May Not Increase the Risk of Postpartum Bleeding

In a retrospective study published in 2020 in the *Journal of Midwifery & Women's Health*, researchers from Columbus, Ohio (USA) examined the usefulness of water immersion during labor and delivery. The cohort consisted of 230 women who were primarily white, married, and college educated. Sixty-one women were in the water labor group; they labored in the water but left the tub to give birth. Fifty-eight women were in the waterbirth group; they labored and gave birth in the tub. Also, 111 women were in neither group. Outcome data from the women and newborns were obtained immediately after birth from the attending certified nurse-midwife. At the six-week postpartum visit, the women were asked to complete a 40-item satisfaction survey. The researchers learned that the women who had a water birth had a shorter second stage of labor. This shortened second stage of labor only achieved significance among multiparous women. These women also tended to have a shorter first stage of labor and a longer third stage of labor. However, it is important to note that more women in the waterbirth group had postpartum hemorrhaging, though the numbers were not clinically significant and did not result in any blood transfusions. And the waterbirth group had one instance of cord avulsion or the tearing of the umbilical cord from its insertion site on the placenta, making the delivery of the placenta more difficult. The researchers concluded that "waterbirth is a reasonable option for low-risk women and their neonates when giving birth with qualified perinatal care providers in the US hospital settings."[9]

Aquatic Exercise Is about as Effective as Land-Based Exercise for Knee Osteoarthritis

In a systematic review and meta-analysis published in 2018 in the journal *Medicine*, researchers from China compared the effectiveness of aquatic exercise to land-based exercise for knee osteoarthritis. The researchers found 8 randomized controlled trials with 579 subjects that met their criteria. The subjects were diagnosed with knee osteoarthritis based on symptoms and radiologic findings without any invasive intervention. All of the trials were published in English between 2001 and 2018, and the main outcomes that were examined included pain relief, physical function, and symptoms and quality of life improvement. The trials were conducted in Brazil, China, Finland, Denmark, Korea, Thailand, and the United States. Although blinding was impossible, 75 percent of the trials were deemed to be of high quality. For all of the outcomes assessed, the researchers found no statistically significant differences between aquatic exercise and land-based exercise over shorter or longer periods of time. Still, the researchers cautioned that "the inclusion of only a small number of studies with limited sample size precluded the ability to draw definitive conclusions."[10]

Water Immersion Seems to Have Little if Any Impact during Labor and Delivery

In a systematic review published in 2018 in the *Cochrane Database of Systematic Reviews*, which was an update of a systematic review published in 2011, researchers from the United Kingdom evaluated the use of water immersion during labor and delivery. The researchers included 15 randomized controlled trials conducted between 1990 and 2015. Eight trials involved water immersion during the first stage of labor; two were during the second stage; four were during the first and second stages; and one compared early versus late immersion during the first stage of labor. All of the trials were held in hospital settings, with varying degrees of medical intervention. The researchers learned that in healthy women at low risk of complications, there is "moderate low-quality evidence" that water immersion may reduce the use of regional analgesia or analgesia that numbs part of the body. For the second stage of labor, the evidence is limited and does not show clear differences. At the same time, labor and birth while immersed in water does not appear to increase adverse effects to the mother or baby. However, "available evidence is limited by clinical variability and heterogeneity across trials."[11]

NOTES

1. Lu, Meili, Youxin Su, Yingjie Zhang, et al. "Effectiveness of Aquatic Exercise for Treatment of Knee Osteoarthritis: Systematic Review and Meta-Analysis." *Zeitschrift für Rheumatogie* 74, no. 6 (August 2015): 543–552.

2. Pires, Diogo, Eduardo Brazete Cruz, and Carmen Caeiro. "Aquatic Exercise and Pain Neurophysiology Education versus Aquatic Exercise Alone for Patients with Chronic Low Back Pain: A Randomized Controlled Trial." *Clinical Rehabilitation* 29, no. 6 (June 2015): 538–547.

3. Abadi, Fariba Hossein, Mohansunder Sankaravel, Fairus Fariza Zainuddin, et al. "The Effect of Aquatic Exercise Program on Low-Back Pain Disability in Obese Women." *Journal of Exercise Rehabilitation* 15, no. 6 (December 31, 2019): 855–860.

4. Dilekçi, Erdal, Kağan Özkuk, and Bariş Kaki. "The Short-Term Effects of Balneotherapy on Pain, Disability and Fatigue in Patients with Chronic Low Back Pain Treated with Physical Therapy: A Randomized Controlled Trial." *Complementary Therapies in Medicine* 54 (November 2020): 102550.

5. Corvillo, Iluminada, Francisco Armijo, Antonio Álvarez-Badillo, et al. "Efficacy of Aquatic Therapy for Neck Pain: A Systematic Review." *International Journal of Biometeorology* 64, no. 6 (June 2020): 915–925.

6. Pérez de la Cruz, S. "Effectiveness of Aquatic Therapy for the Control of Pain and Increased Functionality in People with Parkinson's Disease: A Randomized Clinical Trial." *European Journal of Physical and Rehabilitation Medicine* 53 (2017): 825–832.

7. Pérez-de la Cruz, Sagrario. "Influence of an Aquatic Therapy Program on Perceived Pain, Stress, and Quality of Life in Chronic Stroke Patients: A Randomized Trial." *International Journal of Environmental Research and Public Health* 17 (2020): 4796–4807.

8. Backhausen, Mette G., Ann Tabor, Hanne Albert, et al. "The Effects of an Unspervised Water Exercise Program on Low Back Pain and Sick Leave Among Healthy Pregnant Women—A Randomised Controlled Trial." *PLoS ONE* 12, no. 9 (2017): e0182114.

9. Neiman, Emily, Elizabeth Austin, Alai Tan, et al. "Outcomes of Waterbirth in a U.S. Hospital-Based Midwifery Practice: A Retrospective Cohort Study of Water Immersion During Labor and Birth." *Journal of Midwifery & Women's Health* 65, no. 2 (March 2020): 216–223.

10. Dong, Rui, Yunyao Wu, Shibing Xu, et al. "Is Aquatic Exercise More Effective Than Land-Based Exercise for Knee Osteoarthritis?" *Medicine* (Baltimore) 97, no. 52 (2018): e13823.

11. Cluett, Elizabeth R., Ethel Burns, and Anna Cuthbert. "Immersion in Water During Labour and Birth." *Cochrane Database of Systematic Reviews* 5, no. 5 (May 16, 2018): CD000111.

REFERENCES AND FURTHER READINGS

Abadi, Fariba Hossein, Mohansundar Sankaravel, Fairus Fariza Zainuddin, et al. "The Effect of Aquatic Exercise Program on Low-Back Pain Disability in Obese Women." *Journal of Exercise Rehabilitation* 15, no. 6 (December 31, 2019): 855–860.

Backhausen, Mette G., Ann Tabor, Hanne Albert, et al. "The Effects of an Unsupervised Water Exercise Program on Low Back Pain and Sick Leave Among Healthy Pregnant Women—A Randomised Controlled Trial." *PLoS ONE* 12, no. 9 (2017): e0182114.

Cluett, Elizabeth R., Ethel Burns, and Anna Cuthbert. "Immersion in Water during Labour and Birth." *Cochrane Database of Systematic Reviews* 5, no. 5 (May 16, 2018): CD000111.

Corvilla, Iluminada, Francisco Armijo, Antonio Álvarez-Badillo, et al. "Efficacy of Aquatic Therapy for Neck Pain: A Systematic Review." *International Journal of Biometeorology* 64, no. 6 (June 2020): 915–925.

Dilekçi, Kağan Özkuk, and Bariş Kaki. "The Short-Term Effects of Balneotherapy on Pain, Disability and Fatigue in Patients with Chronic Low Back Pain Treated with Physical Therapy: A Randomized Controlled Trial." *Complementary Therapies in Medicine* 54 (November 2020): 102550.

Dong, Rui, Yunyao Wu, Shibing Xu, et al. "Is Aquatic Exercise More Effective Than Land-Based Exercise for Knee Osteoarthritis?" *Medicine* (Baltimore) 97, no. 52 (2018): e13823.

Lu, Meili, Youxin Su, Yingjie Zhang, et al. "Effectiveness of Aquatic Exercise for Treatment of Knee Osteoarthritis." *Zeitschrift für Rheumatogie* 74, no. 6 (August 2015): 543–552.

Neiman, Emily, Elizabeth Austin, Alai Tan, et al. "Outcomes of Waterbirth in a US Hospital-Based Midwifery Practice: A Retrospective Cohort Study of Water Immersion during Labor and Birth." *Journal of Midwifery & Women's Health* 65, no. 2 (March 2020): 216–223.

Pérez de la Cruz, S. "Effectiveness of Aquatic Therapy for the Control of Pain and Increased Functionality in People with Parkinson's Disease: A Randomized Clinical Trial." *European Journal of Physical and Rehabilitation Medicine* 53 (2017): 825–832.

Pérez de la Cruz, S. "Influence of an Aquatic Therapy Program on Perceived Pain, Stress, and Quality of Life in Chronic Stroke Patients:

A Randomized Trial." *International Journal of Environmental Research and Public Health* 17 (2020): 4796–4807.

Pires, Diogo, Educardo Brazete Cruz, and Carmen Caeiro. "Aquatic Exercise and Pain Neurophysiology Education Versus Aquatic Exercise Alone for Patients with Chronic Low Back Pain: A Randomized Controlled Trial." *Clinical Rehabilitation* 29, no. 6 (June 2015): 538–547.

Lidocaine, Topical

INTRODUCTION

Topical lidocaine is a local anesthetic or numbing medication. Like all anesthetics, topical lidocaine blocks nerves from sending pain signals to the brain. That is why topical lidocaine is good for a wide variety of medical needs, such as applying stitches, needle pokes, IV insertion, catheter insertion, laser treatments, open wounds, minor burns, poison ivy rash, and bug bites.

The compound that is now known as lidocaine was discovered in 1942 by two Swedish chemists, Nils Löfgren and Bengt Lundquist. A tertiary amine synthesized from xylidine, lidocaine, which was initially known as xylocaine, was clinically introduced by Dr. Torsten Gordh, the first physician in Sweden to specialize in anesthesiology. In 1943, Astra AB, a small Swedish pharmaceutical company, acquired the rights. The U.S. patent was granted in 1948, and Astra's Worcester, Massachusetts (USA), manufacturing facility opened in 1951. It was the first amide-type local anesthetic, which meant it broke down in the liver rather than the bloodstream, reducing the risk of allergic reactions. Because lidocaine had a better safety profile than the other older anesthetic agents, it rapidly gained in popularity. Lidocaine is often used with epinephrine, which acts as a vasoconstrictor and extends lidocaine's duration of action.

ADMINISTRATION AND REGULATION

Topical lidocaine is available in several different forms, such as gels, sprays, creams, lotions, ointments, liquids, swabs, solutions, powders, plasters, and skin patches. During an office visit, medical providers may administer topical lidocaine before they begin a potentially uncomfortable or painful procedure. Also, they may prescribe lidocaine for the patient to use at home.

Small amounts of lidocaine are sometimes found in over-the-counter products designed to treat pain. For example, over-the-counter pain patches may have lidocaine. Larger amounts require a prescription, but there are no special requirements. Lidocaine is not a controlled medication. Normally, health insurance should cover a lidocaine prescription, though a copayment may be required. There is no reliable way to know how often lidocaine, in its many different forms, is used.

It is important to apply topical lidocaine exactly as directed on the label or as your medical provider has indicated. Never use extra. If a dose is missed, it should be applied as soon as possible. However, if it is almost time for the next dose, skip the missed dose and resume your regular schedule. Lidocaine should be stored in a closed container at room temperature. Keep it out of reach of children and pets.

No more than three lidocaine patches should be used per day, and they should remain on the skin for no more than 12 hours. Using too many patches or leaving them on too long may cause serious side effects. Since the viscous lidocaine is a thick liquid, it should be shaken before use. Lidocaine viscous should be used as needed, but not more often than every three hours, with a maximum of eight doses in 24 hours. (Though it is not addressed in this entry, in clinical settings, injectable lidocaine may be used to control pain.)

BENEFITS AND RISKS

Since topical lidocaine blocks the signals at the nerve endings in the skin, it may be used on different parts of the body to cause numbness or a loss of feeling. It relieves pain and itching from a wide variety of medical problems. Before using on the skin, clean and dry the affected area. Apply a thin layer of medication to the area, as directed.

Lidocaine viscous topical solution is used to treat a sore mouth or throat that is often associated with chemotherapy and to reduce gagging during x-ray procedures and dental impressions. It is not normally used for sore throats related to colds and coughs. Lidocaine skin patches relieve the stabbing nerve pains or aches caused by herpes zoster or shingles. This type of pain may continue for months or years after a shingles infection. However, the lidocaine patches may also be used for other medical problems.

Lidocaine has excellent painkilling properties. For most people, it is safe and well tolerated and may be used for an extended period of time without developing a tolerance, physical dependence, or addiction.

Still, there are many potential risks. If too much lidocaine is absorbed through the skin, an overdose may occur. This has the potential to cause serious medical problems or death. Symptoms of an overdose include lightheadedness, nervousness, inappropriate happiness, confusion, dizziness, drowsiness, ringing in the ears, blurred or double vision, vomiting, feeling hot, cold or numb, twitching or shaking that is not controllable, uneven breathing, seizures, slowed breathing, coma, or respiratory failure (breathing stops). In addition, lidocaine has been associated with several side effects. These include irritation, burning, numbness, or stinging at the application site, swelling, redness, dizziness, drowsiness, confusion, blurred vision, and ringing in the ears. A more serious side effect is an allergic reaction. Symptoms of an allergic reaction include difficulty breathing, swelling of the face, lips, tongue, or throat.

Fatal overdoses have occurred when medications with lidocaine have been used without the advice of a medical professional, as during a cosmetic procedure such as laser hair removal. But, they have also happened when women were treated with topical lidocaine before a mammogram. Topical lidocaine should not be applied to areas of the skin that are swollen or on deep puncture wounds. It should not be used on skin that is raw or blistered. Never use two doses at the same time. Topical lidocaine should not be ingested; it should be used only on the skin. Also, it is important to keep topical lidocaine out of the reach of children and pets. They may be harmed by ingesting even small amounts. If such ingestion occurs, seek emergency assistance.

Lidocaine products must not come into contact with eyes. They may cause severe irritation. And, avoid touching the sticky side of a lidocaine skin patch. After removing a used lidocaine patch, fold the patch in half with the sticky sides together. On occasion, the skin under a patch may swell or burn. Don't place heat near a patch; no heating pads, electric blankets, tanning lamps, or other sources of heat. It may increase the rate of absorption into the body. Lidocaine should be used with extreme caution in children under the age of three years.

It is not recommended that lidocaine be used in combination with a long list of medications. Hence, be prepared to discuss all of your medications and supplements with your medical provider. Also, if possible, people with certain medical conditions should avoid lidocaine. These include heart problems, lung or breathing problems, large sores, liver disease, sepsis, or traumatized mucosa. Before and after using lidocaine, it is important to wash your hands with soap and water. Be careful not to get any lidocaine in your eyes. If this accidentally occurs, immediately rinse the eyes with water for at least 15 minutes.

Lidocaine has the potential to cause a rare but serious blood problem known as methemoglobinemia. More likely to occur in the elderly, infants under six months, or people with certain medical problems, symptoms of this condition are pale, gray, or blue-colored skin, lips or nails; confusion; headache; lightheadedness; rapid heartbeat; or unusual tiredness or weakness.

Lidocaine viscous may affect the ability to swallow. That is why it is important to wait at least an hour after use before eating, and when using lidocaine viscous, avoid chewing gum; you may unintentionally bite yourself.

RESEARCH FINDINGS

Lidocaine Patch Reduces the Pain Associated with Cannula and Propofol

In a randomized, double-blind, placebo-controlled trial published in 2016 in the *Korean Journal of Anesthesiology*, researchers from Korea wanted to learn if a lidocaine 5 percent patch would reduce the pain associated with the use of cannula (tubing with needle) to administer propofol, a drug used during surgical procedures to decrease the levels of consciousness and memory. The initial cohort consisted of 126 patients between the ages of 18 and 70 years who were having elective surgery. The patients were divided into three groups. The subjects in Group A had pretreatment with a lidocaine 5 percent patch before propofol; the subjects in Group B had pretreatment with a placebo patch before propofol; and the subjects in Group C had pretreatment with a placebo patch and 2 ml of 2 percent lidocaine before propofol. Pain severity was evaluated on a four-point verbal rating scale during intravenous cannulation, propofol injection, and 24 hours after the operation. Four patients were excluded from Group A, five were excluded from Group B, and four were excluded from Group C. Altogether, 113 patients were in the statistical analyses. Eighteen patients in Group A (47.4%) complained of cannula-induced pain compared with 35 (94.6%) in Group B and 36 (94.7%) in Group C. The researchers concluded that "preoperative transdermal administration of 5% lidocaine patch is an effective and simple method in reducing propofol-induced pain as well as cannula-induced pain."[1]

Lidocaine Medicated Plaster Seems to Be Clinically Useful for Postsurgical Neuropathic Pain

In a randomized, double-blind, placebo-controlled, multicenter clinical trial published in 2019 in the journal *Current Medical Research and Opinion*, researchers from Brazil, Germany, and France evaluated the ability of a 700 mg lidocaine-medicated plaster to relieve postsurgical localized neuropathic pain. The cohort consisted of 363 subjects who experienced postsurgical neuropathic pain for a minimum of 3 months and a maximum of 36 months. The trial consisted of a one-week enrollment period, a 12-week double-blind treatment period, and a follow-up visit 7 to 17 days after the trial ended. The subjects applied their lidocaine plasters ($n = 180$) or matching placebo patches ($n = 183$) once a day for 12 weeks, for no longer than 12 hours. During the trial, the subjects had four scheduled visits, about every four weeks, and they kept records of their pain intensity. One hundred forty-seven subjects in each group completed the entire trial. The researchers learned that the subjects with the lidocaine plasters had a clinically relevant reduction in pain, but it was not statistically significant. The researchers commented that "the largest differences between lidocaine and placebo were observed in patients who did not use concomitant pain medication, and in patients who had undergone surgery more than 1 year before enrollment in the trial."[2]

In a single-center, randomized, single-blind, placebo-controlled clinical trial published in 2017 in the journal *Pain Management*, researchers from Italy assessed the efficacy of topical 5 percent lidocaine-medicated plaster for the treatment of chronic post-thoracotomy neuropathic pain. Sixty-three patients received either 5 percent lidocaine medicated plasters ($n = 33$) or nonmedicated placebo plasters ($n = 30$) for 12 hours per day for eight weeks. The subjects, who were all 18 years or older, had a thoracotomy no less than three months and no more than three years from baseline. Pain intensity was recorded at baseline, at four weeks, and when the trial ended. The researchers learned that the subjects with the lidocaine medicated plasters experienced significant reductions in pain at four and eight weeks. They also had reductions in sleep disturbances and improvements in quality-of-life issues. The researchers noted that their findings "clearly demonstrated the efficacy of 5% lidocaine medicated plaster in the treatment of patients with chronic post-thoracotomy pain."[3]

Lidocaine Patches Reduce Post-Thoracotomy Pain

In a double-blind, placebo-controlled, prospective trial published in 2019 in the journal *Thoracic Cancer*, researchers from Naples, Italy wanted to learn if using a lidocaine 5 percent patch would improve the effect of systematic morphine analgesia for controlling acute post-thoracotomy pain. The focus was on studying pain during the first 72 postoperative hours. The initial cohort consisted of 90 patients. During the three days before their thoracotomy for small cell lung cancer, they used either a lidocaine 5 percent patch ($n = 45$) or a placebo ($n = 45$). The patch, which contained 700 mg of lidocaine, was applied at night for 12 hours over the planned skin incision area and removed during the 12 hours of daytime. All of the patients had the same length of skin incision and a standard muscle-sparing thoracotomy. They also had the same chest closures. Periodic assessments were conducted. The researchers learned that the subjects in the lidocaine patch group had better control of postoperative pain, less need for morphine, and a faster recovery of respiratory function. The researchers concluded that "pre-emptive skin analgesia using a lidocaine patch is a safe, quick, and simple procedure for controlling post-thoracotomy pain." Moreover, "it improves pain relief while reducing morphine requirements and morphine-related adverse effects."[4]

Application of Lidocaine Appears to Alleviate the Discomfort of the Insertion of a Nasogastric Tube

In a systematic review and meta-analysis published in 2018 in the journal *Medicine*, researchers based in Taiwan examined the ability of lidocaine to ease the pain associated with the insertion of a nasogastric tube. According to the researchers, all too often, the tube is inserted without the use of any pain relievers. The researchers located 10 randomized controlled trials with 734 subjects who met their criteria; all of the trials were of moderate to high quality. One of the trials was conducted on children. The mean age of the treatment groups was 49 years, and the mean age of the control groups was 50 years. Five of the studies were completed in Asia, two in Australia, two in the United States, and one in Israel. Six studies were in English, three were in Chinese, and one was in Korean. The researchers learned that applying lidocaine before inserting the nasogastric tube reduced levels of pain and discomfort by 26 percent. The researchers conclude that "current evidence confirms the clinical benefit of lidocaine in reducing pain associated with NG tube insertions."[5]

When Combined with Traditional Analgesics, Lidocaine Patches Do Not Appear to Offer Additional Pain Relief after Cardiac Surgery

In a single-center, retrospective cohort evaluation published in 2019 in the journal *Critical Care Nurse*, researchers from New London, Connecticut, and New Haven, Connecticut (USA), compared the use of topical lidocaine 5 percent patches and standard care (opioid and nonopioid analgesics) to standard care alone for patients having a new sternotomy or thoracotomy (types of heart surgery). The trial took place in an 18-bed adult cardiothoracic intensive care unit from January 1, 2015, to December 31, 2015. The average census of the intensive care unit was 15 patients per day. Of the 151 patients enrolled in the trial, 72 received at least one lidocaine 5 percent patch and 79 did not receive any lidocaine 5 percent patches. After exclusion criteria were applied to both groups, the final cohort had 91 patients; 47 patients were in the lidocaine and standard care group and 44 were in the standard care alone group. The primary reason for exclusion in both groups was a lack of documentation of pain ratings for more than one day after patch placement. The researchers found no significant differences between the pain ratings, length of stay in intensive care or hospital, or use of other analgesics between patients treated with the lidocaine 5 percent patches and patients treated with standard care. The researchers concluded that "adjunctive lidocaine 5% patches did not reduce acute pain in post-thoracotomy and poststernotomy patients in the cardiothoracic intensive care unit."[6]

Lidocaine Patches Are Useful for the Pain Associated with Traumatic Rib Fractures

In a randomized, double-blind trial published in 2016 in the journal *Medical Principles and Practice*, a researcher from Taiwan investigated the ability of lidocaine patches to help people dealing with traumatic isolated rib fractures. The cohort consisted of 44 trauma patients with isolated rib fractures; they had a mean age of 56.8 years. There were 23 men and 21 women, and they had between one and five rib fractures. The 27 patients in the intervention group used a Lidopat® 5 percent skin patch at the trauma site and an oral opioid/acetaminophen medication; the 17 patients in the placebo group used a placebo patch and the same oral medication. The skin patch was applied within 12 hours of admission. During the first four days of treatment, there were no significant differences in pain scores between the groups. After the fifth day, the subjects in the patch group had significantly less pain. The subjects in the patch group used significantly less medication and had significantly shorter hospital stays. Using the skin patches in patients with isolated rib fractures "alleviated pain and shortened the hospital stay, and a lower dose of pain-relieving medication was used."[7]

Lidocaine Patches Seem to Be Helpful for Pain Following a Total Knee Arthroplasty

In a retrospective, cohort study published in 2017 in the journal *MedicalExpress*, researchers from Brazil examined the usefulness of lidocaine patches for the pain associated with a total knee arthroplasty or the reconstruction or replacement of the knee. The initial cohort consisted of 48 subjects who had total knee arthroplasty. Twenty-four subjects were treated with standard analgesia and lidocaine patches with 700 mg lidocaine applied to the sides of the surgical incision, and 24 only had the standard analgesia. Forty-five subjects completed the trial; there were 22 in the intervention group and 23 in the control group. The researchers learned that postoperative pain was less intense in the subjects using the lidocaine patch as adjunctive therapy. There was a statistically significant reduction in the amount of opioid required and applied to the lidocaine treated subjects in 15 out of 25 postoperative days. Although the researchers expected that up to 16 percent of the subjects would have an adverse reaction to the patches, during the first 72 hours, there were none. On the other hand, while 4.5 percent of the patches group experienced nausea, 26 percent of the control group had nausea. This was most likely a result of their higher intake of opioid medication. The researchers concluded that "adjuvant treatment after total knee arthroplasty using lidocaine patches was effective in reducing pain and decreasing the use of opioids in the period analyzed, and represents a good addition to multimodal analgesic therapy."[8]

Lidocaine Patches Did Not Help Patients with Acute or Persistent Pain from Robotic Thoracic Surgery

In a randomized, placebo-controlled, double-blind trial published in 2015 in the journal *Pain Medicine*, researchers from Cleveland, Ohio, and Winston-Salem, North Carolina (USA), wanted to assess the ability of lidocaine 5 percent patches to treat acute pain after robotic cardiac valve surgery. In addition, they hoped to learn if the patches could prevent persistent incisional pain. The initial cohort consisted of 80 subjects who had robotic cardiac valve surgery. They were treated with 5 percent lidocaine patches or identical appearing placebo patches. The patches, which contained 700 mg of lidocaine, were applied around each incision 12 hours per day until the pain resolved or for six months. Postoperative opioid analgesia was also used. As two patients had open-heart surgery instead of robotic surgery, the analyses were conducted on 78 subjects. Although the researchers expected the patches to play a key role in pain control, they found them to be ineffective for both the acute and chronic pain that was associated with robotic cardiac valve surgery. The researchers noted that their findings were "consistent with studies showing no benefit of lidocaine patches in treating certain types of postoperative pain."[9]

Lidocaine Patches Do Not Appear to Be Useful for Acute or Postoperative Pain Management

In a systematic search and meta-analysis published in 2015 in the journal *Current Medical Research and Opinion*, researchers from China, Durham, North Carolina (USA), and Singapore investigated the use of lidocaine patches for acute pain. They located four randomized controlled trials and one prospective cohort study, with 251 subjects, which compared the use of lidocaine patches to no treatment or placebos for acute or postoperative pain management. All five studies included information on pain scores at 24 hours; there were no significant differences in pain intensity between the lidocaine and control groups. All five studies also had information on hospital stays; there were no significant differences in hospital stays between the lidocaine and control groups. Three of the studies reported on opioid use. Combined data from these studies showed no difference in opioid consumption between the groups. And in all five studies, the lidocaine patches were not associated with adverse events. The researchers concluded "that the application of a lidocaine patch may not be an effective adjunct for postoperative pain or acute pain management."[10]

Topical Lidocaine May Offer Little Help for Neuropathic Pain in Adults

In a review published in 2014 in the *Cochrane Database of Systematic Reviews*, researchers from the United Kingdom evaluated the use of topical lidocaine for neuropathic pain. They included 12 randomized, double-blind studies with 508 participants; all of the studies had a placebo or active control, and they all had a duration of at least two weeks. Six studies enrolled subjects with moderate or severe postherpetic neuralgia; the remaining studies had different or mixed neuropathic pain conditions. Four different formulations were used: 5 percent medicated patch, 5 percent cream, 5 percent gel, or 8 percent spray. Most of the studies had a crossover design, and the studies tended to be small. Study duration ranged from a single dose to 12 weeks of continuous treatment. All of the studies were considered to have a high risk of bias. Adverse effects were primarily local site reactions, and they were generally said to be mild or moderate in intensity and transient. Though the researchers noted that individual studies found topical lidocaine to be useful for pain relief, they indicated that there was no evidence from good-quality randomized controlled studies that topical lidocaine relieved neuropathic pain. Unfortunately, the quality of the studies "was generally poor by current standards." As a result, the researchers concluded that "several large ongoing studies of adequate duration, with clinically useful outcomes should provide more robust conclusions about both efficacy and harm."[11]

NOTES

1. Hong, Jung-Min, Hyeon Jeong Lee, Ah Reum Cho, et al. "Pretreatment with 5% Lidocaine Patch Reduces Cannula-Induced and Propofol-Induced Pain: A Randomized, Double-Blind, Placebo-Controlled Study." *Korean Journal of Anesthesiology* 69, no. 5 (October 2016): 468–473.

2. Palladini, Mariana, Irmgard Boesl, Simone Koenig, et al. "Lidocaine Medicated Plaster, and Additional Potent Treatment Option for Localized Post-Surgical Neuropathic Pain: Efficacy and Safety Results of

a Randomized, Placebo-Controlled Trial." *Current Medical Research and Opinion* 35, no. 5 (May 2019): 757–766.

3. Sansone, Pasquale, Maria Beatrice Passavanti, Alfonso Fiorelli, et al. "Efficacy of the Topical 5% Lidocaine Medicated Plaster in the treatment of Chronic Post-Thoracotomy Neuropathic Pain." *Pain Management* 7, no. 3 (May 2017): 189–196.

4. Fiorelli, Alfonnso, Caterina Pace, Roberto Cascone, et al. "Preventive Skin Analgesia with Lidocaine Patch for Management of Post-Thoracotomy Pain: Results of a Randomized, Double Blind, Placebo Controlled Study." *Thoracic Cancer*10 (2019): 631–641.

5. Lor, You-Chen, Pei-Ching Shih, Hsin-Hao Chen, et al. "The Application of Lidocaine to Alleviate the Discomfort of Nasogastric Tube Insertion." *Medicine* 97, no. 5 (February 2018): e9746.

6. Liu, Michael, Mabel Wai, and James Nunez. "Topical Lidocaine Patch for Postthoracotomy and Poststernotomy Pain in Cardiothoracic Intensive Care Unit Adult Patients." *Critical Care Nurse* 39, no. 5 (October 2019): 51–57.

7.Cheng, Yu-Cheng. "Lidocaine Skin Patch (Lidopat® 5%) Is Effective in the Treatment of Traumatic Rib Fractures: A Prospective Double-Blinded and Vehicle-Controlled Study." *Medical Principles and Practice* 25 (2016): 36–39.

8. Sadigursky, David, Mariana de Castro Oliveira, João Gilberto Gomes Macedo, et al. "Effectiveness of Lidocaine Patches for Pain Treatment after Total Knee Arthroplasty." *MedicalExpress* 4, no. 6 (2017): M170603.

9. Vrooman, Bruce, Leonardo Kapural, Sheryar Sarwar, et al. "Lidocaine 5% Patch for Treatment of Acute Pain after Robotic Cardiac Surgery and Prevention of Persistent Incisional Pain: A Randomized, Placebo-Controlled, Double-Blind Trial." *Pain Medicine* 16 (2015): 1610–1621.

10. Bai, Yaowu, Timothy Miller, Mingjuan Tan, et al. "Lidocaine Patch for Acute Pain Management: A Meta-Analysis of Prospective Controlled Trials." *Current Medical Research and Opinion* 31, no. 3 (March 2015): 575–581.

11. Derry, Sheena, Philip J. Wiffen, R. Andrew Moore, et al. "Topical Lidocaine for Neuropathic Pain in Adults." *Cochrane Database of Systematic Reviews* 7 (2014): CD010958.

REFERENCES AND FURTHER READINGS

Bai, Yaowu, Timothy Miller, Mingjuan Tan, et al. "Lidocaine Patch for Acute Pain Management: A Meta-Analysis of Prospective Controlled Trials." *Current Medical Research and Opinion* 31, no. 3 (March 2015): 575–581.

Cheng, Yu-Jen. "Lidocaine Skin Patch (Lidopat® 5%) Is Effective in the treatment of Traumatic Rib Fractures: A Prospective Double-Blinded and Vehicle-Controlled Study." *Medical Principles and Practice* 25 (2016): 36–39.

Derry, Sheena, Philip J. Wiffen, R. Andrew Moore, et al. "*Topical* Lidocaine for Neuropathic Pain in Adults." *Cochrane Database of Systematic Reviews* 7 (July 2014): CD010958.

Fiorelli, Alfonso, Caterina Pace, Roberto Cascone, et al. "Preventive Skin Analgesia with Lidocaine Patch for Management of Post-Thoracotomy Pain: Results of a Randomized, Double-Blind, Placebo Controlled Study." *Thoracic Cancer* 10 (2019): 631–641.

Hong, Jung-Min, Hyeon Jeong Lee, Ah Reum Cho, et al. "Pretreatment with 5% Lidocaine Patch Reduces Cannula-Induced and Propofol-Induced Pain: A Randomized, Double-Blind, Placebo-Controlled Study." *Korean Journal of Anesthesiology* 69, no. 5 (October 2016): 468–473.

Liu, Michael, Mabel Wai, and James Nunez. "Topical Lidocaine Patch for Postthoracotomy and Poststernotomy Pain in Cardiothoracic Intensive Care Unit Adult Patients." *Critical Care Nurse* 39, no. 5 (October 2019): 51–57.

Lor, You-Chen, Pei-Ching Shih, Hsin-Hao Chen, et al. "The Application of Lidocaine to Alleviate the Discomfort of Nasogastric Tube Insertion: A Systematic Review and Meta-Analysis." *Medicine* 97, no. 5 (February 2018): e9746.

Palladini, Mariana, Irmgard Boesl, Simone Koenig, et al. "Lidocaine Medicated Plaster, an Additional Potent Treatment Option for Localized Post-Surgical Neuropathic Pain: Efficacy and Safety Results of a Randomized, Placebo-Controlled Trial." *Current Medical Research and Opinion* 35, no. 5 (May 2019): 757–766.

Sadigursky, D., Mariana de Castro Oliveira, João Gilberto Gomes Macedo, et al. "Effectiveness of Lidocaine Patches for Pain Treatment after Total Knee Arthroplasty." *MedicalExpress* 4, no. 6 (2017): M170603.

Sansone, Pasquale, Maria Beatrice Passavanti, Alfonso Fiorelli, et al. "Efficacy of the Topical 5% Lidocaine Medicated Plaster in the Treatment of Chronic Post-Thoracotomy Neuropathic Pain." *Pain Management* 7, no. 3 (May 2017): 189–196.

Vrooman, Bruce, Leonardo Kapural, Sheryar Sarwar, et al. "Lidocaine 5% Patch for Treatment of Acute Pain after Robotic Cardiac Surgery and Prevention of Persistent Incisional Pain: A Randomized, Placebo-Controlled, Double-Blind Trial." *Pain Medicine* 16 (2015): 1610–1621.

Massage Therapy

INTRODUCTION

Massage therapy, which has been used for thousands of years and dates back to the ancient writings in China, Japan, India, Egypt, and Greece, encompasses several different techniques. It is considered one of the earliest tools that people used to relieve pain. Massage therapists usually use their hands, fingers, forearms, or elbows to manipulate therapeutically the muscles and soft tissues of the body. In some instances, they may use their feet or mechanical tools applied to the body's surfaces.

During the renaissance in Europe, massage was widely used. It was introduced to the United States during the 1850s by two American physicians who had studied in Sweden. Though it fell out of favor in the 1930s and 1940s, massage was reintroduced in the 1970s. It appeared to be particularly popular among athletes.

There are several different types of massage. With Swedish massage, which is the most common type, the massage therapist uses long strokes, kneading, deep circular movements, vibration, and tapping. Similar to Swedish massage, sports massage focuses on the specific needs and areas of concern for each athlete. Deep-tissue massage and trigger point massage direct attention to myofascial trigger points or muscle knots. In hot stone massage, the therapist places smooth heated stones on the back, as the subject lies on his or her stomach. The hot stones send soothing heat to the muscles and tissues. However, the therapist may also use cold stones, which may be useful for exercise-related injuries or swelling. Still another form of massage therapy is reflexology. It is based on the belief that pressure on particular areas of the hands and feet will trigger healing in other parts of the body.

According to the American Massage Therapy Association, in 2005, massage therapy was projected to be a \$6 to \$ 11 billion annual industry. However, in 2018, it was already a \$18 billion annual industry. Between

July 2017 and July 2018, roughly 47.5 to 63.6 million adult Americans, or 19 to 28 percent, had at least one massage.[1]

ADMINISTRATION AND REGULATION

As might be expected, massage therapists work in a wide variety of settings, including private offices, hospitals, clinics, rehabilitation and nursing facilities, and sports, beauty salons, spas, and fitness centers. Some massage therapists travel to the homes and offices of clients, but that convenience often means a higher fee. Massage therapists try to create a calming, relaxing atmosphere.

A typical first session will begin with a health assessment. Clients will be asked about symptoms, medical history, and desired results. Subsequent sessions will start with a brief health updates. Normally, clients lie on a massage table in loose-fitting clothing or undressed and covered with a sheet or blanket. Sometimes, massage is administered while a client sits in a massage chair. Massage tables and chairs have special headrests. An oil or lotion is normally used to reduce skin friction. Sessions may be relatively brief, especially those in a chair, or last for an hour or more. In the United States, the average cost of a one-hour massage is $75. Of course, that figure varies according to the location of the massage. It is more costly in the big, expensive cities and their surrounding suburbs and less costly in less expensive cities, suburbs, and rural areas.

Most people, especially those with an acute or chronic problem, would probably love to have a massage every week or two. However, because of costs or time commitments, that is often not possible. Many people do give massage therapy gift certificates as presents for a variety of special events and holidays.

There are about 1,500 massage therapy schools and training programs in the United States. The training includes massage techniques as well as information about the body, business practices, and ethics. These programs are usually approved by the state boards, and some may be accredited by independent agencies, such as the Commission on Massage Therapy Accreditation. Almost all of the states and the District of Columbia have laws that regulate the practice of massage therapy. The National Certification Board for Therapeutic Massage and Bodywork certifies practitioners who pass a national examination. States that license massage therapists tend to require them to have at least 500 hours of training at an accredited institution, pass a national exam, meet certain educational requirements, and have malpractice insurance.

BENEFITS AND RISKS

In addition to helping to reduce pain, especially low back pain, neck and shoulder pain, hand pain, and knee pain, massage therapy seems to be useful for sports injuries, stress, relaxation, arthritis, osteoarthritis of the knee, reducing pain and stiffness, improving range of motion in joints, promoting restful sleep, headaches, anxiety, depression, and general health. When administered by a trained massage professional, massage therapy appears to have few risks. Still, there are a few potential side effects, such as temporary pain or discomfort, bruising, swelling, and an allergic reaction to the massage lotion or oil. People with bleeding disorders should be sure to mention their condition before a massage begins. Massage therapists should avoid any part of the body with blood clots, fractures, wounds, open sores, weakened bones, or skin infections. Cancer patients and pregnant women may want to check with their medical providers before having massages.

RESEARCH FINDINGS

Massage Therapy May Have a Short-Term Benefit for People with Common Musculoskeletal Disorders

In a systematic review published in 2015 in the *Journal of Physiotherapy*, researchers from the Netherlands examined the usefulness of massage therapy for people with musculoskeletal disorders. The most affected areas of the body are the lower back, neck, shoulders, and the knees. The researchers located 26 randomized trials that met their criteria; these trials had a total of 2,565 participants. Sample sizes ranged from 16 to 579 people; 10 studies were considered to be at low risk for bias. Eight studies included subjects with chronic low back pain. Other studies included people with shoulder pain, fibromyalgia, osteoarthritis of the knee, chronic musculoskeletal pain, neck pain or chronic patellar tendinopathy ("jumper's knee"), carpal tunnel syndrome, hand pain, and hand osteoarthritis. The studies included a broad variety of massage techniques, durations, and frequencies. When compared to no treatment, the researchers found that massage therapy had low to moderate benefit levels. And they noted that massage therapy may be "a viable treatment option for several musculoskeletal disorders."

These improvements were generally seen immediately after treatments. The researchers commented that "the results—especially the ones where massage is compared to no treatment—are clinically relevant, mainly in people with low back pain, shoulder pain, or osteoarthritis of the knee."[2]

Massage Therapy May or May Not Be Useful for People with Osteoarthritis or Rheumatoid Arthritis

In a systematic review published in 2017 in the *American Journal of Physical Medicine & Rehabilitation*, researchers from Jacksonville, Florida (USA), wanted to learn more about the effects of massage therapy as a stand-alone therapy for people with osteoarthritis or rheumatoid arthritis. According to the researchers, arthritis and chronic joint stiffness are very common problems affecting more than 50 million people in the United States. The review consisted of seven randomized, controlled trials, which were published between 1997 and 2015; they represented 352 participants who satisfied the inclusion criteria. Four of the seven studies were from the same research group, the Touch Research Institute. Sample sizes ranged from 20 to 125 people, and the length of the massage therapy interventions ranged from 4 to 12 weeks. One study included only females. The areas massaged were described as the whole body, the neck, the wrist and hand, and the knee. Also, there was a high level of heterogeneity across all of the studies with regard to patient population structures treated, type of massage therapy, and reported outcomes. However, only two of the studies were deemed high quality, and all but two studies had a high risk of bias. The researchers found "limited evidence" that massage therapy alone was more effective than nonactive controls in reducing pain and improving function in people with arthritis. At the same time, massage therapy was well tolerated; there was only one report of an adverse effect. The researchers concluded that they were unable to determine if massage therapy is more effective than other forms of treatment. "There is a need for large, methodologically rigorous randomized controlled trials investigating the effectiveness of massage therapy as an intervention for individuals with arthritis."[3]

Massage Therapy May Provide Some Relief to People with Fibromyalgia

In a systematic review and meta-analysis published in the online journal *PLoS ONE*, researchers based in China wanted to learn more about the use of massage therapy for the symptoms associated with fibromyalgia, such as pain, anxiety, depression, and sleep disturbances. Nine randomized, controlled trials with 404 subjects met the inclusion criteria. They were conducted in China, Spain, Sweden, Turkey, and the United States. Sample sizes ranged from 19 to 90 subjects. Massage therapy sessions ranged from 25 to 90 minutes, and total sessions ranged from one to 20. The researchers found that massage therapy sessions that continued for five weeks significantly reduced pain as well as anxiety and depression. The researchers concluded that massage therapy "should be one of the viable complementary and alternative treatments for FM."[4]

Massage Therapy May Be Beneficial for People Dealing with Cancer-Related Pain

In a systematic review and meta-analysis published in 2016 in the journal *Pain Medicine*, researchers based in Alexandria, Virginia (USA), wanted to learn if massage therapy would help the pain associated with cancer. Researchers have found that more than 50 percent of people undergoing cancer treatments experience pain, and up to 90 percent of people with advanced cancer have pain. The researchers located 12 high-quality and four low-quality studies that met their requirements. Treatment doses varied from one single 10-minute session to 15 daily 45-minute sessions over a three-week period of time. In the 16 studies, 31.5 percent were male, and 68.5 percent were female; there was a mean age of 57.2 years. The researchers determined that massage therapy was "relatively" safe and had infrequent adverse events. And, it appeared to be more useful than other active treatments for reducing pain intensity and severity. The researchers concluded that "patients should consider massage therapy as a therapeutic option to help manage their cancer pain."[5]

In another systematic review and meta-analysis published in 2015 in the journal *Integrative Cancer Therapies*, researchers from Korea also investigated the association between massage therapy and cancer-related pain relief. The researchers included 12 randomized and nonrandomized controlled trials with 559 subjects in their analysis. Each study had an intervention and control, and the subjects had different types of cancer. The studies, which were conducted in the United States, South Korea, Taiwan, and the United Kingdom, had a mean duration time of 23.6 days. Sessions ranged from 10 to 50 minutes; the subjects had between one and 12 sessions. When compared to no treatment or conventional care, the researchers learned that massage therapy was effective in reducing pain in people with the various types of cancer. In three studies, it was especially useful for pain after surgery. Interestingly, foot reflexology appeared to be the most effective type of massage. The researchers noted that they "found that massage therapy has significant positive effects for cancer pain relief, particularly for the short-term."[6]

Massage Therapy May Be Useful for Postsurgery Pain

In a systematic review and meta-analysis published in 2017 in the journal *Pain Management Nursing*, researchers from Japan assessed the ability of massage therapy to help with postoperative pain or anxiety. The researchers located ten randomized controlled trials that met their criteria; they included 1,157 subjects who had undergone cardiac, thoracic, colorectal, gynecologic, and vitrectomy (eye) surgery. The mean age range of the subjects was between 54 and 68 years. All of the trials included control groups; the subjects in the control groups received routine care or routine care plus social visits or rest time. Studies were completed in the United States, the United Kingdom, Australia, and Japan. Most of the trials used Swedish massage, and the massages were administered by a massage therapist. In a few trials, nurses completed the massages. The massages continued for 10, 20, or 45 minutes and were given once or twice daily until discharge or twice daily for seven days. While the researchers found that massage therapy was useful for postoperative pain, the effects were not long-lasting. Nevertheless, the researchers suggested that massage therapy could be part of a "multimodal pain management regimen" for postoperative patients. Furthermore, they concluded that "nurses hold an important role in introducing and maintaining the massage therapy program because collaborative work is necessary for its success."[7]

Massage Therapy May or May Not Be Useful for Arthritis of the Knee

In a trial published in 2015 in the journal *Complementary Therapies in Clinical Practice*, researchers based in Miami, Florida (USA), investigated the use of massage therapy for knee arthritis pain. They recruited 48 medical school staff and faculty members, with an average age of 47 years, who had physician-diagnosed knee arthritis pain. They were then randomly placed into a massage group or waitlist control group; each group had 24 subjects. The subjects in the massage group were massaged by a licensed massage therapist once per week for four weeks; each massage lasted a total of 30 minutes. The massages involved moderate pressure, moving the skin on the quadriceps, the hamstrings, and the tendons and ligaments surrounding the patella. Twenty-three women in the massage group and 17 in the control group completed the trial. The women in the massage group had an immediate post-massage improvement in range of motion and a decrease in range of motion-associated pain. By the end of the trial, the massage group had greater increases in range of motion and decreases in range of motion pain as well as less self-reported pain and sleep disturbances than the control group. The researchers concluded that "these data highlight the effectiveness of moderate pressure massage therapy" for the problems associated with knee arthritis.[8]

In a blind, randomized, controlled pilot trial published in 2014 in the *Journal of Back and Musculoskeletal Rehabilitation*, researchers based in Spain assessed the effectiveness of massage therapy as a co-adjuvant treatment for osteoarthritis of the knee. The initial cohort consisted of 18 women, between the ages of 67 and 91 years, who were diagnosed with osteoarthritis of the knee. They were placed in one of two groups. For six weeks, the women in group A were treated with massage therapy and participated in a lower limb exercise program; the women in group B only had the lower limb exercise program. Seventeen women completed the trial. The researchers learned the outcomes between the two groups were not significantly different; the women who received massage therapy did not have significantly better outcomes. Although the researchers acknowledged that their sample size was quite small, they nevertheless concluded that "the incorporation of massage to the exercise program is not relevant in the treatment of KOA [osteoarthritis of the knee]."[9]

Massage May Help People Who Participate in Strenuous Exercise

In a systematic review and meta-analysis published in 2017 in the journal *Frontiers in Physiology*, researchers from China and Australia wanted to learn more about the ability of massage therapy to help people who participate in strenuous exercise. The researchers found 11 randomized, controlled trials with 504 participants that met their criteria. The trials were conducted in the United States, China, Canada, India, and Iran. Nine trials had a low risk of bias. When compared to no intervention, the subjects who received massage intervention following strenuous exercise had significant reductions in muscle soreness and improved muscle performance recovery. In addition, massages lowered levels of creatine kinase (CK), a marker of inflammation and skeletal muscle damage. Interestingly, "the highest efficacy was achieved at 48 h [hours] post-exercise."[10]

Massage Appears to Be Useful for Ankylosing Spondylitis, a Progressive Inflammatory Rheumatic Disease

In a randomized, clinical pilot trial published in 2017 in the journal *Evidence-Based Complementary and Alternative Medicine*, researchers from Poland and the Czech Republic compared the effectiveness of deep-tissue massage and therapeutic massage for the management of ankylosing spondylitis. Thirty-one male rheumatology patients with ankylosing spondylitis were placed in either the deep-tissue massage group or the therapeutic massage group. All of the subjects had 30-minute massage sessions daily for two weeks—a total of 10 sessions. Twenty-seven men completed the trial. The researchers found that both types of massage provider pain relief to the men. Still, "the lack of a control group with no massage in the present study does not allow us to make the conclusions on the usefulness of any kind of massage for AS patients as a self-care for pain relief."[11]

Massage Therapy May Be Useful for Hypertrophic Burn Scars

In a systematic review published in 2018 in the journal *Burns*, researchers from Australia wanted to evaluate the efficacy of massage for hypertrophic burn scars. They located eight studies with 258 human subjects and 15 animal studies that met their criteria. Five of the studies were randomized, controlled trials. The studies were conducted on outpatients and inpatients; five had adults, two had children, and one had rodents. The mean age of the adults was 40.4 years, and the mean age of the children was 7.2 years. All of the studies were single center. The mean time since the initial injury was 143 days, with one study including subjects more than two years after the injury. There were variations in treatment protocols, massage techniques, time to intervention commencement, frequency of massages, and the inconsistent use of outcome measures. The majority of the studies were rated low to medium quality. Still, the researchers determined that massage was beneficial for a number of symptoms associated with burn scars including pain. However, they underscored the need for more research. "Further controlled, clinical trials using valid and standardized outcome measures are required to investigate the important variables outlined above and to develop evidence-based guidelines for the use of massage in the management of hypertrophic scars after burn."[12]

Massage Therapy May Have a Slight Edge over Physical Therapy for Low Back Pain

In a trial published in 2014 in the *Journal of Back and Musculoskeletal Rehabilitation*, researchers from Iran compared the ability of massage therapy and physical therapy to relieve low back pain, a very common medical problem. The cohort consisted of 30 volunteer female subjects, between the ages of 20 and 55 years, with subacute or chronic nonspecific low back pain. They were randomly placed in a massage therapy or routine physical therapy group. The massage therapy group received deep stroking, pulling, friction, rolling, and wringing. The subjects in this group received ten 15-minute massage sessions. Sessions were followed by muscle stretching and stabilizing exercises. The subjects in the routine physical therapy group received ten sessions of a variety of modalities, such as deep tissue heating, TENS, and vibrators, as well as exercises. The subjects in both groups experienced improvements in pain. "However, massage was more effective than other electrotherapy modalities, and it can be used alone or with electrotherapy for the treatment of patients with low back pain."[13]

NOTES

1. American Massage Therapy website. www.amtamassage.org.

2. Bervoets, D. D., P. A. Luijsterburg, J. J. Alessie, et al. "Massage Therapy Has Short-Term Benefits for People with Common Musculoskeletal Disorders Compared to No Treatment: A Systematic Review." *Journal of Physiotherapy* 61, no. 3 (July 2015): 106–116.

3. Nelson, N. L., and J. R. Churilla. "Massage Therapy for Pain and Function in Patients with Arthritis: A Systematic Review of Randomized Controlled Trials." *American Journal of Physical Medicine & Rehabilitation* 96, no. 9 (September 2017): 665–672.

4. Li, Y-H., F-Y. Wang, C-Q. Feng, et al. "Massage Therapy for Fibromyalgia: A Systematic Review and Meta-Analysis of Randomized Controlled Trials." *PLoS ONE* 9, no. 2 (2014): e89304.

5. Boyd, Courtney, Cindy Crawford, Charmagne F. Paat, et al. "The Impact of Massage Therapy on Function in Pain Populations—A

Systematic Review and Meta-Analysis of Randomized Controlled Trials: Part II, Cancer Pain Populations." *Pain Medicine* 17 (2016): 1553–1568.

6. Lee, S. H., J. Y. Kim, S. Yeo, et al. "Meta-Analysis of Massage Therapy on Cancer Pain." *Integrative Cancer Therapies* 14, no. 4 (July 2015): 297–304.

7. Kukimoto, Yukiko, Noriko Ooe, and Norio Ideguchi. "The Effects of Massage Therapy on Pain and Anxiety after Surgery: A Systematic Review and Meta-Analysis." *Pain Management Nursing* 18, no. 6 (December 2017): 378–390.

8. Field, Tiffany, Miguel Diego, Gladys Gonzalez, and C. G. Funk. "Knee Arthritis Pain is Reduced and Range of Motion Is Increased Following Moderate Pressure Massage Therapy." *Complementary Therapies in Clinical Practice* 21 (2015): 233–237.

9. Cortés Godoy, Virginia, Tomás Gallego Izquierdo, Irene Lázaro Navas, and Daniel Pecos Martín. "Effectiveness of Massage Therapy as Co-Adjuvant Treatment to Exercise in Osteoarthritis of the Knee: A Randomized Control Trial." *Journal of Back and Musculoskeletal Rehabilitation* 27, no. 4 (2014): 521–529.

10. Guo, Jianmin, Linjin Li, Yuxiang Gong, et al. "Massage Alleviates Delayed Onset Muscle Soreness After Strenuous Exercise: A Systematic Review and Meta-Analysis." *Frontiers in Physiology* 8 (September 2017): Article 747.

11. Romanowski, Mateusz Wojciech, Maja Špiritovi, Radoslaw Rutkowski, et al. "Comparison of Deep Tissue Massage and Therapeutic Massage for Lower Back Pain, Disease Activity, and Functional Capacity of Ankylosing Spondylitis Patients: A Randomized Clinical Pilot Study." *Evidence-Based Complementary and Alternative Medicine* 2017 (2017): Article ID 9894128.

12. Ault, P., A. Plaza, and J. Paratz. "Scar Massage for Hypertropic Burns Scarring—A Systematic Review." *Burns* 44 (2018): 24–38.

13 Kamali, Fahimeh, Fatemeh Panahi, Samaneh Ebrahimi, and Leila Abbasi. "Comparison Between Massage and Routine Physical therapy in Women with Sub Acute and Chronic Nonspecific Low Back Pain." *Journal of Back and Musculoskeletal Rehabilitation* 27 (2014): 475–480.

REFERENCES AND FURTHER READINGS

Ault, P., A. Plaza, and J. Paratz. "Scar Massage for Hypertonic Burns Scarring—A Systematic Review." *Burns* 44 (2018): 24–38.

Bervoets, D. C., P. A. Luijsterburg, J. J. Alessie, et al. "Massage Therapy Has Short-Term Benefits for People with Common Musculoskeletal Disorders Compared to No Treatment: A Systematic Review." *Journal of Physiotherapy* 61, no. 3 (July 2015): 106–116.

Boyd, Courtney, Cindy Crawford, Charmagne F. Paat, et al. "The Impact of Massage Therapy on Function in Pain Populations—A Systematic Review and Meta-Analysis of Randomized Controlled Trials: Part II, Cancer Pain Populations." *Pain Medicine* 17 (2016): 1553–1568.

Cortés Godoy, Virginia, Tomás Gallego Izquierdo, Irene Lázaro Navas, and Daniel Pecos Martín. "Effectiveness of Massage Therapy as Co-Adjuvant Treatment to Exercise in Osteoarthritis of the Knee: A Randomized Controlled Trial." *Journal of Back and Musculoskeletal Rehabilitation* 27 (2014): 521–529.

Field, Tiffany, Miguel Diego, Gladys Gonzalez, and C. G. Funk. "Knee Arthritis Pain is Reduced and Range of Motion Is Increased Following Moderate Pressure Massage Therapy." *Complementary Therapies in Clinical Practice* 21 (2015): 233–237.

Guo, Jianmin, Linjin Li, Yuxiang Gong, et al. "Massage Alleviates Delayed Onset Muscle Soreness After Strenuous Exercise: A Systematic Review and Meta-Analysis." *Frontiers in Physiology* 8 (September 2017): Article 747.

Kamali, Fahimeh, Fatemeh Panahi, Samaneh Ebrahimi, and Leila Abbasi. "Comparison between Massage and Routine Physical Therapy in Women with Sub Acute and Chronic Nonspecific Low Back Pain." *Journal of Back and Musculoskeletal Rehabilitation* 27 (2014): 475–480.

Kukimoto, Yukiko, Noriko Ooe, and Norio Ideguchi. "The Effects of Massage Therapy on Pain and Anxiety after Surgery: A Systematic Review and Meta-Analysis." *Pain Management Nursing* 18, no. 6 (December 2017): 378–390.

Lee, S. H., J. Y. Kim, S. Yeo, et al. "Meta-Analysis of Massage Therapy on Cancer." *Integrative Cancer Therapies* 14, no. 4 (July 2014): 297–304.

Li, Y-H., F-Y. Wang, C-Q. Feng, et al. "Massage Therapy for Fibromyalgia: A Systematic review and Meta-Analysis of Randomized Controlled Trials." *PLoS ONE* 9, no. 2 (2014): e89304.

Nelson, Nicole L., and James R. Churilla. "Massage Therapy for Pain and Function in Patients with Arthritis." *American Journal of Physical Medicine & Rehabilitation* 96, no. 9 (September 2017): 665–672.

Romanowski, Mateusz Wojciech, Maja Špiritovi, Radoslaw Rutkowski, et al. "Comparison of Deep Tissue Massage and Therapeutic Massage for Lower Back Pain, Disease Activity, and Functional Capacity of Ankylosing Spondylitis Patients: A Randomized Clinical Pilot Study." *Evidence-Based Complementary and Alternative Medicine* 2017 (2017): Article ID 9894128.

Meditation

INTRODUCTION

Meditation is a set of techniques that are designed to improve focus and foster a heightened state of attentiveness. During meditation, people are encouraged to learn to appreciate their feelings without judgment.

A truly ancient tradition, meditation has been practiced in cultures throughout the world. Although it has ties to various religious practices and teachings, meditation is less about faith and more about altering consciousness, finding awareness, and achieving peace. During meditation, people direct their attention and eliminate the endless number of thoughts that crowd the mind. It is believed that this process enhances physical and emotional well-being.

There are several different types of meditation. All of them involve a quiet location with few distractions, a specific, comfortable posture, a focus of attention, and an open attitude. Probably the best-known type of meditation is mindfulness meditation, which originates from Buddhist teachings. With this type of meditation, people pay attention to their thoughts and observe any patterns. Combining concentration and awareness, people focus on an object or their breath, as well as bodily sensations, thoughts, or feelings. This type of meditation is easily practiced alone. The vast majority of studies on pain and meditation deal with mindfulness meditation.

Spiritual meditation is similar to prayer. People who practice this type of meditation, which is often accompanied by essential oils, seek a stronger connection to God or the universe. Spiritual meditation may be practiced at home or in a house of worship or any place one wishes. Another type of meditation, known as focused meditation, involves using any of the five senses to concentrate. Beginners may find it difficult to focus for longer than a few minutes, but it is important to keep refocusing. For example, people may focus on their breath or stare at a candle flame.

Movement meditation consists of gentle forms of moving such as walking in the woods and gardening. It is best for people who prefer to keep moving while their minds wander. With mantra meditation, people clear their minds by repeating a word, phrase, or sound. The continuous repetition enables people to reach deeper levels of consciousness. Similar to mantra meditation, with transcendental meditation, people repeat a specific word or set of words. This type of meditation has a calming effect and appeals to people who gravitate toward more structure.

Progressive relaxation involves slowly tightening and relaxing one muscle group at a time throughout the body. This is a good bedtime stress reliever. Loving-kindness meditation focuses on accepting oneself and others and giving and receiving love. It should be particularly useful for people with feelings of anger or resentment. With visualization meditation, which is also known as guided meditation, people mentally form positive images or think of situations they find relaxing, peaceful, and calming. Using all five senses, they must view the images in as much detail as possible.

There is no way to know how many people practice meditation. However, one can safely assume that it is a relatively common practice, and millions of Americans meditate.

ADMINISTRATION AND REGULATION

Although there are many types of meditation classes, and some people prefer individual meditation instruction, it is also possible to meditate alone at home. Meditation is simple and easy and does not require any special equipment; meditation should be practiced in a quiet, relaxed setting, without any phones. It is best to begin with 5 or 10 minutes of meditation and slowly increase the amount. Many people try different types of meditation until they find one or a combination of types that meet their individual needs. Periods of trial and error are not uncommon. Some people carve out a specific time of the day to meditate, such as the first thing in the morning. Others break up their days with shorter periods of meditation. One can easily meditate at home for no cost. Attending a group session at a local community center or house of worship should be very inexpensive. However, a private meditation instructor may be fairly pricey.

There are no national meditation regulations or guidelines, and there is no generally recognized certification, although that may vary by individual location. People who wish to become certified in mediation should check the requirements of their state and locality, as well as the credibility of the educational facility offering instruction.

BENEFITS AND RISKS

Meditation is thought to be useful for a wide variety of medical problems, particularly those that are exacerbated by stress. In addition to improving pain, especially chronic pain, meditation may lower blood pressure, relieve tension headaches, reduce anxiety, ease symptoms of depression, and improve sleep.

However, meditation is not a universal panacea for everyone. In some instances, it may increase pain and anxiety. Some people are uncomfortable with the hypersensitivity that meditation may trigger. In addition, there have been reports of increases in anxiety and depression, panic attacks, physical pain, and dizziness. Furthermore, mediation is never a replacement for traditional medical treatment.

RESEARCH FINDINGS

Both Group-Based Mindfulness-Based Stress Reduction and Cognitive Behavior Therapy Appear to Be Useful for Chronic Pain

In a systematic review and network meta-analysis published in 2019 in the journal *Evidence-Based Mental Health*, researchers from Canada examined the effectiveness of group-based, mindfulness-based stress reduction and cognitive behavioral therapy for chronic pain. The researchers located 21 studies that met their criteria. Seven of the studies (n = 545) compared mindfulness-based stress reduction to a control; 13 of the studies (n = 1095) compared cognitive behavioral therapy to a control; and one study examined mindfulness-based stress reduction to cognitive behavior therapy and both of these methods (n = 341) to a control. Eighty-one percent of the studies reported that 60 percent or more of their subjects were women, with an average age between 35 and 65 years old. Though 12 studies provided no information on ethnicity, 9 noted that more than 60 percent of their participants were Caucasian. Twelve of the studies were believed to be of fair or good quality. Most of the studies focused on musculoskeletal pain, and nine addressed fibromyalgia. Eight studies dealt with pain duration of more than 10 years; nine studies had pain duration from 3 to 9 years. The researchers found that, when compared to controls, both mindfulness-based stress reduction and cognitive behavioral therapy provided pain relief. Still, the researchers emphasized that the number of mindfulness-based stress-reduction studies was relatively small. The researchers concluded that mindfulness-based stress reduction demonstrated "promise in improving pain severity and reducing pain interference and psychological distress."[1]

Used Together, Mindfulness Meditation and Cognitive Behavioral Therapy Appear to Help People with Chronic Low Back Pain

In a parallel-arm, randomized, controlled pilot trial published in 2016 in the journal *Pain Medicine*, researchers from Wisconsin and Utah (USA) assessed the ability of mindfulness meditation and cognitive behavioral therapy to provide relief to people dealing with chronic low back pain. The cohort consisted of 35 subjects who had been taking at least 30 mg per day of morphine-equivalent medication for chronic low back pain for a minimum of three months. Eighty percent were women; the average age of the subjects was 51.8 years. About one-third were unemployed, and the majority were receiving disability related payments from the Social Security Administration. Despite taking higher doses of medication, they had profound levels of persistent pain. Twenty-one subjects were placed in the intervention group, and 14 served as controls. The subjects in the intervention group received eight weekly group two-hour training sessions of meditation and cognitive behavioral therapy by two experienced psychologists. The subjects were told to meditate at home 30 minutes per day, six days per week. All of the subjects were provided their usual care and opioid therapy management. Outcome results were obtained at baseline; at week 8, when the trial ended; and during a week 26 follow-up. The researchers determined that the combination of meditation and cognitive behavioral therapy was an effective addition to the subjects' treatment, and it significantly reduced levels of pain severity. And, as might be expected, the subjects who consistently practiced more obtained better benefits. The researchers concluded that "mindfulness meditation and CBT [cognitive behavioral therapy]-based interventions have the potential to safely reduce pain severity and sensitivity in patients with opioid-treated CLBP [chronic low back pain]."[2]

Mindfulness Meditation Seems to Offer Modest Relief for Chronic Pain

In a randomized, controlled clinical trial published in 2015 in *Pain Medicine*, researchers from a pain center in Copenhagen, Denmark, investigated the effects of mindfulness meditation on chronic pain. The cohort consisted of 109 subjects with nonspecific chronic pain. Physicians who specialized in treating pain diagnosed the subjects, and the subjects all received standard care at the pain clinic before, during, and after the intervention. The subjects were placed in one of three treatment groups or one of three control (waitlist) groups. Baseline demographic information was collected from the subjects' medical records. During an eight-week period of time, the subjects participating in the intervention attended weekly group meetings and spent 45 minutes per day meditating at home. They also completed questionnaires. A follow-up session was held after the trial ended. (The waitlist subjects were subsequently offered the mindfulness treatments.) Eleven subjects dropped out of the intervention groups, and eight left the waitlist groups, resulting in an overall completion rate of 82 percent. At least two of the subjects experienced temporary strong feelings of anger toward their pain, and at least two had increased anxiety. The researchers learned that practicing mindfulness meditation led to small improvements in pain, but these did not reach statistical significance. Still, the researchers noted that some subjects used less pain medication during the trial. "It is noteworthy that both pain scales showed less pain at the 6-month follow-up."[3]

There May Be Insufficient Evidence to Know if Mindfulness Meditation Is Useful for Chronic Pain

In a systematic review and meta-analysis published in 2015 in the *British Journal of General Practice*, researchers from Scotland reviewed randomized controlled trials on the use of mindfulness meditation to relieve chronic nonmalignant pain. The researchers found 11 studies that met their criteria; all of the trials had active or inactive control groups. The chronic pain conditions included fibromyalgia, rheumatoid arthritis, musculoskeletal pain, failed back surgery syndrome, and mixed etiology, and the primary outcomes reported were pain intensity, depression, physical functioning, quality of life, and pain acceptance. The methodological quality of the trials varied. Eight trials were conducted in the United States, and one each came from Germany, Hong Kong, and the United

Kingdom. With the exception of two trials with older subjects, who had a mean age of 75 years, the mean age of the subjects ranged from 47 to 52 years. The researchers noted that they found limited evidence that mindfulness meditation was effective for chronic pain. However, the trials tended to be small, and many of the results were not statistically significant. From their meta-analysis, the researchers learned that mindfulness interventions may affect perceived pain control, "but there was no evidence of a benefit in terms of clinical outcomes."[4]

Mindfulness-Base Interventions May Provide Relief for Only Certain Aspects of Acute Pain

In a systematic review and meta-analysis published in 2020 in the journal *Pain*, researchers from Australia examined the use of mindfulness-based interventions for acute pain (pain that lasts less than three months). The researchers located 22 randomized, controlled trials with 1964 subjects that met their criteria. The types of pain included acute musculoskeletal injury pain, postoperative pain, clinically induced or procedural pain such as venipuncture, or experimental pain such as cold-pressor test. The trials, which all had at least 20 subjects, were published in peer-reviewed journals in the English language up until January 28, 2020. The primary outcome measured was pain severity either in a numerical rating scale or a visual analogue scale; the secondary outcomes were pain tolerance, pain threshold, and pain-related distress. Because of the varied approaches used by the studies, there was considerable heterogeneity. There were different types of mindfulness, different doses, different modes of delivery, and different control groups. As a result, only 10 trials were included in the meta-analysis. Nevertheless, the researchers were unable to find any evidence that mindfulness-based interventions had any effect on pain severity or pain-related distress. On the other hand, mindfulness-based interventions did appear to impact pain tolerance and pain threshold. The researchers cautioned that the "evidence for pain severity in clinical samples, pain threshold, and pain-related distress was low to very low." So, it is possible that future research may negate these results. "This review highlights that there is a need for further research into the specific effect of different types of MBIs [mindfulness-based interventions] and their optimal dosage to maximize their effectiveness in the management of acute pain."[5]

People with Chronic Low Back Pain May Wish to Try Mindfulness Meditation

In a qualitative analysis published in 2018 in the journal *Pain Medicine*, researchers from Pittsburgh, Pennsylvania (USA) examined the ability of mindfulness meditation to help people with chronic low back pain. The cohort consisted of 25 adults who were at least 65 years old who had a mean age of 76.6 years; 72 percent were white, and 60 percent were women. The subjects completed an eight-week mindfulness meditation program and participated in monthly "booster sessions." They were divided into four focus groups. Each group, which had six or seven members, devoted 90 minutes to discussion about their mindfulness meditation experiences. Included in the discussion were the many ways that mindfulness meditation had impacted their lives, such as relieving pain and enabling them to live with the pain and increase their level of activity. However, others noted that they had little if any pain relief. In general, most of the pain discussion focused one of three topics: overcoming fear of pain, pain awareness, and pain significance. The researchers concluded that their findings "support a mind-body as well as medical approach to patients with chronic pain disorders and underscores the potential for mindfulness to not only improve pain coping skills, but to also decrease pain intensity and pain-related disability."[6]

Mindfulness Meditation Appears to Work Better for the Psychological Components of Pain

In a systematic review published in 2017 in the journal *Current Opinion in Obstetrics and Gynecology*, researchers from the United Kingdom evaluated the ability of mindfulness meditation to offer relief from chronic pain. The researchers located 13 randomized, controlled trials that met their criteria. The types of pain included musculoskeletal pain, back pain, fibromyalgia, diabetic neuropathy pain, general chronic pain, headache, and medically unexplained pain. Length of mindfulness meditation program ranged from 7 to 12 weeks. Three of the trials ($n = 183$) looked at the effect of mindfulness meditation on the reduction of affective pain, and three ($n = 183$) reviewed the reduction of sensory pain. Six trials ($n = 374$) examined the reduction of pain intensity, and three ($n = 251$) studied pain acceptance. Four trials ($n = 368$) reported the effect of mindfulness meditation on depression, and three ($n = 278$) dealt with the effect on anxiety. All of the included trials lacked a suitable control group—a group that received "sham" mindfulness meditation. Yet, the researchers learned that mindfulness meditation did not appear to improve the perception of pain. Rather, it did improve the psychological aspects of living with chronic pain, specifically, depression and quality of life. The researchers concluded that mindfulness meditation "should be considered as an evidence-based adjunct in the treatment of chronic pain."[7]

Both Mindfulness-Based Meditation and Progressive Relaxation Meditation Seem to Help Older People with Diabetic Nerve Pain

In a clinical trial published in 2019 in the *Journal of Evidence-Based Integrative Medicine*, researchers from Abu Dhabi (United Arab Emirates) compared treating women who had diabetic neuropathy with mindfulness-based meditation and progressive relaxation meditation. The initial cohort consisted of 105 women who were all over the age of 55 years; they were recruited from a diabetes clinic in Pakistan from July 2018 to January 2019. Most of the women had annual incomes of $10,000 or less and education levels below high school. On average, they had diabetes for 13 years. The women were randomly placed in one of three groups—mindfulness meditation ($n = 36$), progressive relaxation meditation ($n = 32$), and meditation (control, $n = 37$). (Women in the control meditation group met for the same number of sessions. Each time, they had 15 minutes of discussion followed by 20 minutes of sitting quietly and relaxing.) During an eight-week period of time, the women attended twice weekly 30-minute meditation sessions. Pain assessments were conducted, and no adverse effects were reported by any of the women. By the end of the trial, the women in both intervention groups believed that they had significant improvement in their pain. However, the women in the mindfulness group had greater improvement than the women in the progressive relaxation group. The researchers concluded that "neuromodulatory treatments such as mindfulness meditation need to be conceptualized by health-care providers as low-risk tools that can contribute to the overall benefit of the patient's health."[8]

Mindfulness Meditation May Offer Limited Relief for People Dealing with Migraines

In a randomized clinical trial published in 2021 in *JAMA Internal Medicine*, researchers from Winston-Salem, North Carolina, Boston, Massachusetts, and La Jolla, California (USA), evaluated the effectiveness of mindfulness meditation and headache education for treating migraine headaches. The cohort consisted of 89 adults who experienced between 4 and 20 migraine days per month. Ninety-two percent of the subjects were women, with a mean age of 43.9 years, a mean of 7.3 migraine days per month, and 9.6 headache days per month. For eight weeks, the subjects received two hours per week of either group mindfulness meditation instruction or group headache education. There was also an optional retreat day. The subjects in the mindfulness group were given electronic audio files for home practice and were encouraged to meditate at home 30 minutes per day. Follow-up study visits were held at 12, 24, and 36 weeks. The researchers determined that the subjects in both groups had a reduction in migraine days per month; both groups had "clinically meaningful decreases." Yet, those in the mindfulness program had better improvements in other factors such as headache-related disability, quality of life, depression scores, and self-efficacy. And, the researchers concluded that "mindfulness may help treat the total burden of migraine."[9]

People with Primary Headache Pain May Obtain Limited Benefits from Mindfulness Meditation

In a systematic review and meta-analysis published in 2018 in the *Chinese Medical Journal*, researchers from China analyzed the use of mindfulness meditation for primary headache pain. The researchers located 10 randomized controlled trials and one controlled clinical trial that met their criteria; in total, there were 315 subjects. Four of these studies were conducted in the United States, three in Australia, three in Iran, and one in India. In 10 studies, the mean age of the subjects ranged from 30 to 45 years; in one study, the mean age of the subjects was 19.1 years. One study dealt with migraines; seven studies addressed tension-type headaches, and three studies examined migraines and tension-type headaches. Control groups included pharmacotherapy, waitlist, delayed treatment, relaxation, and education. The methodological quality of the studies varied. Yet, though mindfulness meditation may lower the intensity of pain, the researchers found little evidence that it reduced primary headache pain. "However, a sensitivity analysis to the studies at low risk of bias may suggest a possible overestimation of pain intensity improvement in all studies."[10]

People with Fibromyalgia May or May Not Benefit from Meditation Training

In a randomized, prospective clinical trial published in 2015 in the *Annals of Behavioral Medicine*, researchers from Kentucky, North Carolina (USA), and the United Kingdom analyzed the ability of mindfulness meditation to help with several symptoms of fibromyalgia including pain. The initial cohort consisted of 91 women with fibromyalgia who were at least 18 years old. The women, who tended to be perimenopausal, usually had other medical problems such as arthritis, headaches, chronic fatigue, and respiratory symptoms. In total, 63.7 percent used antidepressants and 23.1 percent used anxiolytic medication. Fifty-one women received sessions of mindfulness-based stress reduction (MBSR), and 40 women were placed on a waitlist. (When the follow-up of the trial was completed, all of these women were offered the MBSR.) The weekly 2½ hour sessions were held for 8 weeks. They included both formal and informal mindfulness practices such as an attention-focusing technique, sitting meditation, and a series of simple yoga positions. The subjects were encouraged to practice these techniques 45 minutes per day, six days a week. A half-day meditation retreat was offered to participants between the sixth and seventh week of the program. There were three assessments—baseline, following the eight-week intervention, and two months after the program ended. The researchers found that the frequency of home mindfulness practice was associated with greater symptom relief. Moreover, while meditation improved some symptoms of fibromyalgia, the improvements in pain failed to reach significance. Thus, while women with fibromyalgia who meditate should expect some relief from their symptoms, they should not anticipate a significant reduction in pain.[11]

Negative Experiences May Occur during Meditation

In an article published in 2017 in the online publication *PLoS*, researchers from Spain and Brazil described the results of an online survey to address some of the negative effects of meditation. The survey was disseminated from April 2013 to July 2015 through several websites in Spanish, English, and Portuguese. The researchers collected comments from 342 people who had at least two months of experience with meditation; of these, 87 reported varying types of "unwanted events." The majority of the responders were women (68.4%) from Spain who had a university level of education (54.4%). The participants noted that they tended to meditate informally every day. Among the symptoms reported were pain, anxiety, "depersonalization," depression, emotional liability, and dizziness. These were more likely to occur during individual, not group, meditation; during focused attention meditation; and when a person meditated for more than 20 minutes. Fortunately, most of these unwanted events were transitory and did not result in discontinuing meditation or require medical assistance. It is important to note that in about 50 percent of the cases, the reports of unwanted events were incomplete. The researchers commented that there is a need for more research on the unwanted events associated with meditation.[12]

NOTES

1. Khoo, Eve-Ling, Rebecca Small, Wei Cheng, et al. "Comparative Evaluation of Group-Based Mindfulness-Based Stress Reduction and Cognitive Behavioural Therapy for the Treatment and Management of Chronic Pain: A Systematic Review and Network Meta-Analysis." *Evidence-Based Mental Health* 22 (2019): 26–35.

2. Zgierska, Aleksanra E., Cindy A. Burzinski, Jennifer Cox, et al. "Mindfulness Meditation and Cognitive Behavioral Therapy Intervention Reduces Pain Severity and Sensitivity in Opioid-Treated Chronic Low Back Pain: Pilot Findings from a Randomized Controlled Trial." *Pain Medicine* 17 (2016): 1865–1881.

3. la Cour, Peter, and Marian Peterson. "Effects of Mindfulness Meditation on Chronic Pain Randomized Controlled Trial." *Pain Medicine* 16, no. 4 (April 2015): 641–652.

4. Bawa, Fathima L. Marikar, Stewart W. Mercer, Rachel J. Atherton, et al. "Does Mindfulness Improve Outcomes in Patients with Chronic Pain? Systematic Review and Meta-Analysis." *British Journal of General Practice* 65, no. 635 (June 2015): e387–e400.

5. Shires, Alice, Louise Sharpe, Jonathan N. Davies, and Toby R. O. Newton-John. "The Efficacy of Mindfulness-Based Interventions in Acute Pain: A Systematic Review and Meta-Analysis." *Pain* 161 (2020): 1698–1707.

6. Luiggi-Hernandez, J. G., J. Woo, M. Hamm, et al. "Mindfulness for Chronic Low Back Pain: A Qualitative Analysis." *Pain Medicine* 19 (2018): 2138–2145.

7. Ball, Elizabeth F., Emira Nur Shafina Muhammad Sharizan, Genny Franklin, and Ewelina Rogozińska. "Does Mindfulness Meditation Improve Chronic Pain: A Systematic Review." *Current Opinion in Obstetrics and Gynecology* 29, no. 6 (December 2017): 353–366.

8. Hussain, Nadia, and Amira S. A. Said. "Mindfulness-Based Meditation versus Progressive Relaxation Meditation: Impact on Chronic Pain in Older Female Patients with Diabetic Neuropathy." *Journal of Evidence-Based Integrative Medicine* 24 (2019): NA.

9. Wells, Rebecca Erwin, Nathaniel O'Connell, Charles R. Pierce, et al. "Effectiveness of Mindfulness Meditation vs. Headache Education for Adults with Migraine." *JAMA Internal Medicine* 181, no. 3 (2021): 317–328.

10. Gu, Qiang, Jin-Chao Hou, and Xiang-Ming Fang. "Mindfulness Meditation for Primary Headache Pain: A Meta-Analysis." *Chinese Medical Journal* 131, no. 7 (April 5, 2018): 829–838.

11. Cash, Elizabeth, Paul Salmon, Inka Weissbecker, et al. "Mindfulness Meditation Alleviates Fibromyalgia Symptoms in Women: Results of a Randomized Clinical Trial." *Annals of Behavioral Medicine* 49, no. 3 (June 2015): 319–330.

12. Cebolla, A., M. Demarzo, P. Martins, et al. "Unwanted Effects: Is There a Negative Side of Meditation? A Multicentre Survey." *PLoS One* 12, no. 9 (2017): e0183137.

REFERENCES AND FURTHER READINGS

Ball, Elizabeth F., Emira Nur Shafina Muhammad Sharizan, Genny Franklin, and Ewelina Rogozińska. "Does Mindfulness Meditation Improve Chronic Pain: A Systematic Review." *Current Opinion in Obstetrics and Gynecology* 29, no. 6 (December 2017): 359–366.

Bawa, Fathima L. Marikar, Stewart W. Mercer, Rachel J. Atherton, et al. "Does Mindfulness Improve Outcomes in Patients with Chronic Pain? Systematic Review and Meta-Analysis." *British Journal of General Practice* 65, no. 635 (June 2015): e387–e400.

Cash, Elizabeth, Paul Salmon, Inka Weissbecker, et al. "Mindfulness Meditation Alleviates Fibromyalgia Symptoms in Women: Results of a Randomized Clinical Trial." *Annals of Behavioral Medicine* 49, no. 3 (June 2015): 319–330.

Cebolla, A., M. Demarzo, P. Martins, et al. "Unwanted Effects: Is There a Negative Side of Meditation? A Multicentre Survey." *PLoS One* 12, no. 9 (2017): e0183137.

Gu, Qiang, Jin-Chao Hou, and Xiang-Ming Fang. "Mindfulness Meditation for Primary Headache Pain: A Meta-Analysis." *Chinese Medical Journal* 131, no. 7 (April 5, 2018): 829–838.

Hussain, Nadia, and Amira S. A. Said. "Mindfulness-Based Meditation versus Progressive Relaxation Meditation: Impact on Chronic Pain in Older Female Patients with Diabetic Neuropathy." *Journal of Evidence-Based Integrative Medicine* 24 (2019): NA.

Khoo, Eve-Ling, Rebecca Small, Wei Cheng, et al. "Comparative Evaluation of Group-Based Mindfulness Stress Reduction and Cognitive Behavioural Therapy for the Treatment and Management of Chronic Pain: A Systematic Review and Network Meta-Analysis." *Evidence-Based Mental Health* 22 (2019): 26–35.

la Cour, Peter, and Marian Petersen. "Effects of Mindfulness Meditation on Chronic Pain: A Randomized Controlled Trial." *Pain Medicine* 16, no. 4 (April 2015): 641–652.

Luiggi-Hernandez, J. G., J. Woo, M. Hamm, et al. "Mindfulness for Chronic Low Back Pain: A Qualitative Analysis." *Pain Medicine* 19 (2018): 2138–2145.

Shires, Alice, Louise Sharpe, Jonathan N. Davies, and Toby R. O. Newton-John. "The Efficacy of Mindfulness-Based Intervention in Acute Pain: A Systematic Review and Meta-Analysis." *Pain* 161 (2020): 1698–1707.

Wells, Rebecca Erwin, Nathaniel O'Connell, Charles R. Pierce, et al. "Effectiveness of Mindfulness Meditation vs. Headache Education for Adults with Migraine: A Randomized Clinical Trial." *JAMA Internal Medicine* 181, no. 3 (2021): 317–328.

Zgierska, Aleksandra E., Cindy A. Burzinski, Jennifer Cox, et al. "Mindfulness Meditation and Cognitive Behavioral Therapy Intervention Reduces Pain Severity and Sensitivity in Opioid-Treated Chronic Low Back Pain: Pilot Findings from a Randomized Controlled Trial." *Pain Medicine* 17 (2016): 1865–1881.

Muscle Relaxants

INTRODUCTION

Also known as muscle relaxers, muscle relaxants are medications used to treat muscle spasms or muscle spasticity. Muscle spasms or cramps are sudden, involuntary contractions of a muscle or group of muscles. With a variety of reasons, such as excessive muscle strain, muscle spasms may occur with back pain, neck pain, and fibromyalgia and may be exceedingly painful. In contrast, muscle spasticity is a continuous muscle spasm that causes stiffness, rigidity, or tightness. It may interfere with normal, everyday activities, such as walking, talking, or basic movements. Muscle spasticity is caused by an injury to the parts of the brain or spinal cord involved with movement. Several conditions, such as multiple sclerosis and cerebral palsy, may cause muscle spasticity.

There are two main groups of prescription muscle relaxant medications: antispasmodics and antispastics. Antispasmodics, which are also known as skeletal muscle relaxants, are used to treat muscle spasms; antispastics are used to treat muscle spasticity. A few antispasmodics may be used to treat muscle spasticity, but antispastics are not used to treat muscle spasms. Antispasmodics are believed to have a sedative effect; they are thought to prevent nerves from sending pain signals to the brain. There are two types of antispasmodics: benzodiazepines and nonbenzodiazepines. Benzodiazepines block certain chemicals in the brain, and nonbenzodiazepines act on both the brain and spinal cord. Antispastics directly affect the spinal cord or the skeletal muscles, improving muscle tightness and spasms.

One of the best-known prescription muscle relaxants is lorazepam (Ativan), a benzodiazepine. By increasing the level of a neurotransmitter, lorazepam relieves muscle spasms caused by inflammation, trauma, or muscle spasticity. Another common prescription muscle relaxant is cyclobenzaprine (Flexeril, Amrix, and Rexmid) a nonbenzodiazepine; it is useful for acute muscle conditions.

Although there is no way to know how many people use and misuse muscle relaxants, a cross-sectional, retrospective study published in 2020 used data from the National Ambulatory Medical Care Survey (NAMCS) to assess the prescribing of muscle relaxants in the United States from 2005 to 2016. This analysis included 314,970, 308 office visits of people with a mean age of 53.5 years. Of these, 194,621,102 were men, and 120,349,206 were women. Patients in these visits were most frequently female, white, and aged 45 to 64 years. During the study period, office visits with a prescribed skeletal muscle relaxants nearly doubled from 15.5 million in 2005 to 30.7 million in 2016. Although visits for new skeletal muscle relaxants remained stable, visits for the continued use of this type of medication tripled from 8.5 million in 2005 to 24.7 million in 2016.[1]

ADMINISTRATION AND REGULATION

All of the prescriptive muscle relaxants must be prescribed by a medical provider, and because of their many side effects, they should be prescribed with caution. Administration varies according to the specific medication. Thus, diazepam, a benzodiazepine, is available in tablets or injections. Diazepam in tablet form is administered in 2 to 10 mg doses three or four times per day. An initial intravenous dose of diazepam may be 5 to 10 mg, and a second dose may be administered three or four hours later. Cyclobenzaprine, a nonbenzodiazepine, is sold in two forms: an immediate-release tablet and an extended-release capsule. Medical providers usually prescribe 5 mg three times per day. Sometimes, medical providers prescribe higher amounts, such as 7.5 to 10 mg three times per day. The maximum is 30 mg per day. The extended-release formula should be taken the same time every day. Prices of muscle relaxants vary according to the medication. They tend to range from relatively inexpensive to more than a dollar per pill.

As the FDA regulates all prescription medications, it also regulates muscle relaxants.

BENEFITS AND RISKS

Muscle relaxants provide relief for a host of different painful muscular problems, from the muscle spasms associated with low back pain to the spasticity related to spinal injury. For countless numbers of people, they represent reductions in pain levels and disability. Yet, because they have so many risk factors, they are often considered a second line of defense, behind nonsteroidal anti-inflammatory drugs and acetaminophen. Sometimes, they are used only after these other alternatives have failed.

Antispasmodics are associated with a number of different side effects and serious risk factors. These include drowsiness, fatigue, muscle weakness, dizziness, headache, nervousness, dry mouth, irritability, confusion, reddish-purple or orange urine, lightheadedness, and lowered blood pressure upon standing. That is why antispasmodics should not be used for more than two or three weeks. Also, they need to be used with extra care by the elderly. Antispastics also have side effects such as drowsiness, dizziness, weakness, fatigue, lightheadedness, and muscle weakness, but they are taken for longer periods of time.

Prescription muscle relaxants may be habit forming, and they may have withdrawal symptoms such as seizures or hallucinations. Never suddenly discontinue muscle relaxant medications, even if you have been using them for a long time. In addition, muscle relaxants depress the central nervous system, making it more difficult to pay attention and stay awake. People taking muscle relaxants should avoid activities that require mental alertness, such as using heavy machinery and driving. Muscle relaxants should not be mixed with alcohol, central nervous system depressant drugs such as opioids, psychotropics, sleeping medications, and certain herbal supplements such as St. John's wort. Muscle relaxants may slow breathing, and overdoses may be fatal.

RESEARCH FINDINGS

Clonazepam Seems to Help the Pain Associated with Burning Mouth Syndrome

In a retrospective, single-center study published in 2017 in the *International Journal of Oral & Maxillofacial Surgery*, researchers from France compared the use of clonazepam, a benzodiazepine, and amitriptyline, a tricyclic antidepressant, for treating burning mouth syndrome (BMS), a illness characterized by a burning sensation inside the mouth for more than two hours per day for more than three months. The cohort consisted of 39 subjects, with a mean age of 65 years; 84.6 percent were women. Twenty-three were treated with clonazepam, and 16 were treated with amitriptyline. Both medications were administered at bedtime. The minimum duration of treatment was three months. After six weeks of treatment, both groups had significant reductions in pain; the differences in pain relief between the two groups were not significant. The pain relief in both groups remained significant after three months. No serious adverse reactions were reported with either treatment. "Clonazepam as well as amitriptyline may be an effective treatment for BMS."[2]

In a systematic review and meta-analysis published in 2016 in the journal *Oral Diseases*, researchers from China examined three randomized, controlled trials and two high-quality case-control studies on the use of clonazepam for symptom remission in primary or secondary BMS. The five studies, which were published between 1998 and 2012, had a total of 195 subjects. Duration of interventions ranged from two weeks to 29 months. There were two different modes of administration: swallowing the tablet and topical administration, which entailed sucking on the tablet near the pain site, retaining saliva without swallowing for three minutes, and then spitting out the saliva. In three studies, the doses of clonazepam were gradually increased. The researchers found that the short-term and long-term use of both types of clonazepam resulted in "significant remission" of symptoms, and the medication demonstrated "therapeutic efficacy." They further concluded that "clonazepam is effective in inducing symptom remission in patients with BMS."[3]

When Combined with Ibuprofen, Chlorzoxazone Provides Relief for Acute Low Back Pain

In an open-label, prospective, parallel-group, multicenter trial published in 2019 in the journal *Pain Therapy*, researchers from India evaluated the ability of muscle relaxants and ibuprofen to treat acute low back pain. The cohort consisted of 406 subjects between the ages of 18 and 60 years with acute low back pain. Two hundred three subjects were treated with a single tablet of the fixed-dose combination of chlorzoxazone 500 mg and ibuprofen 400 mg, and 203 subjects were treated with ibuprofen 400 mg. Both medications were administered three times per day, 30 minutes after meals, for up to seven days. The subjects visited one of the four centers included in the study at baseline and on days three and seven. The researchers conducted various pain and functioning assessments, and all of the subjects completed the trial. Minor adverse events, such as gastritis and stomach pain, were reported by nine subjects in the combination treatment group and six subjects in the ibuprofen group. The researchers learned that there was a 78.2 percent reduction in pain with the combination medication and a 72.3 percent reduction with ibuprofen alone. The subjects on the combination medication also had better improvements in functioning. The researchers concluded that "chlorzoxazone is a useful adjunct to ibuprofen in the treatment of LBP [low back pain] in general practice."[4]

Use of Benzodiazepines May Increase the Risk of Developing Alzheimer's Disease

In a cross-control study published in 2014 in the journal *BMJ*, researchers from Bordeaux, France, and Montreal, Canada, investigated the association between past use of benzodiazepines and the risk of Alzheimer's disease. Why is this important? According to the researchers, elderly individuals frequently use benzodiazepines. Estimates of their use among the elderly range from 7 to 43 percent. The cohort consisted of 1,796 people with a first diagnosis of Alzheimer's disease; they were matched to 7,184 controls. Both groups consisted of people over the age of 66 years who lived in the Quebec, Canada, community from 2000 to 2009. The researchers only included subjects who used benzodiazepines at least five years before their Alzheimer's diagnosis. During the study, 894 people with Alzheimer's disease (49.8%) and 2,873 controls (40.0%) had ever used benzodiazepines; the treatment was still being used at the date of Alzheimer's diagnosis in 64.8 percent of the cases and 60.6 percent of controls. The researchers learned that the long-term use of benzodiazepines was associated with "markedly" higher rates of Alzheimer's disease—32.9 percent versus 21.8 percent among controls. Moreover, the use of benzodiazepines at any time was significantly associated with an increased risk of Alzheimer's disease; the association was stronger for long-acting benzodiazepines than for the short-acting ones and for those who use these medications for longer periods of time. "In view of the evidence, it is now crucial to encourage physicians to carefully balance the benefits and risks when initiating or renewing a treatment with benzodiazepines and related products in older patients."[5]

In the United States, the Use and Misuse of Benzodiazepines Is Relatively Common

In a cross-sectional analysis published in 2019 in the journal *Psychiatry Services*, researchers from Ann Arbor, Michigan (USA), used data from the 2015 and 2016 National Survey of Drug Use and Health (NSDUH) to calculate the rates of use and misuse of benzodiazepines in the United States. The 50-state survey had a portion that was conducted by an interviewer and a section that was completed without any assistance "to increase the likelihood of honest reporting of illicit drug use." For each medication class, NSDUH collected information on the past year's use and misuse. The subjects were asked to describe how they misused the medication, such as without a prescription, as well as their reasons for misuse, such as to relax or experiment. Finally, they were questioned about their source for medication. The researchers learned that an estimated 30.6 million adults reported the past year use of benzodiazepines. That is an overall prevalence of 12.6 percent. Use among adults 50 to 64 years was the highest. Of the 30.6 million users, 25.3 million reported using as prescribed by their clinicians, and 5.3 million reported misuse. Misuse was highest among younger adults between the ages of 18 and 25 years and decreased as people aged; misuse was just 0.6 percent in adults 65 years or older. Yet, relative to younger adults, older respondents were more likely to use their benzodiazepines more often than prescribed. Older adults were likely to use (misuse) their medication to sleep, whereas younger adults misused to "get high." The respondents obtained 70 percent of their misused benzodiazepine from a friend or relative. The researchers concluded that "benzodiazepine use in the U.S. is higher than previously reported and misuse accounted for nearly 20% of use overall." As a result, "clinicians should monitor patients also prescribed stimulants or opioids for benzodiazepine misuse."[6]

Use of Nonbenzodiazepine Medication for Low Back Pain May Result in a Small and Not Clinically Important Reduction in Pain Intensity

In a systematic review published in 2021 in *BMJ*, researchers from Australia investigated the use of nonbenzodiazepines and other medications for nonspecific low back pain. The researchers located 49 randomized, controlled trials that met their criteria. Of these, 35 were peer-reviewed journal articles, 2 were conference abstracts, and 12 were trail registry records. Thirty-one trials, with 6,505 subjects, were included in the meta-analysis. The muscle relaxants used in 29 of the trials were nonbenzodiazepines. In 35 trials, the muscle relaxant was administered orally, and in 32 trials, the muscle relaxant was compared to a placebo. Of the 39 trials assessed for risk of bias, 28 had high risk, 3 had moderate risk, and 8 had low risk. The researchers found very low certainty evidence that nonbenzodiazepine medication may reduce pain at two weeks or less for people with acute low back pain. The effect was only 8 out of a scale of 100 and was not clinically meaningful. Further, these medications had little to no effect on pain from 3 to 13 weeks, though the certainty of evidence ranged from moderate to very low. Low- and very low–certainty evidence showed that nonbenzodiazepines might increase the risk of adverse events and might have little to no effect on treatment discontinuation. The researchers concluded that "large, high quality, placebo controlled trials are urgently needed to resolve uncertainties about the efficacy and safety of muscle relaxants for low back pain."[7]

Use of Methocarbamol, a Nonbenzodiazepine, for Acute Pain after Traumatic Injury May Not Help

In a retrospective, matched cohort study published in 2017 in the *American Journal of Therapeutics*, researchers from Tucson, Arizona (USA), and Jeddad, Saudi Arabia, examined the use of methocarbamol for acute pain after a traumatic injury. The cohort consisted of adults who were consecutively admitted to a hospital between June 1, 2012, and June 30, 2013, for traumatic injury. Data were abstracted from medical records until 100 patients who were treated with methocarbamol for pain were included; the control group also had 100 patients. Overall, the mean age of the cohort was 49 years; 67 percent were men, and 56 percent were white. In the treatment group, the most common daily dose of methocarbamol was 2,250 mg. The researchers learned that the use of methocarbamol during the first three days after traumatic injury did not improve pain control or reduce opioid intake. The researchers concluded that "the use of methocarbamol as part of a multimodal analgesic regimen is not supported."[8]

However, the Use of Methocarbamol May Help Young Adults with Acute Pain from Traumatic Rib Fractures

In an observational, retrospective, single-center study published in 2021 in the journal *Annals of Pharmacotherapy*, researchers from Charleston, South Carolina (USA), evaluated the use of methocarbamol for the treatment of younger adults with acute pain from traumatic rib fractures. The cohort consisted of 50 patients between the ages of 18 and 39 years; they were all admitted with three or more rib fractures to a level-1 trauma center between July 2014 and July 2018. As part of their pain regime, which included opioids, 28 patients received methocarbamol, and 22 received no methocarbamol. Methocarbamol usually began with a single dose of 500 mg every six hours, and it titrated up to a maximum of 1,500 mg every six hours. (The two groups were generally comparable in baseline demographics and injury characteristics.) During the first two days of hospitalization, there were no differences in opioid requirements between the two groups. On the third day, the patients taking methocarbamol required significantly less opioid medication, and they stayed in the hospital three rather than four days. Methocarbamol was not associated with any serious side effects. The researchers concluded that "given the adverse effect profile and risk of dependence associated with opioids, use of methocarbamol as an anesthesia-optimizing, opioid-sparing multimodal agent may be reasonable."[9]

Outpatient Use of Benzodiazepines Appears to Have Markedly Increased

In a serial cross-sectional study published in 2019 in *JAMA Network Open*, researchers from Boston, Massachusetts (USA), used data from the National Ambulatory Medical Care Survey to analyze the outpatient use of benzodiazepines. (The National Ambulatory Medical Care Survey is an annual population-based sample of adult outpatient visits.) Of the 386,457 ambulatory care visits calculated from 2003 to 2015, a total of 919 benzodiazepine visits occurred in 2003 and 1,672 in 2015, representing 27.6 million visits and 62.6 million visits, respectively. The benzodiazepine visit rate increased from 3.8 percent to 7.4 percent. About half of all benzodiazepines visits were to primary care physicians. The researchers learned that the use of benzodiazepines for back and chronic pain as well as undefined conditions had increased substantially. The researchers wondered if this trend reflected "an underappreciation of the risk associated with benzodiazepines and an overappreciation of the benefits." Furthermore, coprescribing had increased for benzodiazepines and opioids and also for benzodiazepines and nonbenzodiazepine sedative hypnotics, muscle relaxants, and antipsychotics. The researchers concluded that "in light of increasing death rates related to benzodiazepine overdose, addressing prescribing patterns may help curb the growing use of benzodiazepines."[10]

Use of Benzodiazepines and Opioids Together May Be Risky

In a cross-sectional study published in 2019 in the journal *Pain Medicine*, researchers from Portland, Oregon (USA), examined the problems associated with the intake of benzodiazepine and opioids in patients with chronic pain. The study, which was conducted at Kaiser Permanente Northwest and VA Portland Health Care System, included 517 adults with musculoskeletal pain; all of the subjects were on long-term opioid therapy. The subjects were interviewed either in person or on the phone. In addition to their opioid medication, 24.6 percent of the 517 subjects had also taken benzodiazepines during the previous year. The mean number of polypharmacy months was 7.6. The researchers learned that the subjects taking both medications were more likely to fall and to have more visits to emergency departments. Further, they were more often diagnosed with depression, post-traumatic stress disorder, and bipolar disorder, and they were more likely to be taking sedatives/hypnotics and antidepressants. As a result, the researchers advised the "need for better risk screening before initiating either benzodiazepines or opioids and . . . clinically addressing overlapping areas of risk." The researchers concluded that "clinicians need additional tools and strategies to treat their patients' pain and psychiatric conditions while simultaneously keeping their patients safe from harm."[11]

When Veterans Who Are Taking an Opioid Also Take a Benzodiazepine Medication, Their Risk of Death Increases

In a case-cohort study published in 2015 in *BMJ*, researchers from Providence, Rhode Island, Boston, Massachusetts, and Ann Arbor, Michigan (USA), examined the incidence of deaths among veterans who were prescribed a benzodiazepine medication in addition to their opioid medication. The cohort consisted of 422,786 veterans. Of these, 112,069 (27%) had filled at least one prescription for benzodiazepines during the study period. Those who received benzodiazepines were more likely to be women, middle-aged, white, and live in wealthier areas, and they were more likely to have a diagnosis of substance abuse or several psychiatric disorders, both of which have their own risks of death from overdose. Of the 2,400 veterans in the study who died from a drug overdose while receiving opioid analgesics, 1,185 (49%) died during a period in which they had been prescribed concurrent benzodiazepines. Veterans taking lorazepam and temazepam had lower rates of death from overdose than those on other types of benzodiazepines. There also appeared to be an association between the dose of benzodiazepine and the risk of death, and the subjects currently using benzodiazepines had a higher risk of death than those who used the medication in the past. The researchers commented that clinicians need "to be aware of the increased risk among patients currently receiving benzodiazepines and opioids and that the risk might be higher among those receiving higher doses of either or both drugs." Clinicians must be even more cautious when prescribing benzodiazepines to these patients.[12]

Some People May Underestimate the Risk of Mixing Opioid Pain Medication with Benzodiazepines

In a cross-sectional study published in 2020 in the journal *Substance Use & Misuse*, researchers from Detroit, Michigan, and New Brunswick, New Jersey (USA), wanted to learn more about the perceptions people have about mixing opioid medications with benzodiazepines. During July and August 2018, the researchers used Facebook to recruit 639 adults; sometimes, they only targeted men or residents of specific zip codes. The subjects completed a 15-minute online survey with a variety of questions about opioids, alcohol, and benzodiazepines. The researchers found that older people were more likely to note the potential hazard of combining opioids with benzodiazepines, whereas younger people were less likely to acknowledge this risk. Likewise, people who had used opioids for nonmedical reasons in the past year or in their lifetime were less likely to view the combined use of opioids and benzodiazepines to be risky. And, medical providers need to educate both themselves and their patients. "A national record review found that around half of patients who received an opioid with a benzodiazepine received both prescriptions from the same prescriber on the same day."[13]

Benzodiazepine Use May Be Detrimental to People with Chronic Pain

In a clinical trial published in 2017 in the *Journal of Pain Research*, researchers from Rochester, Minnesota, examined the association between benzodiazepine and opioid use in adults with chronic pain who were admitted to an outpatient interdisciplinary pain rehabilitation program (IPR). The cohort consisted of 847 consecutive patients admitted to a three-week outpatient IPR program from January 2013 to December 2014 (Mayo Comprehensive Pain Rehabilitation Center). Upon admission, 248 (29%) patients were taking benzodiazepines, and 62 percent of these patients were taking both a benzodiazepine and an opioid. The primary diagnoses of patients admitted to this program were low back pain, fibromyalgia, and chronic headaches. These patients were more likely to be female and on opioid medication. Also, they reported greater perceived pain severity, depressive symptoms, and "pain catastrophizing." The researchers realized that upon admission, there was a direct association between women and depression and the use of benzodiazepines. Further, this association placed these women at a higher risk for overdoses. The researchers concluded that providers should weigh the risks versus benefits when prescribing benzodiazepines for people in chronic pain, especially in combination with opioids, and providers should work with patients to taper and eliminate benzodiazepines.[14]

Taking Benzodiazepines before Surgery Increases the Risk of Filling an Opioid Prescription after Hand Surgery

In a clinical trial published in 2019 in the journal *Clinical Orthopaedics and Related Research*, researchers from Philadelphia, Pennsylvania (USA), investigated the association between the preoperative use of benzodiazepines or sedative/hypnotics and the risk of filling opioid prescriptions after hand surgery. The researchers enrolled 290 patients undergoing upper extremity surgery, such as carpal tunnel release and trigger release, at one academic outpatient surgical center. The researchers learned that a preoperative exposure to benzodiazepines and sedative/hypnotics was associated with the increased number of filled opioid prescriptions. Patients who used more than one controlled substance had more filled opioids prescriptions than those not using more than one controlled substance. Thus, the preoperative prescribing of benzodiazepines may contribute to an increased postoperative use of opioids, and, as a result, these patients "require much greater scrutiny, a more-detailed discussion regarding expectations, and a plan regarding postoperative pain management."[15]

NOTES

1. Soprano, Samantha E., Sean Hennessy, Warren B. Bilker, and Charles E. Leonard. "Assessment of Physician Prescribing of Muscle Relaxants in the United States, 2005–2016." *JAMA Network Open* 3, no. 6 (2020): e207664.

2. Fenelon, M., E. Quinque, E. Arrive, et al. "Pain-Relieving Effects of Clonazepam and Amitriptyline in Burning Mouth Syndrome: A Retrospective Study." *International Journal of Oral & Maxillofacial Surgery* 46 (2017): 1503–1511.

3. Cui, Y., H. Xu, F. M. Chen, et al. "Efficacy Evaluation of Clonazepam for Symptoms Remission in Burning Mouth Syndrome: Mata-Analysis." *Oral Diseases* 22 (2016): 503–511.

4. Patel, Himanshu D., R. B. Uppin, A. Ramakrishnam, et al. "Efficacy and Safety of Combination of NSAIDs and Muscle Relaxants in the Management of Acute Low Back Pain." *Pain Therapy* 8, no. 1 (2019): 121–132.

5. Billioti de Gage, Sophie, Yola Moride, Thierry Ducruet, et al. "Benzodiazepine Use and Risk of Alzheimer's Disease: A Case-Control Study." *BMJ* 349 (2014): g5205.

6. Maust, Donovan T., Lewel A. Lin, and Frederic C. Blow. "Benzodiazepine Use and Misuse among Adults in the United States." *Psychiatry Services* 70, no. 2 (February 1, 2019): 97–106.

7. Cashin, Aidan G., Thiago Folly, Matthew K. Bagg, et al. "Efficacy, Acceptability, and Safety of Muscle Relaxants for Adults with Non-Specific Low Back Pain: Systematic Review and Meta-Analysis." *BMJ* 374 (July 7, 2021): n1446.

8. Aljuhani, Ohoud, Brian J. Kopp, and Asad E. Patanwala. "Effect of Methocarbamol on Acute Pain after Traumatic Injury." *American Journal of Therapeutics* 24, no. 2 (March–April 2017): e202–e206.

9. Deloney, Lindsay P., Melanie Smith Condeni, Cassandra Carter, et al. "Efficacy of Methocarbamol for Acute Pain Management in Young Adults with Traumatic Rib Fractures." *Annals of Pharmacotherapy* 55, no. 6 (June 2021): 705–710.

10. Agarwal, Sumit D., and Bruce E. Landon. "Patterns in Outpatient Benzodiazepine Prescribing in the United States." *JAMA Network Open* 2, no. 1 (2019): e187399.

11. Yarborough, Bobbi Jo H., Scott P. Stumbo, Ashley Stoneburner, et al. "Correlates of Benzodiazepine Use and Adverse Outcomes among Patients with Chronic Pain Prescribed Long-Term Opioid Therapy." *Pain Medicine* 20, no. 6 (2019): 1148–1155.

12. Park, T. W., R. Saitz, D. Ganoczy, et al. "Benzodiazepine Prescribing Patterns and Deaths from Drug Overdose among U.S. Veterans Receiving Opioid Analgesics; Case Cohort Study." *BMJ* 350 (2015): h2698.

13. Ellis, Jennifer D., Stella M. Resko, Rachel Kollin, et al. "Public Perceptions of Risk Associated with Mixing Opioid Pain-Relievers with Alcohol and Benzodiazepines." *Substance Use & Misuse* 55, no. 7 (2020): 1189–1193.

14. Cunningham, Julie L., Julia R. Craner, Michele M. Evans, and W. Michael Hooten. "Benzodiazepine Use in Patients with Chronic Pain in an

Interdisciplinary Pain Rehabilitation Program." *Journal of Pain Research* 10 (2017): 311–317.

15. Hozack, Bryan A., Michael Rivlin, Kevin F. Lutsky, et al. "Preoperative Exposure to Benzodiazepines or Sedative/Hypnotics Increases the Risk of Greater Filled Opioid Prescriptions after Surgery." *Clinical Orthopaedics and Related Research* 477 (2019): 1482–1488.

REFERENCES AND FURTHER READINGS

Agarwal, Sumit D., and Bruce E. Landon. "Patterns in Outpatient Benzodiazepine Prescribing in the United States." *JAMA Network Open* 2, no. 1 (2019): e187399.

Aljuhani, Ohoud, Brian J. Kopp, and Asad E. Patanwala. "Effect of Methocarbamol on Acute Pain after Traumatic Injury." *American Journal of Therapeutics* 24, no. 2 (March–April 2017): e202–e206.

Billioti de Gage, Sophie, Yola Moride, Thierry Ducruet, et al. "Benzodiazepine Use and Risk of Alzheimer's Disease: A Case-Control Study." *BMJ* 349 (2014): g5205.

Cashin, Aidan G., Thiago Folly, Matthew K. Bagg, et al. "Efficacy, Acceptability, and Safety of Muscle Relaxants for Adults with Non-Specific Low Back Pain: Systematic Review and Meta-Analysis." *BMJ* 374 (July 7, 2021): n1446.

Cui, Y., H. Xu, F. M. Chen, et al. "Efficacy Evaluation of Clonazepam for Symptom Remission in Burning Mouth Syndrome: A Meta-Analysis." *Oral Diseases* 22 (2016): 503–511.

Cunnningham, Julie L., Julia R. Craner, Michele M. Evans, and W. Michael Hooten. "Benzodiazepine Use in Patients with Chronic Pain in an Interdisciplinary Pain Rehabilitation Program." *Journal of Pain Research* 10 (2017): 311–317.

Ellis, Jennifer D., Stella M. Resko, Rachel Kollin, et al. "Public Perceptions of Risk Associated with Mixing Opioid Pain-Relievers with Alcohol and Benzodiazepines." *Substance Use & Misuse* 55, no. 7 (2020): 1189–1193.

Deloney, Lindsay P., Melanie Smith Condeni, Cassandra Carter, et al. "Efficacy of Methocarbamol for Acute Pain Management in Young Adults with Traumatic Rib Fractures." *Annals of Pharmacotherapy* 55, no. 6 (June 2021): 705–710.

Fenelon, M., E. Ouinque, E. Arrive, et al. "Pain-Relieving Effects of Clonazepam and Amitriptyline in Burning Mouth Syndrome: A

Retrospective Study." *International Journal of Oral & Maxillofacial Surgery* 46 (2017): 1503–1511.

Hozack, Bryan A., Michael Rivlin, Kevin F. Lutsky, et al. "Preoperative Exposure to Benzodiazepines or Sedative/Hypnotics Increases the Risk of Greater Filled Opioids after Surgery." *Clinical Orthopaedics and Related Research* 477 (2019): 1482–1488.

Maust, Donovan T., Lewel A. Lin, and Frederic C. Blow. "Benzodiazepine Use and Misuse among adults in the United States." *Psychiatry Services* 70, no. 2 (February 1, 2019): 97–106.

Park, T. W., R. Saitz, D. Ganoczy, et al. "Benzodiazepine Prescribing Patterns and Deaths from Drug Overdose Among US Veterans Receiving Opioid Analgesics: Case-Cohort Study." *BMJ* 350 (2015): h2698.

Patel, HImanshu D., R. B. Uppin, A. Ramakrishnam Naidu, et al. "Efficacy and Safety of Combination of NSAIDs and Muscle Relaxants in the Management of Acute Low Back Pain." *Pain Therapy* 8, no. 1 (2019): 121–132.

Soprano, Samantha E., Sean Hennessy, Warren B. Bilker, and Charles E. Leonard. "Assessment of Physician Prescribing of Muscle Relaxants in the United States, 2005–2016." *JAMA Network Open* 3, no. 6 (2020): e207664.

Yarborough, Bobbi Jo H., Scott P. Stumbo, Ashley Stoneburner, et al. "Correlates of Benzodiazepine Use and Adverse Outcomes among Patients with Chronic Pain Prescribed Long-Term Opioid Therapy." *Pain Medicine* 20, no. 6 (2019): 1148–1155.

Music Therapy

INTRODUCTION

It is well known that music is able to soothe, inspire, energize, and uplift. What is probably less well known is that music has the potential—at least in some instances—to relieve both acute and chronic pain.

Pain affects the entire body—physically, psychologically, mentally, and emotionally. In addition, pain is exacerbated by stress and anxiety. Music reaches out to all of these aspects of the body. Music therapists use all types of music to reduce the perception of pain and suffering. During their therapeutic music sessions, patients and clients increase their motivation to participate in treatment and improve.

Music has been incorporated into medicine for thousands of years. It is at least as old as the writings of Aristotle and Plato. However, it did not become an integral part of care in the United States until the soldiers returned from the two world wars. Both professional and amateur community members sang for the soldiers receiving care in veterans' hospitals. It soon became obvious that the veterans responded to the music, and a demand developed for a college curriculum to train music therapists. Music therapists maintain that almost anyone dealing with pain may benefit from music therapy. This includes children, adolescents, adults, and the elderly.

ADMINISTRATION AND REGULATION

Music therapy for the treatment of pain is offered in many pain centers and cancer centers, but it may well be available in other health-care and wellness environments. Currently, there are music therapists in the United States who work with patients in pain management centers, hospitals, senior and community centers, rehabilitation facilities, and drug and alcohol programs. Some music therapists provide their services in the home. Music therapy may be delivered to an individual client or to a group of people.

Music therapists design musical interventions for people with chronic pain based on their specific likes and needs. The therapy may include listening to music, singing along to songs, composing songs, discussing music and lyrics, meditating with background music, and using music to form images in the minds.

Music therapy is an accredited health-care profession. Music therapists use music as a tool to meet the unique needs of each patient or client. More than 70 colleges and universities offer music therapy degree programs approved by the American Music Therapy Association. Music therapists have a minimum of a bachelor's degree; they must complete 1,200 hours of clinical training, including an internship at a health-care or education facility, and pass an independently administered national board certification examination to become board-certified music therapists. Among other subjects, they study psychology, counseling, physiology, and anatomy, and they must become proficient in four instruments—piano, guitar, voice, and a fourth instrument that they select. There are approximately 5,000 music therapists in the United States. Fees for their services vary, but they tend to be about $90 for 45 minutes and $150 for 90 minutes. Music therapy may or may not be covered by insurers. It is best to check before therapy begins and obtain preapproval for the services. It has been estimated that about 20 percent of music therapists receive third-party reimbursement. Though music therapists tend to be accomplished musicians, their patients or clients are not required to have any musical experience or ability.

BENEFITS AND RISKS

Music therapy, which provides sensory stimulation that evokes a response in people, may benefit in several different ways. Music therapy may lower the amount of perceived pain. It may promote relaxation, rhythmic breathing, and rest, and it may relieve anxiety and stress. And, music therapy may improve mood. People dealing with chronic pain who participate in music therapy may require less pain medication; experience improvements in respiration, blood pressure, heart rate, and muscle relaxation; and have a better quality of life.

Still, there are a few risks associated with music therapy. Music therapy may trigger the release of repressed emotions, which some may find unsettling. Also, if the patient or client is uncomfortable with the music therapy experience, it may cause anxiety or dissatisfaction. And sometimes, as in people with cognitive impairment, listening to music results in overstimulation and confusion.

RESEARCH FINDINGS

Music Therapy May Be Useful for Pregnant Women in Labor

In a trial published in 2018 in the journal *Complementary Therapies in Clinical Practice*, researchers from Turkey wanted to learn if music therapy would be useful for labor pains and anxiety among women having their first baby. Twenty-five women were placed in the music therapy group and 25 in the control group. The sociodemographic characteristics of the two groups were similar, and both groups of women had "very high levels of fear" concerning labor. The women in the music therapy group were asked if they would like to listen to music; none of the women refused. All of the women noted that they liked listening to music. Music was played during the active phase of the labor. Different assessments were conducted. The researchers found that the women who listened to music had lower levels of pain. In fact, after the first hour of labor, the women listening to music had statistically less pain, and their labors progressed faster. Interestingly, when the women who listened to music were asked if the music helped their pain, 88 percent noted that it was "partially effective" and 12 percent said that it was "not effective." The researchers concluded that "musicotherapy, a non-pharmacological method is an effective, simple and economical method" that helps women dealing with labor.[1]

In a systematic review and meta-analysis published in 2019 in the *Journal of Advanced Nursing*, researchers from Taiwan and Oklahoma (USA) examined randomized controlled trials or quasi-experimental trials on the use of music therapy on primiparous women in labor. The cohort consisted of five studies with 197 women in music therapy groups and 195 women in control groups; all of the studies were conducted in Asia, and they all applied a visual analog scale to measure the pain. However, they used different types of music therapy, and there was the potential for "treatment effect bias." In addition, in these studies, music was administered by physicians and nurses rather than certified music therapists, and the methodological quality of the studies was not high. Pain measurements were taken before and after music therapy and routine care or routine care alone. The researchers learned that music therapy lowered labor pain levels, but the results were not statistically significant. The researchers concluded that "music intervention may prove an effective intervention for the management of pain and anxiety for primiparous women during labour."[2]

Music Therapy May Help People with Chronic Pain

In a systematic review and meta-analysis published in 2017 in the journal *Pain Medicine*, researchers from Mexico and Denmark examined the use of music therapy as an adjuvant for chronic pain. The researchers identified 14 randomized, controlled trials that met their criteria; the trials used any type of music therapy, such as active music playing or the more passive listening to music. The mean music duration in the included studies was 30 minutes. Eleven trials investigated pain reduction as a primary outcome, and three assessed pain as a secondary outcome. The trials ranged in size between 25 and 200 subjects; there were a total of 1,178 subjects. The mean age of the included subjects was 55 years, and their mean length of pain condition was 7.3 years. The majority of the trials had subjects with pain from cancer or fibromyalgia, but the causes of pain also included palliative care, osteoarthritis, multiple sclerosis, chronic nonmalignant pain, and inflammatory bowel disease. Seven of the 11 trials with recorded music used headphones for delivery, and the others used CD players. The types of music varied widely, including Chinese classical music, Swedish songs, Taiwanese folk songs, jazz, pop, and classical Western music. The quality of the studies was considered adequate, and they had an overall low risk of bias. The researchers learned that music therapy moderately reduced levels of chronic pain. Furthermore, "the analgesic effects of music were greater for patient-chosen than researcher-chosen music." In all of the reviewed studies, music therapy reduced pain, "and, in general, these effects were significant."[3]

Music Therapy May Help Manage Pain in Adult Intensive Care Units

In systematic review and meta-analysis published in 2020 in the *Journal of Pain and Symptom Management*, researchers from Canada and Minnesota (USA) examined the ability of music therapy to reduce pain in adult patients in intensive care units (ICUs). The researchers located 18 randomized, controlled trials with a total of 1,173 subjects who met their criteria for a qualitative synthesis. Ten studies were included in the meta-analysis. The 18 trials were mostly in English, but some were in German,

Spanish, Portuguese, French, Greek, Turkish, and Chinese. Sample sizes ranged from 17 to 156, and the subjects had a mean age of 60 years, with 60 percent being male and 40 percent female. Eight studies had subjects who had cardiac surgeries, four studies had subjects with various types of surgeries, and five had subjects with a variety of medical diagnoses. Although 15 studies had subjects who could communicate, 3 studies had subjects who were unable to communicate. Eight trials reported low mean baseline pain scores, and five reported moderate pain scores. The types of music interventions varied widely across the trials. For example, the music interventions ranged from 10 to 90 minutes, with most administering music for 30 minutes. In 5 trials, the same music was used for all subjects, whereas in the other 13 trials, the subjects had a choice of at least two selections. Interestingly, eight subjects in three trials were so dissatisfied with the music that they withdrew from their studies. The music was usually delivered by headphones or earphones. The researchers determined that, when compared to standard care and noise reduction, music was "significantly efficacious" in reducing pain scores, and no adverse effects were reported. Twenty to 30 minutes of music intervention "can decrease pain by almost two points on a 0–10 scale for ICU adults able to self-report."[4]

Music Therapy May Benefit Intensive Care Patients in Many Ways, Including Pain Management

In a clinical trial published in 2019 in the *American Journal of Critical Care*, researchers from Virginia and California (USA) wanted to learn if music therapy would benefit patients in a medical-surgical intensive care unit in a suburban community hospital. A total of 52 English-speaking adults were recruited to participate in the trial; the most common diagnoses were ST-elevation myocardial infarction (classic heart attack), cardiac arrest, gastrointestinal bleeding, respiratory failure, renal failure, and stroke. Forty of the patients were white, and 33 were female. The median age was 62 years. Participants were offered a single, 30-minute music therapy session with a board-certified music therapist. Nearly half of the patients had been in the ICU for only one day when they received the therapy. Before and after the session, the therapist recorded vital signs and assessed levels of pain and anxiety. The researchers learned that reductions in pain were achieved after the music sessions. The researchers concluded that "the presence of a music therapist, who can tailor an intervention to the patient's immediate physiological and psychological needs, may be an important variable in the differential effects of these interventions."[5]

Music Therapy May Be Useful for People Having Spine Surgery

In a trial published in 2017 in the *American Journal of Orthopedics* (Belle Mead, New Jersey), researchers from New York City wanted to determine if music therapy would help people recovering from spine surgery. It is well known that patients recovering from spine surgery tend to have a good deal of pain. The cohort consisted of 60 patients (35 females and 25 males) who had anterior, posterior, or anterior-posterior spinal fusions; they ranged in age from 40 to 55 years. The patients received either music therapy plus standard care ($n = 30$) or standard care alone ($n = 30$). Patients in the music therapy group received one 30-minute music therapy session during an 8-hour period within 72 hours after surgery. For both groups, measurements were taken before and after the study window. After completion of the postintervention surveys, the control patients were offered music therapy. Also, the patients in both groups were given the option of receiving follow-up music therapy for the remainder of their hospital stay. The researchers learned that music therapy was significantly beneficial in reducing pain levels. Other measurable benefits included "increased comfort, reduced pain, improved gait, increased range of motion, endurance, and ability to relax."[6]

Music Therapy May Help People Having All Types of Surgery

In a systematic review and meta-analysis published in 2018 in the *British Journal of Surgery*, researchers from the Netherlands and Boston, Massachusetts (USA), evaluated the use of music therapy for the pain and anxiety associated with different types of surgery in different types of populations. The researchers located 92 randomized, controlled trials (7385 subjects) that were included in their systematic review; 81 of these trials were included in their meta-analysis. The subjects in the trials had a mean age of 51.7 years, and 57 percent of the subjects were female. Music therapy was offered at various times, such as before surgery, during surgery, after surgery, or multiple times. Sometimes, no specific time frames were noted.

The included studies had a moderate to high risk of bias, and many studies did not adequately address methodological considerations. Still, the researchers learned that music therapy before, during, or after surgery statistically reduced levels of pain. However, the most reduction in pain was seen in the postoperative delivery of music. The researchers noted that their findings "provide evidence for the implementation of music interventions before, during and after surgery." Why is this so important? "Pain relief after surgery continues to be an important medical challenge."[7]

Music Therapy May Be Useful for People Having a Nasal Bone Fracture Reduction Procedure

In a randomized, controlled trial published in 2019 in the journal *Otolaryngology—Head and Neck Surgery*, researchers from Chile wanted to determine if music therapy would reduce the pain and anxiety associated with nasal bone fracture reduction, a painful procedure performed under local anesthesia. In the United States, nasal fractures have an incidence of 53.2 out of 100,000 people, and they are most common in men between the ages of 20 and 40 years. The cohort consisted of 36 patients; there were 25 men and 11 women, with a median age of 30.5 years. The median time from the initial face trauma to the reduction procedure was 10.7 days. Seventeen patients received music therapy through headphones before, during, and after their procedures, and 19 did not. No adverse effects were observed in either of the groups. The researchers learned that the patients in the music group had lower pain scores, "showing a positive effect of the use of music for this procedure." They also concluded that "music therapy appears to be an easy-to apply, widely available, and safe tool to improve the care of patients who undergo this procedure."[8]

Music Therapy May Help Manage the Discomfort and Pain Associated with a Colonoscopy

In a randomized, controlled trial published in 2020 in *Complementary Therapies in Clinical Practice*, researchers from Turkey investigated the ability of music therapy to help with the discomfort and pain associated with a colonoscopy, a procedure used to view the entire large intestine. The trial was conducted between October 15, 2015, and September 16, 2016, in the endoscopy unit of the general surgical clinics of a hospital located in the west of Turkey. The cohort consisted of 112 patients; there were 56 in the music therapy group and 56 in the control group. The patients in the music therapy group had 30 minutes of music therapy during their colonoscopies; the patients in the control group only had their colonoscopies. The same researchers performed all of the procedures; the data were collected before, during, and after the colonoscopy. The researchers determined that music therapy during the colonoscopy reduced pain and anxiety and increased comfort. "Since music therapy is an inexpensive, simple, noninvasive, and nonpharmacological method without any side effects, it might be used as an adjunct to analgesics and sedatives for patients undergoing colonoscopy."[9]

Music Therapy May or May Not Help People with the Pain after Cardiac Surgery

In a review published in 2019 in the journal *Interactive CardioVascular and Thoracic Surgery*, researchers from the United Kingdom wanted to learn if postoperative treatment with music therapy would help people dealing with the pain and anxiety of cardiac surgery. The researchers located seven studies that met their criteria; six of these were randomized trials. The specific music therapy protocols varied widely, ranging from one postoperative session given the day after surgery to several music therapies per day for a 72-hour period of time. Most of the therapies involved relaxing music. Four studies found that music therapy resulted in a statistically significant reduction in pain. However, in only one of these studies did the music therapy result in a statistically significant reduction in the opioid medication requirement. Moreover, the number of subjects in each of the studies was small, ranging from only 19 to 50 subjects, with a mean of 33 subjects in the intervention groups. The researchers concluded that there was insufficient evidence to support the use of music therapy after cardiac surgery. "The current best available evidence fails to support the benefits of music therapy as an effective non-pharmacological option in reducing pain and anxiety following open-heart surgery."[10]

Live Music May or May Not Reduce the Distress and Pain Associated with Wound Care Treatments for Burns in Children

In a randomized, assessor-blinded, controlled trial published in 2018 in the journal *Burns*, researchers from the Netherlands, South Africa, and

Boston, Massachusetts (USA), examined the ability of live music therapy to ease the distress and pain associated with wound care treatments for burns in children. The trial took place at the burns unit of a children's hospital in Cape Town, South Africa. It included newly admitted children, no older than 13 years, with a median age of 22.6 months, who were having their first or second wound care procedure. Most of the burns were scalds. Twenty-three patients were older than five years and eligible to report distress and pain. The cohort consisted of 135 children. Seventy-one children received the three- to five-minute live music interventions after the wound care procedure; 64 were controls and received only wound care. Assessments were conducted by independent researchers. Three different music therapists offered the therapy. The researchers learned that the distress and pain scores were not significantly different between the music and control groups. However, in a "small group" of children over five years old, the scores were lower for those in the music group. These children "seemed to have benefited from this intervention."[11]

NOTES

1. Gokyildiz Surucu, Sule, Melike Ozturk, Burcu Avcibay Vurgec, et al. "The Effect of Music on Pain and Anxiety of Women during Labour on First Time Pregnancy: A Study from Turkey." *Complementary Therapies in Clinical Practice* 30 (February 2018): 96–102.

2. Chuang, Ching-Hui, Po-Cheng Chen, ChihChen Sophia Lee, et al. "Music Intervention for Pain and Anxiety Management of the Primiparous Women During Labour: A Systematic Review and Meta-Analysis." *Journal of Advanced Nursing* 75, no. 4 (April 2019): 723–733.

3. Garza-Villarreal, Eduardo A., Victor Pando, Peter Vuust, and Christine Parsons. "Music-Induced Analgesia in Chronic Pain Conditions: A Systematic Review and Meta-Analysis." *Pain Physician* 20 (2017): 597–610.

4. Richard-Lalonde, Melissa, Céline Gélinas, Madalina Boitor, et al. "The Effect of Music on Pain in the Adult Intensive Care Unit: A Systematic Review of Randomized Controlled Trials." *Journal of Pain and Symptom Management* 59, no. 6 (June 2020): 1304–1319.e6.

5. Golino, Amanda J., Raymond Leone, Audra Gollenberg, et al. "Impact of An Active Music Therapy Intervention on Intensive Care Patients." *American Journal of Critical Care* 28, no. 1 (January 2019): 48–55.

6. Moondanaro, John F., Peter Homel, Baron Lonner, et al. "Music Therapy Increases Comfort and Reduces Pain in Patients Recovering from

Spine Surgery." *American Journal of Orthopedics* (Belle Mead, New Jersey) 46, no. 1 (January–February 2017): E13–E22.

7. Kühlmann, A. Y. R., A. de Rooij, L. F. Kroese, et al. "Meta-Analysis Evaluating Music Interventions for Anxiety and Pain in Surgery." *British Journal of Surgery* 105, no. 7 (June 2018): 773–783.

8. Ortega, Alvaro, Felipe Gauna, Daniel Munoz, et al. "Music Therapy for Pin and Anxiety Management Nasal Bone Fracture Reduction: Randomized Controlled Clinical Trial." *Otolaryngology—Head and Neck Surgery* 161, no. 4 (October 2019): 613–619.

9. Çelebi, Dilruba, Emel Yilmaz, Semra Tutcu Şahin, and Hakan Baydur. "The Effect of Music Therapy During Colonoscopy on Pain, Anxiety and Patient Comfort: A Randomized Controlled Trial." *Complementary Therapies in Clinical Practice* 38 (2020): 101084.

10. Grafton-Clarke, Ciaran, Laura Grace, and Amer Harky. "Music Therapy following Cardiac Surgery—Is It an Effective Method to Reduce Pain and Anxiety?" *Interactive CardioVascular and Thoracic Surgery* 28 (2019): 722–727.

11. van der Heijden, Marianne J. E., Johannes Jeekel, Heinz Rode, et al. "Can Live Music Therapy Reduce Distress and Pain in Children with Burns after Wound Care Procedures? A Randomized Controlled Trial." *Burns* 44, no. 4 (June 2018): 823–833.

REFERENCES AND FURTHER READINGS

Çelebi, Dilruba, Emel Yilmaz, Semra Tutcu Şahin, and Hakan Baydur. "The Effect of Music Therapy during Colonoscopy on Pain, Anxiety and Patient Comfort: A Randomized Controlled Trial." *Complementary Therapies in Clinical Practice* 38 (2020): 101084.

Chuang, Ching-Hui, Po-Cheng Chen, ChihChen Sophia Lee, et al. "Music Intervention for Pain and Anxiety Management of the Primiparous Women during Labour: A Systematic Review and Meta-Analysis." *Journal of Advance Nursing* 75, no 4 (April 2019): 723–733.

Garza-Villarreal, Eduardo A., Victor Pando, Peter Vuust, and Christine Parsons. "Music-Induced Analgesia in Chronic Pain Conditions: A Systematic Review and Meta-Analysis." *Pain Physician* 20 (2017): 597–610.

Gokyildiz Surucu, Sule, Melike Oztruk, Burcu Avcibay Vurgec, et al. "The Effect of Music on Pain and Anxiety of Women during Labour on

First Time Pregnancy: A Study From Turkey." *Complementary Therapies in Clinical Practice* 30 (February 2018): 96–102.

Golino, Amanda J., Raymond Leone, Audra Gollenberg, et al. "Impact of an Active Music Therapy Intervention on Intensive Care Patients." *American Journal of Intensive Care* 28, no. 1 (January 2019): 48–55.

Grafton-Clarke, Ciaran, Laura Grace, and Amer Harky. "Music Therapy following Cardiac Surgery—Is It an Effective Method to Reduce Pain and Anxiety?" *Interactive CardioVascular and Thoracic Surgery* 28 (2019): 722–727.

Kühlmann, A. Y. R., A. de Rooij, L. F. Kroese, et al. "Meta-Analysis Evaluating Music Interventions for Anxiety and Pain in Surgery." *British Journal of Surgery* 105, no. 7 (June 2018): 773–783.

Mondanaro, John F., Peter Homel, Baron Lonner, et al. "Music Therapy Increases Comfort and Reduces Pain in Patients Recovering from Spine Surgery." *American Journal of Orthopedics* (Belle Mead, New Jersey) 46, no. 1 (January–February 2017): E13–E22.

Ortega, Alvaro, Felipe Gauna, Daniel Munoz, et al. "Music Therapy for Pain and Anxiety Management Nasal Bone Fracture Reduction: Randomized Controlled Clinical Trial." *Otolaryngology—Head and Neck Surgery* 161, no. 4 (October 2019): 613–619.

Richard-Lalonde, Melissa, Céline Gélinas, Madalina Boitor, et al. "The Effect of Music on Pain in the Adult Intensive Care Unit: A Systematic Review of Randomized Controlled Trials." *Journal of Pain and Symptom Management* 59, no. 6 (June 2020): 1304–1319.e6.

Van der Heijden, Marianne J. E., Johannes Jeekel, Heinz Rode, et al. "Can Live Music Therapy Reduce Distress and Pain in Children with Burns after Wound Care Procedures? A Randomized Controlled Trial." *Burns* 44, no. 4 (June 2018): 823–833.

Myofascial Release, Foam Rolling, and Structural Integration

INTRODUCTION

Also known as myofascial therapy and trigger point therapy, myofascial release is a form of physical therapy that is used to treat pain, specifically myofascial pain, or the pain associated with the strong membranes—the fascia—that wrap, connect, surround, and support the muscles throughout the body. Generally, the pain originates from specific hypersensitive points within myofascial tissues, called "trigger points." Myofascial release focuses on reducing pain by easing tension and tightness in the trigger points. As it is often hard to locate pain to a specific trigger point, myofascial release is generally used over a wider area of muscles and tissues.

Practitioners trained in myofascial release are able to detect myofascial areas that are tense and stiff and apply the appropriate amount of sustained pressure. These areas are not necessarily near the source of the pain. Though the exact elements of myofascial release vary slightly from practitioner to practitioner, the gentle, sustained pressure that they exert elongates muscles and reduces the pain.

With foam rolling, a type of myofascial release, people place their own body mass on a foam roller. That process exerts pressure on soft tissue, which stretches soft tissue and generates friction. Foam rolling may be considered a type of self-massage. The pressure that the foam roller exerts on the muscles is similar to the pressure during a massage by a professional massage therapist. Though it may be a little uncomfortable, foam rolling helps the body heal.

Created by biochemist Ida Pauline Rolf, PhD (1896–1979), rolfing is a therapy that involves manipulation of the soft tissue and movement education. According to rolfing, which may be referred to as structural integration or rolfing structural integration, fascia tightens around an injury and remains rigid, even after the injury heals. This rigidity causes pain and discomfort. Rolfing manually separates, loosens, and relieves the fascia, thus releasing tension patterns and realigning the legs, torso, shoulders, arms, and head. Once this occurs, the body's natural mechanisms take over and correct the remaining imbalances. In response to the negative forces of gravity on the body, rolfing attempts to improve human biomechanical functioning as a whole, rather than to treat individual symptoms.

Though there is no way to know how many people practice myofascial release, foam rolling, and rolfing, one may assume it is somewhat popular, at least among those who practice complementary and integrative medicine and health care.

ADMINISTRATION AND REGULATION

Myofascial release sessions tend to take place in office settings. Many different professionals may include this practice in their treatment plans. These include osteopathic physicians, chiropractors, physical therapists, occupational therapists, sports medicine and injury specialists, and massage therapists. Most insurance plans probably do not cover the cost of myofascial release alone. However, there is a good chance that it will be covered when combined with another medical visit, such as a visit to a chiropractor or physical therapist. Costs vary widely and are a direct result of the training of the professional; the area of the country; and the specific city, suburban, or rural location.

During a myofascial release treatment, the practitioner feels for tightened areas and gently massages and stretches the fascia. Light manual pressure, but more than is typically used in massage, is then applied on trigger points and surrounding areas and repeated multiple times. The goal is to reduce tension throughout the body, a process that may be slightly uncomfortable. Treatments are performed directly on the skin, without oils or creams.

There are no myofascial release regulations, and while there are a number of certification programs, certification is not required. Myofascial programs tend to be offered at massage and healing arts schools.

When first beginning a foam rolling regimen, it may be desirable to ask for instruction during a visit with a physical therapist or personal trainer. Although a visit with a physical therapist may be covered by insurance, in all probability, a visit with a personal trainer is not. Still, some personal training assistance may be available to people who belong to a gym. If cost is an issue, it is best to check before scheduling an appointment. Most people will probably not receive individual instruction. For them, there are a host of different online videos. There are even foam-rolling online classes. It is a good idea to watch videos made by those with experience in their respective fields.

Normally, foam rollers are cylindrical in shape and made of dense foam. However, they may be found in a range of sizes and in various levels of firmness. Smooth rollers have an even, dense foam surface; textured rollers, which have ridges and knobs, are used for deeper penetration. Foam-covered massage sticks are good for deep massage in the back and legs, and foam massage balls are used for targeted muscle areas, such as knots in the shoulders. It may take a little trial and error to find the right foam roller. Beginners should start with a softer roller and work their way up to a denser one. In some instances, sales personnel at a sporting store may be a resource.

Though there are no regulations regarding foam rolling, it is a good idea to follow these guidelines. Always start with light pressure. At first, slowly roll tender areas for 10 seconds. Work up to 30 to 60 seconds. Sore spots may require a few minutes of foam rolling. After completing a routine, be sure to hydrate properly.

During a rolfing session, which takes place in an office setting, the practitioner systematically addresses areas of strain, misalignment, and restricted movement. After a brief assessment, a typical rolfing session will last for about 75 minutes. Ideally, people should wear a straight-strap sports top and shorts, and they should expect to move on and off the treatment table to standing or seated positions. Rolfing pressure ranges from light to very deep. Techniques vary according to the needs of the individual clients. Practitioners tend to recommend 10 sessions, spaced one week apart.

There do not appear to be any national rolfing regulations, but there may well be individual state requirements, and certification programs are available. Probably the best-known program is offered by the Dr. Ida Rolf Institute in Boulder, Colorado. There is no way to know how many people provide myofascial release, foam rolling, and rolfing, and prices vary by the location and type and training of the practitioner. Expect to spend at least $100 or more per session, and do not assume these treatments are covered by insurers; it is always a good idea to check.

BENEFITS AND RISKS

Myofascial release appears to be particularly useful for people with myofascial pain syndrome, a persistent pain disorder caused by sensitivity and tightness in myofascial tissues. People with chronic headaches may also benefit; the gentle massaging of the neck and head may bring relief. Those with venous insufficiency, a painful condition in which blood collects in the deep veins of the legs, may also obtain help. Likewise, myofascial release is said to be useful for back pain, neck pain, fibromyalgia, repetitive strain injuries, and muscular imbalances.

People with burns, injuries, painful wounds, fractures, fragile or weak bones, deep-vein thrombosis, malignancy, aneurysm, acute rheumatoid arthritis, advanced diabetes, severe osteoporosis, or those taking blood-thinning medications should avoid myofascial release. In very rare instances, myofascial release has been associated with bleeding, temporary paralysis, or difficulty with moving muscles.

Foam rolling may help relieve muscle tightness, soreness, inflammation, and increase the range of motion. Foam rolling appears to be useful for back pain, back tension, and symptoms associated with fibromyalgia, such as pain. Foam rolling breaks up adhesions and scar tissue that prevent muscles from working properly. Many people advise spending a little time foam rolling both before and after a workout. They suggest that people who incorporate foam rolling into their regular workouts tend to have less soreness.

Foam rolling is generally considered safe for most people. However, some people should avoid foam rolling, such as those dealing with a torn muscle or a broken bone. Also, people should not roll over small joints, such as the joints in the knees, elbows, and ankles, which may cause you to hyperextend or damage them.

When performed by a skilled practitioner, rolfing is believed to be safe and effective. It may help people recover from injuries, deal with chronic pain, reduce tingling or numbness, and perform better and hurt less. Any risks associated with rolfing tend to be minimal. Side effects include respiratory symptoms, headaches, soreness, swelling, minor bruising, or nausea. People with circulatory problems, cardiopulmonary disease, musculoskeletal disease, neurological problems, or high levels of psychological stress should check with a medical provider before visiting a rolfing practitioner. Following a rolfing session, be sure to hydrate properly.

RESEARCH FINDINGS

Myofascial Release Appears to Help People with Neck Pain

In a single-blind, randomized, controlled trial published in 2018 in the *American Journal of Physical Medicine & Rehabilitation*, researchers from Spain investigated the usefulness of myofascial release for neck pain.

The cohort consisted of 41 subjects with neck pain who were outpatients at local clinics. Twenty-one subjects were assigned to receive five myofascial sessions over a two-week period of time; 21 subjects were assigned to receive 10 physical therapy sessions, also during a two-week period of time. All of the subjects completed the treatment and the end-of-trial evaluation. One subject in the physical therapy group did not complete the one-month follow-up evaluation. The researchers learned that although the subjects in both groups had improvements in pain, the subjects in the myofascial group experienced a 20 percent greater improvement than the subjects in the physical therapy group. However, because the results were short term, the researchers underscored that the findings "should be interpreted with caution."[1]

Myofascial Release Seems to Be Useful for Chronic Low Back Pain

In a double-blind, randomized, parallel sham, controlled trial published in 2017 in the journal *Spine*, researchers from Spain evaluated the ability of myofascial release to provide relief to people with nonspecific low back pain. The cohort consisted of 54 subjects with chronic low back pain; all of the subjects were between the ages of 18 and 60 years. Twenty-seven subjects (mean age 46.6 years) received four myofascial release treatments, twice a week for two weeks; each session lasted 40 minutes. The other 27 subjects (mean age 46.4 years) received the same treatment schedule, only with sham myofascial release. Pain assessments were conducted at baseline, at the end of the treatments, and at a 12-week follow-up. Although the researchers did not observe differences in pain between the two groups after the treatments, at the 12-week follow-up, the myofascial release group had significantly lower levels of pain. The researchers cautioned that "larger sample size trials are necessary to support the clinical relevance of MFR [myofascial release] as an isolated technique, or its usefulness as a complement of other forms of physiotherapy treatment."[2]

In a systematic review and meta-analysis published in 2021 in the journal *Frontiers in Medicine*, researchers from China also evaluated the use of myofascial release for chronic low back pain. They included eight randomized controlled trials with 375 subjects. There were 187 subjects in the myofascial groups and 188 subjects in the control groups; 212 were female, and 163 were male. Mean age ranged from 24 to 74 years. The trials were conducted in six countries: Brazil, India, Italy, Korea, Spain, and Turkey. In all of the trials, myofascial release was the primary intervention. The researchers learned that myofascial release significantly improved the pain and physical functioning of people with chronic low back pain. However, it appeared to have no significant effect on other aspects such as balance function, pain pressure threshold, and trunk mobility. Still, the researchers were able to include only eight trials that tended to be low quality. "More and more rigorously designed RCTs [randomized controlled trials] should be included in the future to verify these conclusions."[3]

Myofascial Release May or May Not Help Chronic Musculoskeletal Pain

In a systematic review and meta-analysis published in 2018 in the journal *Clinical Rehabilitation*, researchers wanted to determine the utility of myofascial release for chronic musculoskeletal pain. They located eight randomized controlled trials that met their criteria. Two trials focused on lateral epicondylitis (n = 95), also known as "tennis elbow"; two focused on fibromyalgia (n = 145); three dealt with low back pain (152); and one addressed on heel pain (n = 65), for a total of 457 subjects. The risk of bias was deemed low in three trials and high in five trials. The duration of therapy was 30 to 90 minutes, 4 to 24 times, during 2 to 20 weeks. The trials came from three countries and five research groups. Three of the trials were conducted in the outpatient clinic of a myofascial therapy and research foundation, two samples involved members of a fibromyalgia association, one sample was gathered in a physiotherapy outpatient department, and two were from tertiary outpatient clinics. The control procedures included sham myofascial release, sham ultrasound, and sham magnetotherapy. Two trials addressed adding myofascial release to manual or physiotherapy. While the authors of each of the trials concluded that myofascial release was an effective treatment for pain, the researchers found the evidence to be "scarce and inconsistent." They maintained that only three low-quality trials had short-term improvement, either in pain or functioning, and the other five trials did not have clinically significant differences between the intervention and the controls. Only three of the trials had credible control groups enabling the differentiation between myofascial release and manual touching. And, the researchers concluded that the "current evidence on myofascial release therapy is not sufficient to warrant this treatment in chronic musculoskeletal pain."[4]

Foam Rolling Appears to Help Hip Osteoarthritis Pain

In a retrospective propensity-matched cohort study published online in 2020 in the journal *Physiotherapy Theory and Practice* researchers from Japan evaluated the use of foam rolling for the pain associated with hip osteoarthritis. The initial cohort consisted of 115 subjects with hip osteoarthritis and pain around the hip joint for at least three months; all of the subjects were outpatients between January 2017 and March 2019 who received instructions on home exercise programs. Based on these home exercises, the subjects were divided into foam-rolling or non-foam-rolling groups. The subjects in the foam-rolling group had been told to perform foam rolling for more than 10 minutes once per day. After the researchers completed propensity-score matching for both groups, there were 37 well-matched subjects in each group. The researchers learned that the subjects in both groups had significant improvements in pain levels. However, the subjects in the foam-rolling group had better improvements in hip pain, physical function, and quality of life than those in the non-foam-rolling group. Further, the hip pain "improved more effectively" in the foam-rolling group. The researchers concluded that foam rolling "is an effective intervention for hip pain in patients at all stages of hip osteoarthritis, and could therefore become a new conservative therapy for these patients."[5]

Foam Rolling Seems to Help Delayed-Onset Muscle Soreness

In a controlled study published in 2015 in the *Journal of Athletic Training*, researchers from Canada and Australia examined the ability of foam rolling to help with the discomfort following an intense exercise protocol, a problem known as delayed-onset muscle soreness, that is characterized by variable amounts of muscle tenderness, stiffness, and pain. The cohort consisted of eight healthy physically active males, who were recreational resistance trainers, with an average age of 22.1 years. Before participating, they completed a physical activity readiness questionnaire. The subjects performed two protocols, separated by four weeks, involving 10 sets of 10 repetitions of back squats at 60 percent of their single-repetition maximum, followed by either no foam rolling or 20 minutes of foam rolling, immediately, after 24 hours, and after 48 hours. Beginning 24 hours before the trial and throughout the trial, the subjects were told to refrain from heavy exercise. The researchers learned that foam rolling enhanced recovery and reduced physical performance "decrements" (or losses) after the exercise protocol. Specifically, when compared to the controls, foam rolling resulted in an increased pressure-pain threshold. The researchers concluded that "this form of self-induced massage could benefit athletes seeking a recovery modality that is relatively affordable, easy to perform, and time efficient and that enhances muscular recovery."[6]

Foam Rolling Is Useful for Recovery after Exercise Induced Muscle Damage

In a trial published in 2019 in the *Journal of Sports Science and Medicine*, researchers from Spain compared the effects of vibration and nonvibration foam rolling on recovery after exercise induced muscle damage. Thirty-eight healthy volunteers (32 men and 6 women), with an average age of 22.2 years, were randomly assigned to a vibration or nonvibration foam-rolling group. All of the subjects were considered active and free from musculoskeletal disorders, and both groups had no significant differences in age, height, weight, adipose tissue thickness, and training days per week. The subjects, who abstained from any unaccustomed exercise, medications, and dietary supplements for 72 hours before baseline, used a gravity-free training device flywheel to perform a 10 × 10 (sets and repetitions) eccentric squat protocol to induce muscle damage. The administration of foam rolling was the same for both groups, except that one included a roller with vibration. After conducting a variety of assessments, and the researchers determined that the subjects in both groups made substantial improvements in a variety of factors, including pain tolerance. However, vibrating foam rolling appeared to be better for short-term pain perception and passive hip extension range of motion. The researchers cautioned that further studies are "needed to deepen our understanding of the effects of this combination of techniques."[7]

In a trial published in 2020 in the *International Journal of Sports Physical Therapy*, researchers from Salem, Massachusetts (USA), also studied the use of foam rolling to improve recovery after exercise-induced muscle damage. The cohort consisted of 40 subjects; the subjects performed 40 15-meter sprints, designed to induce muscle damage. Nineteen of the subjects, between the ages of 19 and 38 years, completed the foam-rolling protocol, and 21 subjects between the ages of 19 and 30 years served as controls (and did not complete the foam-rolling protocol). The foam-rolling protocol consisted of six foam-rolling movements that targeted four sections of the thigh. Each roll was timed to the tempo of a metronome. In addition to other assessments, levels of muscle soreness of the quadriceps, hamstrings, gluteus maximus, and gastrocnemius muscles were measured. The researchers determined that, when compared to the controls, foam rolling appeared to reduce the perceptions of muscle soreness. However, the results were variable. Some subjects obtained no or minimal effects, whereas others obtained far more notable results. And, the researchers concluded that "foam rolling may be useful for reducing soreness following damaging exercise."[8]

Foam Rolling after Exercise May Impact Pain Perception

In a systematic review and meta-analysis published in 2019 in the journal *Frontiers in Physiology*, researchers from Germany and Australia evaluated the use of pre-exercise and postexercise foam rolling for a number of factors including muscle pain. They also compared the use of a foam roller to a foam massager. The researchers located 21 studies that met their criteria; 14 of these studies used pre-exercise foam rolling as an exercise warm-up routine, and seven used postexercise foam rolling to enhance recovery. In total, there were 454 subjects; none of the studies was considered to be of high risk for bias, except for a high risk of placebo bias. While pre-exercise rolling did not appear to have any notable impact on pain, postexercise rolling reduced muscle pain perception. In one study, a researcher found that the use of postexercise rolling reduced muscle pain in 66 percent of the subjects. Such a reduction is important, as it may affect a person's readiness to participate in physical activity. Though the comparison between foam roller and foam massagers tended to be inconclusive, it did appear that the use of postexercise rolling with foam rollers was more effective than postexercise rolling with foam massagers. Still, the researchers did not discount the use of pre-exercise rolling for pain. "As psychological aspects play an important role in most sports, the fact that an athlete feels less pain after pre-rolling might be sufficient to justify its use despite the absence of measurable physiological benefits."[9]

Rolfing Appears to Reduce Back Pain

In a trial published in 2017 in *The Journal of Physical Therapy Science*, researchers from Austria assessed the ability of rolfing to help people with back pain. The cohort consisted of 19 females and 17 males, with a mean age of 37.9 years. All of the subjects had nonspecific back pain, and only two subjects were not normally active. Eighteen subjects were assigned to receive rolfing, and 18 participated in a physical exercise program known as Fascial Fitness. The 60-minute rolfing sessions were held once weekly for three weeks; the 60-minute fitness classes were also once weekly for three weeks. During the study, the subjects were advised to avoid additional medical or therapeutic treatments. Still, five subjects in each group performed extra back exercise routines. Sixteen subjects in the rolfing group and 17 in the fitness group completed the trial. Using standard questionnaires, the subjects were asked about their pain levels at baseline and when the trial ended. While the subjects in the fitness group experienced a "trend toward improvement," the subjects in the rolfing group achieved significant reductions in pain. The researchers concluded that "the therapeutic technique of structural integration can reduce back pain."[10]

Rolfing Seems to Significantly Help People with Fibromyalgia

In a trial published in 2014 in the journal *Revista Dor*, researchers from Brazil investigated the usefulness of rolfing for the pain associated with fibromyalgia. The cohort consisted of 30 female patients with neurologist-diagnosed fibromyalgia. Although the patients had been under conventional treatment for at least one year, they had not improved. All of the subjects had 10 30-minute rolfing sessions, and they were evaluated at baseline, at the end of their treatments, and three months after the trial ended. Before the treatments, the vast majority of the women reported "unbearable" levels of pain. By the time the treatments ended, the women were markedly improved, and improvements were still evident at the three-month follow-up. In fact, rolfing had a statistically significant effect on pain intensity. The researchers commented that rolfing "has contributed to the recovery of fibromyalgia patients."[11]

Patients with Chronic Nonspecific Low Back Pain May or May Not Benefit from Adding Rolfing to Outpatient Rehabilitation

In a randomized clinical trial published in 2015 in the journal *Evidence-Based Complementary and Alternative Medicine*, researchers from several cities in Massachusetts and Burlington, Vermont (USA), evaluated the addition of rolfing to outpatient rehabilitation for people with chronic nonspecific low back pain. The cohort consisted of 46 Boston-area outpatients with chronic nonspecific low back pain. Twenty-three people were assigned to receive both rolfing and rehabilitation, and 23 received only rehabilitation. The rehabilitation sessions varied, but they were generally one-half to one hour in duration and were held twice weekly for four to six weeks. The subjects in the combined therapy group also received 10 one-hour rolfing sessions. Five subjects were lost to a 20-week follow-up. Any adverse events were deemed mild to moderate, and all were self-limiting. Even though levels of disability improved in the combination group, the researchers learned that there were no significant differences in pain levels between the two groups. Further research should center on comparing rolfing alone to outpatient rehabilitation alone, and "that a direct comparison of the two could control for tine, attention, and cutaneous stimulation across treatment groups."[12]

Rolfing May Help People with Cervical Spine Dysfunction

In a retrospective trial published in 2009 in the *Journal of Bodywork and Movement Therapies*, researchers investigated the usefulness of rolfing for people with cervical spine dysfunction. The cohort consisted of 31 subjects; there were 25 females and 6 males between the ages of 22 and 66 years. They all had 10 rolfing sessions for their symptoms associated with cervical spine dysfunction, such as neck pain and stiffness. The subjects were evaluated before and after they received their sessions. Their medical records revealed that they were treated by other health practitioners, such as chiropractors and acupuncturists, before their rolfing sessions. Sixteen subjects assessed their pain on a scale of 0 to 10, and 15 assessed their pain on a scale of 0 to 5. The researchers learned that the rolfing sessions resulted in lower levels of pain and increased range of neck movement. Also, rolfing appeared to improve pain more effectively in people between the ages of 52 and 66 years than in those 22 to 49 years. "The mean values for pain at best, worst, and now were reduced."[13]

NOTES

1. Rodríguez-Huguet, Manuel, José Luis Gil-Salú, Pablo Rodríguez-Huguet, et al. "Effects of Myofascial Release on Pressure Pain Thresholds in Patients with Neck Pain: A Single-Blind Randomized Controlled Trial." *American Journal of Physical Medicine & Rehabilitation* 97, no. 1 (January 2018): 16–22.

2. Arguisuelas, María D., Juan Francisco Lisón, Daniel Sánchez-Zuriaga, et al. "Effects of Myofascial Release in Nonspecific Chronic Low Back Pain: A Randomized Clinical Trial." *Spine* 42, no. 9 (2017): 627–634.

3. Wu, Zugui, Yi Wang, Xiangling Ye, et al. "Myofascial Release for Chronic Low Back Pain: A Systematic Review and Meta-Analysis." *Frontiers in Medicine* 8 (July 2021): Article 697986.

4. Laimi, Katri, Annika Mäkilä, Esa Bärlund, et al. "Effectiveness of Myofascial Release in Treatment of Chronic Musculoskeletal Pain: A Systematic Review." *Clinical Rehabilitation* 32, no. 4 (April 2018): 440–450.

5. Ikutomo, Hisashi, Koutatsu Nagai, Keiichi Tagomori, et al. "Effects of Foam Rolling on Hip Pain in Patients with Hip Osteoarthritis: A Retrospective Propensity-Matched Cohort Study." *Physiotherapy Theory and Practice* (2020): NA.

6. Pearcey, Gregory E. P., David J. Bradbury-Squires, Jon-Erik Kawamoto, et al. "Foam Rolling for Delayed-Onset Muscle Soreness and Recovery of Dynamic Performance Measures." *Journal of Athletic Training* 50, no. 1 (2015): 5–13.

7. Romero-Moraleda, Blanca, Jaime González-García, Ángel Cuéllar-Rayo, et al. "Effects of Vibration and Non-Vibration Foam Rolling on Recovery after Exercise with Induced Muscle Damage." *Journal of Sports Science and Medicine* 18 (2019): 172–180.

8. D'Amico, Anthony, Jason Gillis, Kelley McCarthy, et al. "Foam Rolling and Indices of Autonomic Recovery Following Exercise Induced Muscle Damage." *International Journal of Sports Physical Therapy* 15, no. 3 (June 2020): 429–440.

9. Wiewelhove, Thimo, Alexander Döweling, Christoph Schneider, et al. "A Meta-Analysis of the Effects of Foam Rolling on Performance and Recovery." *Frontiers in Physiology* 10 (April 2019): Article 376.

10. Baur, Heidi, Hannes Gatterer, Barbara Hotter, and Martin Kopp. "Influence of Structural Integration and Fascial Fitness on Body Image and the Perception of Back Pain." *The Journal of Physical Therapy Science* 29 (2017): 1010–1013.

11. Stall, Paula, and Manoel Jacobsen Teixeira. "Fibromyalgia Syndrome Treated with the Structural Integration Rolfing® Method." *Revista Dor* 15, no. 4 (October–December 2014): 248–252.

12. Jacobsen, Eric E., Alec L. Meleger, Paolo Bonato, et al. "Structural Integration as an Adjunct to Outpatient Rehabilitation for Chronic Nonspecific Low Back Pain: A Randomized Pilot Clinical Trial." *Evidence-Based Complementary and Alternative Medicine* 2015 (2015): 813418.

13. James, Helen, Luis Castaneda, Marilyn E. Miller, and Thomas Findley. "Rolfing Structural Integration Treatment of Cervical Spine Dysfunction." *Journal of Bodywork and Movement Therapies* 13, no. 3 (July 2009): 229–238.

REFERENCES AND FURTHER READINGS

Arguisuelas, María D., Juan Francisco Lisón, Daniel Sánchez-Zurianga, et al. "Effects of Myofascial Release in Nonspecific Chronic Low Back Pain: A Randomized Clinical Trial." *Spine* 42, no. 9 (2017): 627–634.

Baur, Heidi, Hannes Gatterer, Barbara Hotter, and Martin Kopp. "Influence of Structural Integration and Fascial Fitness on Body Image and the Perception of Back Pain." *Journal of Physical Therapy Science* 29 (2017): 1010–1013.

D'Amico, A. D., Jason Gillis, Kelley McCarthy, et al. "Foam Rolling and Indices of Autonomic Recovery following Exercise Induced Muscle Damage." *International Journal of Sports Physical Therapy* 15, no. 3 (June 2020): 429–440.

Ikutomo, Hisashi, Koutatsu Nagai, Keiichi Tagomort, et al. "Effects of Foam Rolling on Hip Pain in Patients with Hip Osteoarthritis: A Retrospective Propensity-Matched Cohort Study." *Physiotherapy Theory and Practice* (2020): NA.

Jacobsen, Eric E., Alec L. Meleger, Paolo Bonato, et al. "Structural Integration as an Adjunct to Outpatient Rehabilitation for Chronic

Nonspecific Low Back Pain: A Randomized Pilot Clinical Trial." *Evidence-Based Complementary and Alternative Medicine* 2015 (2015): Article ID 813418.

James, Helen, Luis Castaneda, Marilyn E. Miller, and Thomas Findley. "Rolfing Structural Integration Treatment of Cervical Spine Dysfunction." *Journal of Bodywork and Movement Therapies* 13, no. 3 (July 2009): 229–238.

Laimi, Katri, Annika Mäkilä, Esa Bärlund, et al. "Effectiveness of Myofascial Release in Treatment of Chronic Musculoskeletal Pain: A Systematic Review." *Clinical Rehabilitation* 32, no. 4 (April 2018): 440–450.

Pearcey, Gregory E. P., David J. Bradbury-Squires, Jon-Erik Kawamoto, et al. "Foam Rolling for Delayed-Onset Muscle Soreness and Recovery of Dynamic Performance Measures." *Journal of Athletic Training* 50, no. 1 (2015): 5–13.

Rodríguez-Huguet, Manuel, José Luis Gil-Salú, Pablo Rodríguez-Huguet, et al. "Effects of Myofascial Release on Pressure Pain Thresholds in Patients with Neck Pain: A Single-Blind Randomized Controlled Trial." *American Journal of Physical Medicine & Rehabilitation* 97, no. 1 (January 2018): 16–22.

Romero-Moraleda, Blanca, Jaime González-Garcia, Ángel Cuéllar-Rayo, et al. "Effects of Vibration and Non-Vibration Foam Rolling on Recovery after Exercise with Induced Muscle Damage." *Journal of Sports Science and Medicine* 18 (2019): 172–180.

Stall, Paula, and Manoel Jacobsen Teixeira. "Fibromyalgia Syndrome Treated with the Structural Integration Rolfing® Method." *Revista Dor* 15, no. 4 (October–December 2014): 248–252.

Wiewelhove, Thimo, Alexander Döweling, Christoph Schneider, et al. "A Meta-Analysis of the Effects of Foam Rolling on Performance and Recovery." *Frontiers in Physiology* 10 (April 2019): Article 376.

Wu, Zugui, Yi Wang, Xiangling Ye, et al. "Myofascial Release for Chronic Low Back Pain: A Systematic Review and Meta-Analysis." *Frontiers in Medicine* 8 (July 2021): Article 697986.

Nerve Blocks, Spinal Cord Stimulation, and TENS

INTRODUCTION

Also known as a neural blockade, a nerve block is a nonsurgical or surgical method of producing anesthesia or the loss of feeling in order to control pain. With nonsurgical nerve blocks, numbing medication is injected around a specific nerve or bundle of nerves. The medication prevents the nerve impulses from reaching the brain, thus replacing pain with a numb or pins-and-needles feeling. The loss of feeling tends to last for 12 to 36 hours. In surgical nerve blocks, physicians cut or destroy certain nerves to prevent them from sending impulses to the brain. The loss of feeling is likely permanent. However, sometimes nerves repair themselves or regrow. If they do, the pain may or may not return. A nerve block may be used alone or in conjunction with other forms of pain relief.

There are three main types of nonsurgical nerve blocks. Probably the best-known type of nerve block, an epidural, is injected outside the spinal cord to numb the abdomen and lower extremities. It is used to ease the pain of labor and delivery. Spinal anesthesia is injected into the fluid surrounding the spinal cord. And, with peripheral nerve blocks, medication is injected around a target nerve that is causing pain. Similarly, there are three main types of surgical nerve blocks. In a rhizotomy, the roots of the nerves that extend from the spine are surgically destroyed. With a neurectomy, a damaged peripheral nerve is surgically destroyed. And a sympathetic blockage blocks pain from the sympathetic nervous system to one specific area.

Spinal cord stimulators are sometimes implanted after nonsurgical methods, such as medications and physical therapy, have failed to provide adequate relief from chronic pain. Using fluoroscopy to determine proper placement, spinal cord stimulators, which consist of electrodes or thin wires and a small generator, are implanted within the epidural space; the stimulators send low levels of electricity directly into the spinal cord, which relieves pain.

There are three main types of spinal cord stimulators. Only two are currently widely used. The conventional implantable pulse generator (IPG) is a battery-operated spinal cord stimulator that is surgically implanted. Unfortunately, when the battery is depleted, it must be surgically replaced. The IPG has a relatively low electrical output and is good for people with pain in one part of the body. A rechargeable IPG works in the same way as a conventional IPG, but it may be recharged without surgery. It emits more electricity and is a good choice for people with low back pain or pain in one or both legs. Also, a radiofrequency stimulator has a battery that is outside the body. Because of improvements in technology, it is now rarely used.

Traditional spinal cord stimulators replace the pain sensation with a tingling feeling or paresthesia. Newer versions of spinal cord stimulators are unable to be felt. Spinal cord stimulators work best when implanted within two years of the onset of pain. They tend to be less successful in people who have been living with pain for many years.

Designed to relieve pain, a transcutaneous electrical nerve stimulator (TENS) unit is a device that sends low-voltage electrical currents to targeted areas of the body. Some TENS units may only be used safely in a medical or rehabilitation facility; others may be used at home. A TENS unit sends electrical pulses through the skin, temporarily or permanently controlling pain signals in the body.

There are two main theories that explain exactly how TENS units relieve pain. One theory contends that electric current stimulates nerve cells that block the transmission of pain signals, thereby altering the perception of pain. The other theory hypothesizes that nerve stimulation raises levels of endorphins, which block the perception of pain.

ADMINISTRATION AND REGULATION

Nerve blocks are administered in an office, clinic, or hospital setting. Before a nerve block, the skin around the injection site will be cleaned. Your physician will use a local injection to numb the area. Once numb, your physician will use an ultrasound, fluoroscope, or some other device to guide the needle to the correct area and then inject the numbing medication. Sometimes, the needle needs to be inserted deeply, which may be briefly uncomfortable. When the procedure is over, you will be monitored for any adverse effects. The entire procedure should take less than

30 minutes. Normally, depending on the type of block, relief lasts between 8 and 36 hours. However, that number is variable. In some instances, as in postsurgery pain relief, a physician may use a nerve catheter to provide continuous relief for a few days. For this process, the physician places a small tube, which is connected to an infusion pump, below the skin near the nerve. Anesthesia is automatically delivered for a specified period of time. It is important to note that while the effects of the shots tend to be immediate, in general, nerve blocks are temporary solutions to pain relief. The contents of the shots are absorbed into the body.

Many physicians limit the number of nerve blocks. For example, they may refuse to administer more than a certain number of nerve blocks per patient during a single year, especially if the injecting formulation contains steroids.

Spinal cord stimulator implantation has two phases. During a trial phase, while in an office, clinic, or hospital setting, a physician carefully inserts electrodes into the epidural space of the spine. The location of the pain determines the exact location of the electrodes. A generator is placed on the outside of the body. For about a week, the patient evaluates the degree of pain relief. If pain is reduced by at least 50 percent, a permanent stimulator will be implanted with sutures to minimize movement, and the generator is placed under the skin, generally near the buttocks or abdomen. The implantation procedure should take between one and two hours, and it is normally performed in an outpatient setting. Patients use a remote control outside of the body to trigger electrical impulses that reduce pain. On the other hand, if the stimulator fails to notably reduce pain, the trial wires may be easily removed.

Before administration of spinal cord stimulators, your physician may order imaging tests and a psychological screening. In fact, some insurance companies require psychological screening to ensure that the pain is not exacerbated by anxiety or depression.

Like other medical devices, spinal cord stimulators are regulated and approved by the FDA. The FDA collects data on the reported problems associated with the implantation of devices, such as inadequate pain relief, pain, unexpected therapeutic effects, infection, and discomfort, as well as problems with the devices themselves, such as charging issues, impedance, migration, and battery malfunctioning.

Though any health-care professional may administer the types of TENS units that are designed to be used in a clinical setting, TENS units tend to be used by chiropractors, physical therapists, and acupuncturists. Some versions are available for home use. The frequency of the units may be adjusted by turning a dial. Professional TENS sessions are short, lasting fewer than 15 minutes, and may be combined with another therapy.

The FDA regulates TENS units that are considered medical devices, as defined by Section 201(h) of the Food, Drug, and Cosmetic Act.

BENEFITS AND RISKS

Nerve blocks are useful for a number of different medical problems that cause pain, including labor and childbirth, surgery, cancer, arthritis, menstrual pain, endometriosis, multiple sclerosis, fibromyalgia, low back pain, severe facial pain, chronic regional pain syndrome, migraines, diabetic neuropathy, spinal cord injury, herniated discs, shingles, blood vessel spasms, and Raynaud's syndrome. In some instances, nerve blocks are used to locate the source(s) or origin(s) of pain.

There are a number of different side effects and risks associated with nerve blocks. These include infection, bruising, bleeding, injection site tenderness, delivery of medication into the bloodstream, blocking the wrong nerve, and Horner's syndrome, which causes a drooping eyelid and decreased pupil size when the nerve between the brain and the eye is affected. Fortunately, nerve damage and overdoses rarely occur, especially when the procedure is conducted by physicians experienced in pain-focused areas of medicine, such as orthopedic surgeons and rheumatologists.

For at least 24 hours before a nerve block, it is important to avoid taking any anti-inflammatory medications or blood-thinning supplements. People who take blood-thinning medications need to share that information with the medical provider who will administer the nerve block.

Although most often used after failed back surgery, spinal cord stimulators are helpful for different types of pain. These include chronic back pain, postsurgery or amputation pain, heart pain, arachnoiditis (or pain in a thin membrane that covers the brain and spinal cord), nerve pain, peripheral vascular disease, complex regional pain syndrome, visceral abdominal pain, and perineal pain. People with spinal cord stimulators are often able to reduce their intake of medications, especially narcotic medications, and have more restful sleep.

The most frequent problem associated with spinal cord stimulators is hardware malfunction. Other risks associated with spinal cord stimulators include infection, bleeding, movement of electrodes, device damage, spinal cord trauma, or the excessively deep insertion of the needle or electrodes resulting in severe headaches. People with spinal cord stimulators should turn off the electricity before X-rays and CT scans, and it may or not may be safe for them to have MRIs. Similarly, the are conflicting views on whether it is safe to have a spinal cord stimulator and a pacemaker or defibrillators. The stimulators may set off airport security detectors; be sure to carry an identification card allowing you to bypass the machine. At the very least, turn off the stimulator before walking into the screening machine. Do not swim or take showers or baths with a temporary stimulator, and turn off the stimulator when driving or operating heavy machinery; sudden changes in stimulation may be distracting.

TENS therapy is believed to be useful for the pain associated with a number of different medical problems including bursitis, arthritis, tendinitis, injuries, fibromyalgia, tendinitis, chronic pelvic pain, peripheral artery disease, open wounds that are not infected, and headaches. TENS therapy may provide instant pain relief, and sometimes the relief is prolonged. In some instances, a series of treatments results in permanent pain relief, but the usefulness of TENS treatments may vary from person to person. High-frequency TENS seems to be more useful for pain than low-frequency TENS. Placing the electrodes on acupuncture points may increase their pain-reduction properties.

For the vast majority of people, TENS therapy is considered safe. In some rare instances, an electrical current may be too intense and may cause irritation or burning to the skin. The electrical impulses may produce a buzzing, tingling, or prickling sensation, which people may find uncomfortable. Some people may have skin reactions to the electrode pads used with the units; they may wish to try hypoallergenic pads. As it is not known what effect electrical currents may have on a fetus, women who are pregnant should not use TENS units. People with heart conditions should check with a medical provider before considering TENS treatments, and people with pacemakers, infusion pumps, or defibrillators must not be exposed to the electrical currents produced by TENS units. People with a bleeding disorder, deep-vein thrombosis, or thrombophlebitis should avoid using these units. TENS therapy may induce seizures in people with epilepsy. TENS should not be used on infected tissues, recently radiated skin, damaged skin, near the reproductive organs or genitals, and areas of the body with lower levels of sensation. Never place the electrode on the front of the neck or the eyes. Such placement on the neck may lower blood pressure and cause spasms, and placing the electrode on the eyes may increase internal eye pressure and cause an injury.

People who use TENS units every day may develop a tolerance to the treatment, and they will no longer experience the same degree of relief. To prevent this from happening, alternate between low-frequency and high-frequency treatments.

RESEARCH FINDINGS

Pectoral Nerve Blocks May Help Patients Having Breast Cancer Surgery

In a systematic review and meta-analysis published in 2020 in the journal *Medicine*, researchers from China evaluated the use of pectoral (breast or chest) nerve blocks for females having breast cancer surgery. The researchers located 13 randomized, controlled trials that met their criteria; in total, there were 940 patients. The majority of the nerve blocks were performed after the induction of anesthesia, and the injections contained ropivacaine or bupivacaine or levobupivacaine. Eleven trials did not have a high risk of bias. One trial had a high risk of detection bias, and one trial had a high risk of attrition bias. Pain scores were reported in all of the trials. The researchers learned that, when compared to the controls, at all time points, patients receiving nerve blocks had significantly lower pain scores up to 24 hours following surgery. In addition, the intraoperative and postoperative administration of nerve blocks reduced the use of opioids, and the women with nerve blocks waited longer before first requesting postoperative pain medication. Patients who had lower intakes of opioids were more satisfied and had shorter hospital stays. The researchers concluded that "further studies are needed to investigate the long-term outcomes such as postoperative chronic pain, tumor recurrence and metastases, and recovery of shoulder function in these patients."[1]

Elders with Hip or Femoral Neck Fractures May Benefit from Nerve Blocks

In a systematic review published in 2016 in the journal *CJEM*, researchers from Canada examined the use of regional nerve blocks for elders with hip or femoral neck fractures. The researchers located nine randomized, controlled trials that met their criteria; the sample sizes ranged from 33 to 154 patients, with two-thirds of the trials enrolling 50 or fewer subjects. In all of the trials, single regional nerve blocks were administered, and pain scores were recorded before surgery and compared to other forms of standard pain management, which was defined as opiates, acetaminophen, or nonsteroidal anti-inflammatory drugs. In five of the nine trials, the nerve blocks were administered by emergency physicians or residents. The researchers learned that in eight of the trials, pain improved when the regional nerve block was used. A significant reduction in parenteral opiate use was seen in five out of six studies. No trial reported any immediate life-threatening complications from the nerve blocks. Because of the variable methods of reporting outcome results, missing statistics, and clinical heterogeneity between the trials, no meta-analysis was performed. Nevertheless, the researchers learned that regional nerve blocks were most likely at least as effective and possibly better at reducing hip or femoral pain than standard pain management. "The performance of regional nerve blocks for hip and femoral neck fractures in the ED [emergency department] can be recommended."[2]

Though They Relieve Pain, Nerve Blocks Do Not Appear to Improve the Outcomes of Ambulatory Shoulder Surgery

In a retrospective, population-based historical cohort study published in 2019 in the journal *Anesthesiology*, researchers from Canada evaluated the association between nerve blocks and health systems outcomes after ambulatory shoulder surgery. Using data from hospitals in Ontario, Canada, the researchers included 59,644 patients who had ambulatory shoulder surgery from April 1, 2009, to December 31, 2016. Of these, 31,073 had nerve blocks. The number of nerve blocks increased every year that was studied, and they added $325 to the overall cost of the surgery. Of the subjects with the nerve blocks, 2,808 (9.0%) had an unplanned admission, readmission, or emergency department visit within seven days of surgery compared to 3,424 (12.0%) of 28,571 patients without a nerve block. The researchers determined that "after multilevel, multivariate adjustment, no significant differences remained." Also, the early pain relief benefits of nerve blocks do not appear to have any meaningful effect after discharge. The researchers underscored the need for additional research. "Pragmatic randomized trials powered for patient-centered post-discharge outcomes, as well as process evaluation, are needed to understand how the early benefits of blocks may extend after discharge and to fully inform anesthetic care."[3]

Spinal Cord Stimulation Is Less Effective for Chronic Spine-Related Pain in Obese People

In a retrospective cohort study published in 2019 in the *Spine Journal*, researchers from Cleveland, Ohio (USA), investigated the association between spinal cord stimulation and body mass index (BMI). Did increases in weight have any adverse effects on the efficacy of spinal cord stimulation implants? Were people with lower weight able to reduce their intake of opioid medication? The cohort consisted of 181 patients who had undergone successful spinal cord stimulation for their chronic spine-related pain and had experienced at least a 50 percent reduction in pain. The group was divided into four subgroups according to BMIs. Thirty-three patients were either underweight or normal weight (BMI ≤ 24.9); 72 were overweight (BMI 25–29.9); 63 were obese (BMI 30–39.9); and 13 were morbidly obese (BMI ≥ 40). The researchers found a statistically significant negative association between increases in BMI and the effectiveness of spinal cord stimulators at 6 and 12 postimplant months, with a notable reduction of around 2 percent in efficacy for every unit increase of BMI. However, it is important to note that the reductions in pain did not coincide with decreases in the use of opioid medications. The subjects continued to take their same doses of narcotic medications. The researchers theorized that the subjects may have "increased physical activity and overall functionality" or were "resistant to decreasing their medication doses."[4]

Percutaneous Spinal Cord Stimulation May Help People Dealing with Failed Back Surgery Syndrome

In a retrospective study published in 2020 in the journal *Turkish Neurosurgery*, researchers from Turkey evaluated the usefulness of spinal cord stimulation for people dealing with the pain associated with failed back surgery syndrome. The initial cohort consisted of 12 women and 4 men whose ages ranged from 35 to 80 years, with a median age of 50 years; they all had a history of at least one spinal operation with postoperative chronic back or leg pain and unsuccessful medical and physical therapy treatments. After trial stimulators were implanted and determined to be effective in reducing pain by at least 50 percent, the actual spinal cord stimulators were implanted from January 2016 to December 2018. (Three subjects did not experience that level of improvement and were excluded from the analyses.) Two serious complications occurred in one patient. Follow-up assessments were conducted annually during outpatient visits. The researchers concluded that percutaneous spinal cord stimulation "is a safe and effective treatment for patients with FBSS [failed back surgery syndrome]."[5]

The Implantation of Implantable Pulse Generators Often Cause Varying Levels of Site Pain

In a retrospective single-center study published in 2020 in the journal *Regional Anesthesia & Pain Medicine*, researchers from the United Kingdom analyzed the prevalence of pain that occurs following the implantation of implantable pulse generators. (Implantable pulse generators, or IPGs, power spinal cord stimulators.) The initial cohort consisted of 775 subjects—361 males and 414 females—who had IPGs implanted between September 2013 and March 2020. The IPGs were implanted in the posterior chest wall ($n = 376$), buttock ($n = 292$), flank ($n = 50$), and abdomen ($n = 46$). Because data were missing on 11 subjects, the final analyses were conducted on 764 subjects—359 males and 405 females. The majority of the subjects had failed back surgery syndrome or postsurgical persistent pain at the cervical spine. Also, the size of the IPGs varied; 396 subjects had large rechargeable IPGs, 250 had small rechargeable IPGs, and 118 had nonrechargeable IPGs. Implantation site pain was reported in 47 males and 80 females, an incident rate of 17 percent. Twenty percent of females reported site pain, as did 13 percent of males. Site pain was lowest for the nonrechargeable IPGs and highest for the large rechargeable IPGs. Nonrechargeable IPGs had the lowest rates of site pain for the posterior chest wall and abdominal implants. For buttock placement, small rechargeable IPGs had the lowest rate of site pain. And, for the flank area, small rechargeable and nonrechargeable IPGs had equally low rates of site pain. The researchers concluded that their study highlights †he importance of placement of IPGs and "the importance of systematically recording and reporting SCS [spine cord stimulator] associated complications."[6]

Patients Who Obtained Pain Relief from Trial Spinal Cord Stimulators Were More Likely to Obtain Pain Relief from Permanent Spinal Cord Stimulators

In a retrospective study published in 2020 in the journal *Neuromodulation*, researchers from Boston, Massachusetts, and Baltimore, Maryland

(USA), analyzed the association between results from trial spinal cord stimulations and the effectiveness of permanent spinal cord stimulations. The researchers identified 88 men and women who had undergone trial and permanent implantation of spinal cord stimulators between 2015 and 2018. Fifty-seven percent were female. All of the trials lasted between 3 and 10 days. Pain scores were obtained at baseline, after the trial, and after the permanent implantation. The researchers determined that 70 subjects (79%) had successful permanent implantation and that decreased pain scores after the trial implants were associated with a higher predictability of successful permanent implants. Specifically, people who had post-trial pain scores of less than or equal to 4.6 out of 10 had a more than 50 percent probability of having a successful permanent implant. Still, the researchers cautioned that pain reduction during the trial period is not always an accurate predictor of implant outcome. "The validity of utilization of pain scores for interventional procedures like spinal cord stimulator implant remains complicated by its subjective nature."[7]

TENS May Help Relieve the Pain Associated with Some Hip Fracture Surgeries

In a randomized, controlled clinical trial published in 2019 in the journal *Clinical Interventions in Aging*, researchers from Israel investigated the ability of TENS therapy to help deal with the pain associated with hip fracture surgery. The cohort consisted of 41 people who had a specific type of hip fracture surgery known as Gamma nail. Beginning 24 hours after surgery, all of the subjects had daily physical therapy sessions. In addition, 23 subjects had daily TENS sessions, and 18 had daily sham TENS sessions, each for five days. Pain levels were assessed during the day and at night. The researchers learned that the pain was most intense during the first two days after surgery, and there were no differences in analgesic use between the two groups during the first four post-operative days. By the fifth day of therapy, the subjects in both groups had significant decreases in pain intensity, and the average amount of non-narcotic use was significantly lower in the TENS group. Meanwhile, the subjects who received TENS treatments had significantly less pain when walking. The researchers commented that the effects of TENS on people who are not mobile appear to be different from the effects on pain in people who are moving, a finding that is consistent with previous studies. The researchers concluded that "the positive effects of TENS on pain during walking and increased walking distance determined in the present study support the integration of TENS with the standard care of elderly patients following Gamma nail surgical fixation of extracapsular hip fractures."[8]

TENS May Provide Some Relief for People with Fibromyalgia

In a randomized, double-blind, sham-controlled clinical trial published in 2021 in the *Journal of Pain Research*, researchers from Massachusetts (USA) evaluated the use of wearable TENS units for people with fibromyalgia. The initial cohort consisted of 119 people with fibromyalgia. For three months, 62 subjects wore an active TENS device, and 57 wore a sham device. The active and sham devices appeared the same but were equipped with standard software or modified software. The subjects, who wore their TENS units on the lower extremity of either leg, typically the upper calf, were told that one device was high density and the other was low density. Each therapy session lasted for 60 minutes; the sham device provided three two-minute periods of stimulation during each session, for a total of six minutes per session. The subjects were told to use their TENS units for at least two one-hour sessions per day. The researchers conducted a variety of assessments. One hundred subjects completed the entire trial; however, one active and three sham participants did not return for the three-month follow-up. During the course of the trial, the subjects continued to take their pain medications; 21.8 percent were taking opioids. The subjects averaged 3.5 sessions per day and used their TENS units an average of 68.9 days and 23.7 nights. The researchers learned that the subjects wearing the active TENS unit had only "modest treatment effects." The subjects with higher pain sensitivity had better results than those with lower pain sensitivity. Still, the researchers concluded that "wearable TENS represents a safe and effective treatment option for people with fibromyalgia."[9]

TENS May Not Be as Useful for Low Back Pain as Many People Believe

In a systematic review and meta-analysis published in 2018 in the journal *Regional Anesthesia and Pain Medicine*, researchers based in Taiwan compared the use of TENS units to a control and to other nerve stimulation therapies for the treatment of chronic low back pain. Control treatments included sham, placebo, or medication, and other nerve stimulation therapies included electroacupuncture, percutaneous electrical nerve stimulation, and percutaneous neuromodulation therapy. Their cohort consisted of 12 randomized controlled trials with 700 subjects; these trials were published between 1986 and 2011. Of the 700 subjects, 350 received TENS therapy, 81 had another type of nerve stimulation therapy, and 269 were in control groups. The mean age reported for all but two trials ranged from 36.6 to 61.5 years. The trials were performed in Hong Kong, Japan, Europe, the United States, Canada, and South America. Trial durations varied from three days to eight months. The researchers learned that the efficacy of pain relief was about the same for TENS as it was for the controls, and other types of nerve stimulation therapy provided better pain relief than TENS. However, two trials found TENS to be better at improving functional disability within six weeks of starting treatment. The researchers emphasized the need for more randomized controlled trials on TENS.[10]

NOTES

1. Sun, Qianchuangm, Shuyann Liu, Huiying Wu, et al. "Clinical Analgesic Efficacy of Pectoral Nerve Block in Patients Undergoing Breast Cancer Surgery." *Medicine* 99, no. 14 (2020): e19614.

2. Ritcey, Brandon, Paul Pageau, Michael Y. Woo, and Jeffrey J. Perry. "Regional Nerve Blocks for Hip and Femoral Neck Fractures in the Emergency Department: A Systematic Review." *CJEM* 18, no. 1 (January 2016): 37–47.

3. Hamilton, Gavin M., Reva Ramlogan, Anne Lui, et al. "Peripheral Nerve Blocks for Ambulatory Shoulder Surgery: A Population-Based Cohort Study of Outcomes and Recourse Utilization." *Anesthesiology* 131, no. 6 (December 2019): 1254–1263.

4. Mekhail, Nagy, Diana Mehanny, Sherif Armanyous, et al. "The Impact of Obesity on the Effectiveness of Spinal Cord Stimulation in Chronic Spine-Related Pain Patients." *The Spine Journal* 19 (2019): 476–486.

5. Harman, Ferhat, Seckin Aydin, Savas Sencan, et al. "Percutaneous Spinal Cord Stimulation for Failed Back Surgery Syndrome: A Retrospective Study." *Turkish Neurosurgery* 30, no. 5 (2020): 739–745.

6. Baranidharan, Ganesan, Beatrice Bretherton, Gemme Richert, et al. "Pocket Pain, Does Location Matter: A Single-Centre Retrospective Study

of Patients Implanted With a Spinal Cord Stimulator." *Regional Anesthesia & Pain Medicine* 45, no. 11 (November 2020): 891–897.

7. Orhurhu, Vwaire, Robert Chu, Mariam Salisu Orhurhu, and Charles A. Odonkor. "Association between Pain Scores and Successful Spinal Cord Stimulator Implantation." *Neuromodulation* 23, no. 5 (July 2020): 660–666.

8. Elboim-Gabyzon, Michal, Sahar Andrawus Najjar, and Haim Shtarker. "Effects of Transcutaneous Electrical Nerve Stimulation (TENS) on Acute Postoperative Pain Intensity and Mobility after Hip Fracture: A Double-Blinded, Randomized Trial." *Clinical Interventions in Aging* 14 (2019): 1841–1850.

9. Jamison, Robert N., Robert R. Edwards, Samantha Curran, et al. "Effects of Wearable Transcutaneous Electrical Nerve Stimulation on Fibromyalgia: A Randomized Controlled Trial." *Journal of Pain Research* 14 (2021): 2265–2282.

10. Wu, Lien-Chen, Pei-Wei Weng, Chia-Hsien Chen, et al. "Literature Review and Meta-Analysis of Transcutaneous Electrical Nerve Stimulation in Treating Chronic Back Pain." *Regional Anesthesia and Pain Medicine* 43 (2018): 425–433.

REFERENCES AND FURTHER READINGS

Baranidharan, G., B. Bretherton, G. Richert, et al. "Pocket Pain, Does Location Matter: A Single-Centre Retrospective Study of Patients Implanted with a Spinal Cord Stimulator." *Regional Anesthesia & Pain Medicine* 45, no. 11 (2020): 891–897.

Elboim-Gabyzon, Michal, Sahar Andrawus Najjar, and Haim Shtarker. "Effects of Transcutaneous Electrical Nerve (TENS) on Acute Postoperative Pain Intensity and Mobility after Hip Fracture: A Double-Blinded, Randomized Trial." *Clinical Interventions in Aging* 14 (2019): 1841–1850.

Hamilton, Gavin M., Reva Ramlogan, Anne Lui, et al. "Peripheral Nerve Blocks for Ambulatory Shoulder Surgery: A Population-Based Cohort Study of Outcomes and Resource Utilization." *Anesthesiology* 131, no. 6 (December 2019): 1254–1263.

Harman, Ferhat, Seckin Aydin, Savas Sencan, et al. "Percutaneous Spinal Cord Stimulation for Failed Back Surgery Syndrome: A Retrospective Study." *Turkish Neurosurgery* 30, no. 5 (2020): 739–745.

Jamison, Robert N., Robert R. Edwards, Samantha Curran, et al. "Effects of Wearable Transcutaneous Electrical Nerve Stimulation on Fibromyalgia: A Randomized Controlled Trial." *Journal of Pain Research* 14 (2021): 2265–2282.

Mekhail, Nagy, Diana Mehanny, Sherif Armanyous, et al. "The Impact of Obesity on the Effectiveness of Spinal Cord Stimulation in Chronic Spine-Related Pain Patients." *Spine Journal* 19, no. 3 (March 2019): 476–486.

Orhurhu, Vwaire, Robert Chu, Mariam Salisu Orhurhu, and Charles A. Odonkor. "Association between Pain Scores and Successful Spinal Cord Stimulator Implantation." *Neuromodulation* 23, no. 5 (July 2020): 660–666.

Ritcey, Brandon, Paul Pageau, Michael Y. Woo, and Jeffrey J. Perry. "Regional Nerve Blocks for Hip and Femoral Neck Fractures in the Emergency Department: A Systematic Review." *CJEM* 18, no. 1 (January 2016): 37–47.

Sun, Qianchuang, Shuyan Liu, Huiying Wu, et al. "Clinical Analgesic Efficacy of Pectoral Nerve Block in Patients Undergoing Breast Cancer Surgery." *Medicine* 99, no. 14 (2020): e19614.

Wu, Lien-Chen, Pei-Wei Weng, Chia-Hsien Chen, et al. "Literature Review and Meta-Analysis of Transcutaneous Electrical Nerve Stimulation in Treating Chronic Back Pain." *Regional Anesthesia and Pain Medicine* 43 (2018): 425–433.

Nonsteroidal Anti-inflammatory Drugs (NSAIDs)

INTRODUCTION

Nonsteroidal anti-inflammatory drugs, which are often referred to as NSAIDs, are a broad group of drugs from a number of different classes. Although their chemical structures differ, they all have the same effects. They reduce pain, inflammation, and fever. Unlike opioids, which are used for the most severe types of pain, NSAIDs are widely used for mild to moderate pain levels. Also, they are the most common pain-relief drugs in the world. Every day, NSAIDs are used by about 30 million Americans. In the USA, more than 70 million prescriptions are written each year, and more than 30 billion doses are consumed annually.

When the body is dealing with an injury or infection, it may respond with inflammation. Signs of inflammation include heat, redness, swelling, and pain. NSAIDs and other anti-inflammatory medications relieve pain by reducing inflammation.

NSAIDs slow the formation of compounds known as prostaglandins, which play a role in the body's inflammatory response. Lowering the levels of prostaglandins reduces inflammation and pain. Specifically, NSAIDs block the effects of COX-1 and COX-2 enzymes, which play a key role in making prostaglandins.

It should be parenthetically noted that NSAIDs are typically divided into groups based on their chemical structure and selectivity. Thus, aspirin is an acetylated salicylate, salsalate is a nonacetylated salicylate, naproxen is a propionic acid, and meloxicam is an enolic acid.

The history of NSAIDs may be traced back about 3,500 years when the Greek physician Hippocrates prescribed an extract from willow bark and leaves for inflammation. In the 17th century, salicin was identified as the active ingredient in willow bark. The Kolbe Company in Germany began mass-producing salicylic acid in 1860, and the Bayer Company in Germany began selling aspirin, a more palatable form of salicylic acid, in 1899. Still, the development of additional NSAIDs did not really gain momentum until later in the 20th century. It was then that researchers learned more about the mechanism of action of these therapeutics. Over time, they determined that while NSAIDs had excellent pain-fighting and anti-inflammatory properties, they had a number of side effects, such as gastrointestinal problems. Even later, it became evident that NSAIDs, except aspirin, could negatively impact the cardiovascular system. That is why, for example, Vioxx was withdrawn from the market in 2004. Another NSAID, Celecoxib, was allowed to remain on the market but with a black box warning.

ADMINISTRATION AND REGULATION

Some NSAIDs are available only by prescription. These include celecoxib, oxaprozin, etodolac, indomethacin, naproxen, nabumetone, diclofenac, and vimovo. Some are available over the counter. These include ibuprofen (Advil, Motrin), aspirin, and naproxen sodium (Aleve). NSAIDs are sold as tablets, capsules, suppositories, creams, gels, and injections. Medical providers tend to start patients on over-the-counter NSAIDs. If they are well tolerated but the pain is not properly controlled, a higher-dose prescription medication may be prescribed. Higher-dose NSAIDs have an increased risk of side effects. Over-the-counter NSAIDs are relatively inexpensive; the generic brands are incredibly inexpensive. Prescription NSAIDs are more costly, but they may be covered by insurance.

Adults 19 years old and older taking over-the-counter aspirin will usually be told to begin with 325 to 650 mg every four to six hours; enteric-coated aspirin is usually administered 650 to 1,300 mg every eight hours, not to exceed 3.9 g/day. (Normally, except in the case of certain illnesses, children and teens should not use aspirin. Before giving a child or teen aspirin, consult with a medical provider.) Adults and children 12 years of age and older taking over-the-counter ibuprofen should begin with an initial dose of 200 or 400 mg. Follow-up doses are 200 to 400 mg every 4 hours, up to a maximum of 1200 per day. Adults and children 12 years and older taking naproxen should begin with doses of 220 or 440 mg. Follow-up doses are 220 mg every 8 to 12 hours. No more than 440 mg should be taken during any 8- to 12-hour period or 660 mg in a 24-hour period. Topical NSAIDs are diclofenac sodium 1.5 percent solution, diclofenac hydroxyethyl pyrrolidine 1.3 percent patch, and diclofenac sodium gel 1 percent. Follow label directions closely. Intravenous ibuprofen, which is a 30-minute infusion, may be administered in a medical setting or, in some cases, in a home setting. For the treatment of pain, the recommendation is 400 to 800 mg every six hours.

As with all over-the-counter medicines, the FDA has determined that over-the-counter NSAIDs are safe and effective for direct consumer use based on the instructions and warnings on the label. The FDA requires a stricter margin of safety for prescription medications. Sometimes, the FDA takes more direct action. For example, during the spring of 2020, when the world was dealing with the first few months of the COVID-19 pandemic, there was concern that the use of NSAIDs would exacerbate the symptoms. The U.S. FDA issued a statement that NSAIDs did not worsen the symptoms of the illness. A few years earlier, in 2015, the FDA issued a warning that the use of nonaspirin NSAIDs increased the incidence of certain cardiovascular problems, such as heart attacks and strokes.

BENEFITS AND RISKS

NSAIDs are useful for a wide variety of painful conditions. These include arthritis, low back pain, colds, flu, headaches, menstrual pain, joint or bone injuries, sprains, strains, muscle or joint complaints, and toothaches.

Still, NSAIDs are not without risks. They have a number of side effects including indigestion, stomachaches, diarrhea, stomach ulcers, headaches, fluid retention, drowsiness, dizziness, and allergic reactions. In rare instances, NSAIDs have caused problems with the liver, kidneys, heart, and circulation. Moreover, NSAIDs interact with several medications, such as other NSAIDs, low-dose aspirin, cyclosporine, diuretics, lithium, methotrexate, and selective serotonin reuptake inhibitors. NSAIDs should not be combined with anticlotting medications; when taken together, they may cause internal bleeding. Drinking higher amounts of alcohol while taking NSAIDs may irritate the gut and increase the risk of stomach bleeding. Long-term or high-dose use of NSAIDs may lead to peptic ulcers or ulcers in the gut. Prostaglandins are known to protect the stomach lining. By reducing the actions of prostaglandins, NSAIDS leave the stomach at increased risk for ulcers. Some people may need to take a separate medication to lower acid production in the stomach.

People with heart, liver, kidney, circulation, or gastrointestinal problems should check with their medical provider before using NSAIDs, as should people over the age of 65 years and women who are pregnant or breastfeeding. People with asthma or stomach ulcers may be told not to use

NSAIDs. Side effects tend to occur more often in people who take higher doses of NSAIDs for longer periods of time. And, as has been noted, non-aspirin NSAIDs may increase the risk of heart attacks and strokes.

People who accidentally or knowingly overdose on NSAIDs may experience a number of different symptoms. Milder symptoms of overdose include tinnitus (ringing in the ear), heartburn, nausea, vomiting, stomach pain, diarrhea, dizziness, blurred vision, rash, and sweating. More serious symptoms include difficult or slow breathing, convulsions, hypotension (low blood pressure), seizures, little to no urine output, severe headache, coma, and death.

RESEARCH FINDINGS

NSAIDs Are Useful in the Treatment of the Pain from Acute Renal Colic or Urinary Stones

In a systematic review and meta-analysis published in 2018 in the journal *European Urology*, researchers from Qatar and Australia evaluated the use of NSAIDs, opioids, and acetaminophen for the acute severe pain associated with urinary stones that block any part of the urinary tract (kidneys, ureters, bladder, and urethra). Their cohort consisted of 36 randomized, controlled trials with 4,887 subjects. The trials, which were from 16 countries, were published between 1982 and 2016. Thirty-two trials compared NSAIDs to opioids, three trials compared NSAIDs to acetaminophen, and one trial included all three treatments. Only three of the trials had 100 subjects or more per treatment arm. Five of the trials were open label, and nine indicated that they had industry sponsorship. The researchers determined that 30 minutes after the administration of NSAIDs, they were at least as useful in the relief of acute renal colic pain as opioids and acetaminophen. In addition, NSAIDs required fewer rescue treatments, they had lower rates of vomiting, and they had a lack of analgesia abuse or addiction properties. As a result, the researchers thought they should become "as the first-line analgesic agents to treat renal colic pain." NSAIDs should be "the preferred analgesic option for patients presenting to the emergency department with renal colic."[1]

Topical NSAIDs Are Useful for Acute Musculoskeletal Pain

In a systematic review published in 2015 in the *Cochrane Database of Systematic Reviews*, researchers from the United Kingdom investigated the ability of topical NSAIDs to help people dealing with acute musculoskeletal pain. This report, which included 61 randomized controlled trials, was an update of a 2010 systematic review. Five thousand three hundred and eleven subjects were treated with topical NSAIDs; 3,470 subjects were treated with a placebo, and 220 were treated with an oral NSAID. This was an increase of 635 in the number of subjects from the 2010 review. The researchers found that several formulations of NSAID (diclofenac, ibuprofen, ketoprofen, piroxicam, and indomethacin) demonstrated significantly higher levels of pain relief than the placebos. Benzydamine did not. The researchers determined that the topical NSAIDs generally provided "good levels of pain relief" for acute conditions such as sprains, strains, and overuse injuries. Gel formulations of diclofenac, ibuprofen, and ketoprofen tend to have the best effects. Adverse effects were minimal. Topical NSIADs are able to relieve pain "without associated systemic adverse events."[2]

Locally Administered Ketorolac Decreased the Pain of Breast Surgery

In a systematic review and meta-analysis published in 2018 in the *Clinical Journal of Pain*, researchers from Taiwan wanted to determine if the local administration of the NSAID ketorolac would help relieve the pain associated with breast surgery. They found four randomized controlled trials with 255 subjects that met their criteria; all of these trials were published from 1996 to 2009. The patient sample sizes ranged from 45 to 100 women. Whereas one trial included women who had a mastectomy or lumpectomy, the other three trials had women having breast augmentation surgery. The ketorolac dosage for all four trials was 30 mg. The researchers learned that the patients who received the locally administered ketorolac or a ketorolac-bupivacaine solution had significantly lower levels of pain than the controls. Interestingly, the breast augmentation patients who received the combined formulation requested more opioids than the controls. Nevertheless, the researchers underscored the need for more research. "Despite the relevant and pragmatic significance of this study, further study with larger sample size is required to obtain a reliable conclusion."[3]

NSAIDs May or May Not Be Useful for Postoperative Endodontic Pain

In a systematic review and meta-analysis published in 2017 in the *Journal of Endodontics*, researchers from Portland, Oregon (USA), wanted to determine if NSAIDs would help patients after their dental surgery for endodontic pain. (Endodontic pain is primarily caused by inflammation of the pulp tissue from dental caries deep in the tooth.) The researchers located 15 randomized, controlled trials that met their criteria. Of these, six were included in the meta-analysis. There were notable differences between the trials including treatment drugs, medication doses, population type, sample size, preoperative diagnosis, time of drug administration, and time of outcome variable measurement. Eight of the trials were deemed to have a high risk of bias. The researchers learned that ibuprofen at a dose of 600 mg was the most common NSAID in the endodontic literature and was found to be more effective than placebo at relieving pain six hours after endodontic treatment. However, the researchers commented that the available evidence was "generally sparse, of low quality, and considered insufficient to draw broad conclusions regarding the comparative effectiveness of NSAIDS." As a result, they noted that they were unable to recommend "the most effective NSAID, dose amount, or dose interval for relieving postoperative endodontic pain."[4]

NSAIDs May or May Not Have Benefits for People with Chronic Low Back Pain

In a systematic review published in 2016 in the *Cochrane Database of Systematic Reviews*, researchers from the Netherlands evaluated the use of NSAIDs for chronic low back pain. They included 13 randomized, controlled double-blind and single-blind trials. Ten of these trials were considered to have low bias. Six studies compared NSAIDs to placebos and included 1,354 subjects; all of these trials reported adverse events, suggesting that people taking NSAIDs are more likely than people taking placebos to have adverse events. Two trials compared ibuprofen to diclofenac and piroxicam to indomethacin. Though the samples were small, no differences were found between these NSAIDs. Six of the trials found that NSAIDs are "slightly more effective" than placebos in reducing pain intensity. Still, "the magnitude of the effects is small," and there was a low level of evidence. The researchers concluded that they were unable "to make firm statements about the occurrence of adverse events or whether NSAIDs are safe for long-term use."[5]

NSAIDs May or May Not Be Useful for the Pain Associated with Cancer

In a systematic review and reappraisal published in 2019 in the *British Journal of Anaesthesia*, researchers from the United Kingdom wanted to learn if NSAIDs would help people dealing with the pain associated with cancer. The researchers identified 30 randomized, controlled trials or double-blind controlled studies that met their criteria. Although only studies with adults were included, the study designs, durations of treatment, durations of follow-up, dosing regimens, routes of administration, underlying cancer diagnoses, and pain phenotypes all varied. The studies examined NSAIDs versus placebos, NSAIDs versus other NSAIDs, NSAIDs versus opioids, NSAIDs and opioids, and the opioid-sparing effects of NSAIDs. The researchers learned that NSAIDs were more effective than placebos in reducing cancer-related pain. There were insufficient data to determine if any of the NSAIDs were better than any others, and, because of heterogeneity and small sample sizes, the researchers were unable to learn if the NSAIDs were better than opioids for pain. The researchers concluded that they had insufficient data to decide if NSAIDs would help people manage cancer pain. "Further work investigating the roles of NSAIDs in cancer pain management is undoubtedly warranted."[6]

Gastroprotective Agents May Help Protect against the Gastrointestinal Bleeding Associated with NSAIDs

In a retrospective, observational study published in 2019 in the journal *Scientific Reports*, researches from South Korea wanted to learn more about the use of gastroprotective agents to protect against gastrointestinal bleeding in people taking NSAIDs. Their cohort consisted of 9,133 people with osteoarthritis or rheumatoid arthritis who used NSAIDs for one month or longer. A total of 6,465 of the subjects took NSAIDs and a gastroprotective agent, and 2,668 took NSAIDs without a gastroprotective agent. The mean age of the subjects was 54.2 years. During a mean follow-up of 5.7 months, occult bleeding developed in 1,191 people (13%). Of these, 82 subjects had endoscopy confirmed gastrointestinal bleeding. Sixty-five subjects had upper gastrointestinal bleeding, and 17 had lower gastrointestinal bleeding. The researchers found that when compared to the subjects who did not take a gastroprotective agent, the subjects who took such an agent had a 36 percent reduction in the risk of gastrointestinal bleeding. In a subanalysis, the researchers found that proton pump inhibitors, H2RAs (H2 blockers), misoprostol, and rebamipide significantly reduced the risk of gastrointestinal injury. On the other hand, there was no significant difference in gastrointestinal bleeding in those using eupatilin. The researcher concluded "that mucoprotective agents, such as rebamipide and misoprostol, as well as acid suppressants, are effective in reducing the risk for GI injury in NSAID users."[7]

Certain Factors Increase the Risk of NSAIDs-Related Gastrointestinal Bleeding

In a retrospective hospital-based study published in 2018 in the journal *Medicine* (Baltimore), researchers from China evaluated the factors that place people at increased risk of NSAIDs-related gastrointestinal bleeding. The cohort consisted of 4728 patients who were 60 years old or older and were taking NSAIDs for at least 14 days. A total of 928 patients experienced gastrointestinal bleeding. Of these, 556 were males with a mean age of 72.46 years and 372 were females with a mean age of 72.58 years. The researchers learned that people 60 years and older with specific medical concerns—peptic ulcer disease, a family history of gastrointestinal bleeding, the use of antiplatelet drugs, a history of cardiovascular and cerebrovascular disease, diabetes mellitus, hypocholesterolemia, and *H. pylori* infection—had an increased risk for gastrointestinal bleeding when they used NSAIDs for two weeks to three months. It appeared that upper gastrointestinal discomfort may be a predictor of the bleeding in people using NSAIDs.[8]

Use of Aspirin before Foot or Ankle Surgery May Not Increase the Risk of Hematoma and Bleeding Complications

In a study published in 2019 in the *Journal of Foot & Ankle Surgery*, researchers from Ohio (USA) noted that it is generally recommended that patients discontinue NSAIDs three to five days before foot or ankle surgery. The researchers wanted to determine if this practice was actually necessary. That is why they reviewed the medical records of 379 consecutive patients who had foot or ankle outpatient surgery over a three-year period of time. The patients ranged in age from 27 to 81 years, with a mean age of 60.77 years. There were 204 women and 175 men. A total of 238 patients were taking 81 mg of aspirin perioperatively, and 141 were not taking any aspirin. The researchers learned that two patients in the aspirin group and one in the no-aspirin group had postoperative hematomas. As a result, the researchers commented that they had too few instances of bleeding to determine the role that aspirin may or may not play in the bleeding. And, they concluded that the "discontinuation of aspirin before any foot and ankle surgery may not be warranted."[9]

Use of NSAIDs Appears to Be Associated with Cardiac Problems

In a case-time-control study published in 2017 in the *European Heart Journal—Cardiovascular Pharmacotherapy*, researchers from Denmark investigated the association between the use of NSAIDs and the risk of an out-of-hospital cardiac arrest (OHCA). The researchers used data from the Denmark Cardiac Arrest Registry to identify people who died of cardiac arrests outside of a hospital setting. In Denmark, all ambulance personnel are required to complete a form whenever a cardiac arrest occurs. They identified 28,947 people who died of OHCA between 2001 and 2010; of these, 3,376 (11.7%) were treated with a NSAID up to 30 days before the fatal heart attack. Comprising 51 percent of the NSAIDs, ibuprofen was the most commonly prescribed NSAID; it was followed by diclofenac, at 21.8 percent. The users of NSAIDs were more likely to be women who had less cardiovascular disease but higher rates of cancer and rheumatic diseases. The researchers learned that the use of any type of NSAID was associated with a significantly increased risk of cardiac arrest. The researchers commented that their findings "call for special awareness in order to balance risks against benefits in treatments with NSAIDs."[10]

In a double-blind, randomized, multicenter, safety trial published in 2017 in the *European Heart Journal*, researchers from several locations in the United States and abroad but based in Switzerland examined the blood pressure effects of ibuprofen, naproxen, and celecoxib in patients who are taking the NSAIDs for arthritis. The cohort consisted of 444 subjects with a mean age of 62 years; 92 percent of the subjects had osteoarthritis, and 8 percent had rheumatoid arthritis. The subjects received either celecoxib (n = 146), ibuprofen (n = 151), naproxen (n = 147), or matching controls. To provide gastric protection, esomeprazole was given to all of the subjects. Many of the subjects were on one or more cardiac medications, and 53 percent took multiple antihypertensive medications. Subjects on low-dose aspirin were allowed to continue their medication. A total of 374 subjects completed the entire four-month trial. Assessments were conducted at baseline, at two months, and when the trial ended. The researchers learned that the subjects taking ibuprofen had consistent increases in ambulatory systolic blood pressure readings. And when compared to the subjects taking naproxen and celecoxib, the subjects taking ibuprofen had more cardiovascular and renal events. The researchers concluded that "clinicians need to weigh the potential hazards of worsening BP [blood pressure] control and its clinical sequelae as well as the risk to gastrointestinal safety when considering the use of these agents, particularly ibuprofen."[11]

In a systematic review and individual patient meta-analysis published in 2017 in the journal *BMJ*, researchers from Canada, Finland, and Germany evaluated the risk of acute myocardial infarctions from the use of NSAIDs. The researchers obtained data from administrative health or medical databases on a total of 446,763 individuals. Of these, 61,460 had acute myocardial infarctions. The researchers learned that taking any dose of NSAIDs for one week, one month, or longer were associated with an increased risk of myocardial infarctions. The risk appears to begin as soon as the NSAID is used. Higher doses were associated with increased risk for acute myocardial infarction, but a longer duration of treatment does not appear to increase risk. Taking a high dose of ibuprofen, naproxen, or rofecoxib for 8 to 30 days was especially harmful. The researchers concluded that "given that the onset risk of acute myocardial infarction occurred in the first week and appeared greatest in the first month of treatment with high doses, prescribers should consider weighing the risks and benefits of NSAIDs before instituting treatment, particularly for higher doses."[12]

Use of NSAIDs in Late Pregnancy May Increase the Risk of Preterm Birth

In a population-based cohort study published in 2018 in the journal *Pain*, researchers from Quebec (Canada) wanted to learn if the use of NSAIDs or COX-2 inhibitors late in pregnancy could increase the risk of preterm birth. The researchers used data from the Quebec Pregnancy Cohort, which enabled them to have a total of 156,531 pregnancies in their cohort. During the three months before their deliveries, 391 pregnancies were exposed to nonselective NSAIDS, 55 were exposed to COX-2 inhibitors (a subclass of NSAIDs), and 12 were exposed to biological agents. Preterm births were defined as births that occurred before 37 completed weeks of gestation. After adjustments for risk factors, such as maternal autoimmune disease, celecoxib was the only medication that was associated with a statistically significant increased risk of premature birth during late pregnancy. In fact, nearly one out of four women taking celecoxib in late pregnancy may have premature birth.[13]

NOTES

1. Pathan, Sameer A., Biswadev Mitra, and Peter A. Cameron. "A Systematic Review and Meta-Analysis Comparing the Efficacy of Nonsteroidal Anti-Inflammatory Drugs, Opioids, and Paracetamol in the Treatment of Acute Renal Colic." *European Urology* 73, no. 4 (April 2018): 583–595.

2. Derry, Sheena, R. Andrew Moore, Helen Gaskell, et al. "Topical NSAIDs for Acute Musculoskeletal Pain in Adults." *Cochrane Database of Systematic Reviews* 6 (June 2015): CD007402.

3. Chen, Jen-Yin, I-Jung Feng, El-Wui Loh, et al. "Analgesic Effects of Locally Administered Ketorolac-Based Analgesics After Breast Surgery: Meta-Analysis of Randomized Controlled Trials." *Clinical Journal of Pain* 34, no. 6 (June 2018): 577–584.

4. Smith, Elizabeth A., J. Gordon Marshall, Shelley S. Selph, et al. "Nonsteroidal Anti-Inflammatory Drugs for Managing Postoperative Endodontic Pain in Patients Who Present with Preoperative Pain: A Systematic Review and Meta-Analysis." *Journal of Endodontics* 43, no. 1 (January 2017): 7–15.

5. Enthoven, Wendy T. M., Pepijn D. D. M. Roelofs, Richard A. Deyo, et al. "Non-Steroidal Anti-Inflammatory Drugs for Chronic Low Back Pain." *Chronic Database of Systematic Reviews* 2, no. 2 (February 2016): CD012087.

6. Magee, D. J., S. Jhanji, G. Poulogiannis, et al. "Nonsteroidal Anti-Inflammatory Drugs and Pain in Cancer Patients: A Systematic Review and Reappraisal of the Evidence." *British Journal of Anaesthesia* 123, no. 2 (2019): e412–e423.

7. Kim, Tae Jun, Eun Ran Kim, Sung Noh Hong, et al. "Effectiveness of Acid Suppressants and Other Mucoprotective Agents in Reducing the Risk of Occult Gastrointestinal Bleeding in Nonsteroidal Anti-Inflammatory Drug Users." *Scientific Reports* 9, no. 1 (August 12, 2019): 11696.

8. Chi, Tian-Yu, Hong-Ming Zhu, and Mei Zhang. "Risk Factors Associated with Nonsteroidal Anti-Inflammatory Drugs (NSAIDs)-Induced

Gastrointestinal Bleeding Resulting on People over 60 Years Old in Beijing." *Medicine* (Baltimore) 97, no. 18 (May 2018): e0665.

9. Hassan, Mohammed K., and Lawrence G. Karlock. "Association of Aspirin Use with Postoperative Hematoma and Bleeding Complications in Foot and Ankle Surgery: A Retrospective Study." *Journal of Foot & Ankle Surgery* 58, no. 5 (September 2019): 861–864.

10. Sondergaard, Kathrine B., Peter Weeke, Mads Wissenberg, et al. "Non-Steroidal Anti-Inflammatory Drug Use Is Associated with Increased Risk of Out-of-Hospital Cardiac Arrest: A Nationwide Case-Time-Control Study." *European Heart Journal—Cardiovascular Pharmacotherapy* 3, no. 2 (April 2017): 100–107.

11. Ruschitzka, Frank, Jeffrey S. Borer, Henry Krum, et al. "Differential Blood Pressure Effects of Ibuprofen, Naproxen, and Celecoxib in Patients with Arthritis: The PRECISION-ABPM (Prospective Randomized Evaluation of Celecoxib Integrated Safety Versus Ibuprofen or Naproxen Ambulatory Blood Pressure Measurement) Trail." *European Heart Journal* 38, no. 44 (November 2017): 3282–3292.

12. Bally, M., N. Dendukuri, B. Rich, et al. "Risk of Acute Myocardial Infarction with NSAIDs in Real World Use: Bayesian Meta-Analysis of Individual Patient Data." *BMJ* 357 (2017): j1909.

13. Bérard, Anick, Odile Sheehy, Sylvie Girard, et al. "Risk of Preterm Birth Following Late Pregnancy Exposure to NSAIDs or COX-2 Inhibitors." *Pain* 159, no. 5 (May 2018): 948–955.

REFERENCES AND FURTHER READINGS

Bally, M., N. Dendukuri, B. Rich, et al. "Risk of Acute Myocardial Infarction with NSIADs in Real World Use: Bayesian Meta-Analysis of Individual Patients Data." *BMJ* 357 (2017): j1909.

Bérard, Anick, Odile Sheehy, Sylvie Girard, et al. "Risk of Preterm Birth Following Late Pregnancy Exposure to NSIADs or COX-2 Inhibitors." *Pain* 159, no. 5 (May 2018): 948–955.

Chen, Jen-Yin, I-Jung Feng, El-Wui Loh, et al. "Analgesic Effects of Locally Administered Ketorolac-Based Analgesics after Breast Surgery: A Meta-Analysis of Randomized Controlled Trials." *Clinical Journal of Pain* 34, no. 6 (June 2018): 577–584.

Chi, Tian-Yu, Hong-Ming Zhu, and Mei Zhang. "Risk Factors Associated with Nonsteroidal Anti-Inflammatory Drugs (NSAIDS)-Induced

Gastrointestinal Bleeding Resulting on People over 60 Years Old in Beijing." *Medicine* (Baltimore) 97, no. 18 (May 2018): e0665.

Derry, Sheena, R. Andrew Moore, Helen Gaskell, et al. "Topical NSAIDs for Acute Musculoskeletal Pain in Adults." *Cochrane Database of Systematic Reviews* 6 (June 2015): CD007402.

Enthoven, Wendy T. M., Pepijn D. D. M. Roelofs, Richard A. Deyo, et al. "Non-Steroidal Anti-Inflammatory Drugs for Chronic Low Back Pain." *Cochrane Database of Systematic Reviews* 2, no. 2 (February 10, 2016): CD012087.

Hassan, Mohammed K., and Lawrence G. Karlock. "Association of Aspirin Use with Postoperative Hematoma and Bleeding Complications in Foot and Ankle Surgery: A Retrospective Study." *The Journal of Foot & Ankle Surgery* 58, no. 5 (September 2019): 861–864.

Kim, Tae Jun, Eun Ran Kim, Sung Noh Hong, et al. "Effectiveness of Acid Suppressants and Other Mucoprotective Agents in Reducing the Risk of Occult Gastrointestinal Bleeding in Nonsteroidal Anti-Inflammatory Drug Users." *Scientific Reports* 9, no. 1 (August 12, 2019): 11696.

Magee, D. J., S. Jhanji, G. Poulogiannis, et al. "Nonsteroidal Anti-Inflammatory Drugs and Pain in Cancer Patients: A Systematic Review and Reappraisal of the Evidence." *British Journal of Anaesthesia* 123, no. 2 (2019): e412–e423.

Pathan, Sameer A., Biswadev Mitra, and Peter A. Cameron. "A Systematic Review and Meta-Analysis Comparing the Efficacy of Nonsteroidal Anti-Inflammatory Drugs, Opioids, and Paracetamol in the Treatment of Acute Renal Colic." *European Urology* 73, no. 4 (April 2018): 583–595.

Ruschutzka, Frank, Jeffrey S. Borer, Henry Krum, et al. "Differential Blood Pressure Effects of Ibuprofen, Naproxen, and Celecoxib in Patients with Arthritis: The PRECISION-ABPM (Prospective Randomized Evaluation of Celecoxib Integrated Study Versus Ibuprofen and Naproxen Ambulatory Blood Pressure Measurement) Trial." *European Heart Journal* 38, no. 44 (November 21, 2017): 3282–3292.

Smith, Elizabeth A., J. Gordon Marshall, Shelley S. Selph, et al. "Nonsteroidal Anti-Inflammatory Drugs for Managing Postoperative Pain in Patients Who Present with Preoperative Pain: A Systematic

Review and Meta-Analysis." *Journal of Endodontics* 43, no. 1 (January 2017): 7–15.

Sondergaard, Kathrine B., Peter Weeke, Mads Wissenberg, et al. "Non-Steroidal Anti-Inflammatory Drug Use Is Associated with Increased Risk of Out-of-Hospital Cardiac Arrest: A Nationwide Case-Time-Control Study." *European Heart Journal—Cardiovascular Pharmacotherapy* 3, no. 2 (April 1, 2017): 100–107.

Occupational Therapy

INTRODUCTION

Occupational therapists use therapeutic everyday activities to treat injured, ill, or disabled children or adults. In so doing, they help people develop, recover, improve, and maintain the skills needed for working and living.

According to occupational therapists, a person's life is made up of occupations or meaningful everyday activities. Occupations are the things people do to occupy themselves; they refer to any purposeful activity and include the areas of self-care, productivity, and leisure, as well as functioning in different roles, such as a parent, friend, or spouse. Occupational therapists try to help people who are having trouble completing their occupations because of a variety of reasons, including pain and disability. For example, if someone suffers a wrist injury or has arthritis in the wrist joints, it may be painful to dress in the morning, prepare meals, carry packages, or drive a car. Thus, wrist pain is disrupting daily occupations. It is the role of the occupational therapist to introduce changes, including environmental modifications and the use of assistive devices, that ease pain and support better functioning of the wrist. Occupational therapy tries to teach individuals and groups of people how to adapt. It enables people to do the things they need and want to do and to be as independent as possible. When dealing with pain, occupational therapists focus primarily on the impact of pain on occupational performance.

ADMINISTRATION AND REGULATION

Most occupational therapists work in hospitals or occupational therapy practices. They may also work in nursing and rehabilitation facilities, schools, prisons, corporate offices, industrial workplaces, outpatient clinics, community centers, physician offices, health-care facilities, and home health services. Though statistics vary, it has been estimated that there are over 100,000 occupational therapists employed in the United States.

A first appointment with an occupational therapist generally begins with an individualized evaluation of patient goals and which of the goals appear to be achievable. This appointment may take place at home, a workplace, or a school. Next, the occupational therapist will devise a customized intervention to improve the person's ability to perform daily activities and to reach specific goals. This may include assessment of a client's home, school, or workplace environment and a recommendation for the inclusion of adaptive equipment. It is a role of the occupational therapist to train the client or caregiver(s) how to use this equipment; the occupational therapist focuses on adapting the environment to fit the needs of the client and to find approaches that minimize pain. During the therapy, there will be periodic evaluations and modifications to ensure that the goals are achieved. On average, a patient will have six to eight occupational therapy sessions. Almost all insurance plans offer some form of occupational therapy. Still, insurance plans usually require a referral from a physician, who indicates that the therapy is medically necessary. People without insurance should discuss costs and payment options before therapy begins.

Occupational therapists earn an undergraduate degree and then a master's degree in occupational therapy. They must pass a national examination administered by the National Board for Certification in Occupational Therapy (NBCOT). However, licensure is conducted at the state level. Some occupational therapists complete additional training to specialize in a specific area, such as hand therapy. Occupational therapists often work in conjunction with physicians, physical therapists, psychologists, or other health professionals. Sometimes, occupational therapists work with occupational therapy assistants, though assistants never assess patients or create therapy plans.

BENEFITS AND RISKS

Occupational therapists help people recover from injury or illness and regain, to the fullest extent, their skills. They may offer support to elders who are experiencing physical and cognitive changes and to children with disabilities, enabling them to participate fully in school and social situations. Occupational therapists may be useful for people with a number of different conditions that cause chronic pain, such as arthritis, spinal cord injury, cancer, multiple sclerosis, and cerebral palsy.

There do not appear to be any significant risks associated with occupational therapy. Occupational therapy interventions seem to offer at least nominal benefits to the lives of most patients, and they have the potential to offer substantial improvements.

RESEARCH FINDINGS

Occupational Therapy Is Able to Play an Important Role in the Management of Chronic Pain

In a systematic review published in 2018 in the journal *Pain Research and Management*, researchers from Quebec (Canada) examined the various roles that occupational therapy may play in caring for people with chronic pain. The researchers located 52 studies that meet their criteria. These included 19 reviews, 13 empirical studies, 7 qualitative studies, 6 documents from the gray literature, 3 descriptive studies, 3 author opinions, and one mixed-method study. The studies originated in the United States, Canada, Sweden, Spain, Australia, France, Ireland, Germany, the Netherlands, Belgium, Denmark, Switzerland, and the United Kingdom. The researchers learned that the primary role of an occupational therapist was to improve activities and participation in adults living with chronic pain. These included actions that enhanced and restored functioning and body mechanics and activity tolerance. As experts in occupations, occupational therapists are particularly useful "in how individuals living with CP [chronic pain] can perform and engage in their daily occupations." Furthermore, "the use of disciplinary models ensures a better emphasis on occupation as an end and as a mean throughout the entire OT [occupational therapy] treatment process."[1]

In a retrospective trial published in 2017 in the *American Journal of Occupational Therapy*, researchers from Los Angeles, California (USA), tested the ability of an occupational therapy program known as Lifestyle Redesign® to help 45 patients suffering from chronic pain. The patients, who all lived in southern California, were referred to the program by their physicians. They had a mean age of 42.6 years, and there were 32 women, 12 men, and one person who did not provide an answer. The most common diagnoses were lumbago, myalgia, and complex regional pain syndrome. The mean number of occupational sessions was slightly over nine, and the mean duration of the therapy was 18 weeks. According to the researchers, Lifestyle Redesign is an occupational therapy method that focuses on the development of "healthy self-care routines and habits to prevent and manage chronic conditions." During individualized weekly sessions, the occupational therapist and patient focused on specific topics, such as physical activity, body mechanics, and planning for pain flare-ups. Working with the occupational therapist, patients learned to solve problems and increase their motivation. Solutions were identified, and healthy habits and daily routines were incorporated into their daily lives. The researchers determined that Lifestyle Redesign had a significant positive effect on the subjects dealing with chronic pain. For example, they had improvements in their functional abilities, self-efficacy, and quality of life. The researchers concluded that their findings "demonstrated the need for more occupational therapist incorporating lifestyle techniques into existing practices," as well as "the need to routinely incorporate occupational therapy into chronic pain management care."[2]

Occupational Therapy Appears to Help People with Rheumatoid Arthritis

In an article published in 2017 in the *American Journal of Occupational Therapy*, researchers from Albuquerque, New Mexico (USA), examined systematic reviews, meta-analyses, and randomized, controlled trials on the ability of occupational therapy to help people dealing with the painful symptoms of rheumatoid arthritis. The cohort consisted of 51 studies published between January 2000 and July 2014; 19 dealt with physical activity and 32 were psychoeducational. The physical activity studies reviewed home exercise and coaching, dynamic exercise, aquatic exercise, aerobic exercise, resistive exercise, Tai Chi, and yoga. The psychoeducational studies addressed patient education and self-management, cognitive behavioral therapy, multidisciplinary approaches, joint protection, assistive devices, emotional disclosure, and comprehensive occupational therapy. The researchers observed that none of the studies reported that the interventions caused adverse events or increased disease activity in the subjects. In fact, they found strong evidence that the interventions improved function, pain, and other symptoms associated with rheumatoid arthritis. A small number of randomized, controlled trials found little difference between the intervention and control groups. However, these trials tended to involve interventions that were short in duration or were very similar. In some studies, the subjects believed that they had improvements, although the measurement of symptoms did not change. Also, the researchers commented that more research is needed to determine ways to better sustain improvements. "Even though laboratory measures of disease activity may not appear to change, improvements in self-efficacy may have positive effects on psychological status, function, and overall well-being."[3]

There Is Room for Improvement on the Quality of Some of the Studies on the Ability of Occupational Therapy to Help People with Chronic Pain

In a systematic review published in 2015 in the journal *Occupational Journal International*, researchers from Sweden assessed the quality of 19 studies on the ability of occupational therapy to help people with chronic pain. The researchers included studies with subjects between the ages of 18 and 65 years who had chronic pain for more than three months. The studies had four main types of design—descriptive, experimental, outcome, and qualitative. A few of the studies were found to have high levels of evidence, and many were thought to have high levels of quality. As occupational therapists may play a role on the ability of a person to return to work, it was notable that seven of the studies focused on work-oriented interventions. And, many of the studies provided advisory or educational sessions including work techniques and management strategies in the performance of activities and adaptations to the environment. Outcome variables and follow-up times differed across the studies, though most had a follow-up before six months, and some had a follow-up between six months and four years. The researchers commented that there were high-quality studies with evidence that is able to guide clinical work. "Nevertheless, most of the studies need to be replicated with a larger number of subjects, as well as more distinct study designs."[4]

Occupational Therapy Appears to Benefit People with Lower-Extremity Musculoskeletal Disorders

In a systematic review published in 2017 in the *American Journal of Occupational Therapy*, researchers from Ithaca, New York (USA), investigated the ability of occupational therapy to help people dealing with lower-extremity musculoskeletal disorders, problems that may seriously impair their ability to carry out daily activities. The cohort consisted of 43 peer-reviewed scientific articles published in English between January 1995 and July 2014. The researchers focused on functional or occupation-based interventions, outcomes that targeted improving function, and other interventions within the scope of the practice of occupational therapy. The most commonly mentioned medical problems were hip fracture, hip or knee replacement, lower-extremity amputation or limb loss, and nonsurgical osteoarthritis and pain. The researchers found strong evidence that occupational therapy, when used in conjunction with a multidisciplinary team, was useful for people with hip fractures and hip or knee replacements. There was moderate evidence that occupational therapy, also when used in conjunction with a multidisciplinary team, was useful for people with lower-extremity amputation or limb loss. There is moderate evidence that occupational therapy is useful for hip and knee osteoarthritis. The researchers concluded that occupational therapy may serve an important function in rehabilitating people with lower-extremity musculoskeletal disorders.[5]

Occupational Therapists May Play an Important Role in Facilitating Pain Management in Children with Burn Injuries

In an article published in 2017 in the *Australian Occupational Therapy Journal*, researchers from Australia noted that it is well known that pain, anxiety, and stress are integral parts of burn injuries, as well as the numerous wound care procedures used to heal them. As a result, burn healing in children may be associated with prolonged healing, poor compliance with rehabilitation, chronic pain, sleep disturbances, poor feeding, and mental health issues. Although caring for children with burns is very much a team effort, the researchers noted that occupational therapists may play an integral role. By supporting children and their families and providing effective pain reduction interventions, occupational therapists help them deal with the painful procedures. These interventions, such as age-appropriate software content and age and injury-appropriate hardware design and usability, have resulted in "substantial reductions to the amount of pain and stress experienced by children and adolescents." In addition, the interventions improve compliance and reduce the time needed to complete wound care procedures. The researchers commented that "the application of these results extends globally with effective treatment of pain and anxiety, improvements to clinical process efficiency, treatment times and rates of healing in burn and other wound care procedures."[6]

Play-Based Occupational Therapy Seems to Help Children Hospitalized with Cancer

In a small pilot trial published in 2017 in the *Asia-Pacific Journal of Oncology Nursing*, researchers from Iran investigated the use of play-based occupational therapy on children hospitalized with cancer. The trial had only two children (a boy who was nine years old and a girl who was seven years old) with acute lymphoblastic leukemia who received at least two courses of chemotherapy. Each child had nine 30 to 40 minute play-based occupational therapy sessions. Play was used as both a means to reduce symptoms, such as pain, and as a way to increase their participation in playful activities. And, it was notably effective. Assessments demonstrated that the children experienced reductions in pain, anxiety, and fatigue scores. The researchers commented that "occupational therapy using both play as a means and play as end in pediatric oncology ward could help children to overcome some discomfort situations in the hospital."[7]

When a Parent Has Chronic Pain, Occupational Therapists May Help Families Cope

In a scientific literature review published in 2019 in the *Scandinavian Journal of Occupational Therapy*, researchers from New Zealand examined research on the role that occupational therapists may play in facilitating open family communication when at least one parent suffers from chronic pain. The review included 24 "items" published between 1978 and 2017. Two of the items were different chapters from the same book. Most of the items were peer-reviewed journal articles written for health professionals by health professionals, living in the United States. The authors were from a range of disciplines, and 12 authors contributed more than one item. The most commonly discussed approach involved health professionals working with the whole family unit. The researchers learned that occupational therapists may help family members find ways to participate in enjoyable shared occupations. Participating in these share occupations, such as eating dinner together, strengthens family bonds, and improves family communication. Additionally, the occupational therapist may teach the parent with pain to use pacing strategies to help manage fatigue. Learning these problem-solving and goal-setting strategies is important. "Therapists can use occupation-centered interventions to create opportunities for family conversations to occur, while also supporting members to develop the motivation, confidence and self-awareness required to clearly express their views to one another."[8]

Occupational Therapists Have Opinions on How to Manage Their Clients' Chronic Pain and the Obstacles That Their Clients Face

In a study published in 2013 in the *Australian Occupational Therapy Journal*, researchers interviewed nine occupational therapists from Australia and New Zealand. The researchers asked them to describe how their clients viewed their chronic pain, a common diagnosis. The study design was qualitative and used a narrative inquiry. The therapists were interviewed once or twice, with interviews lasting from two to three and a half hours; they had worked with chronic pain patients from as little as three years to over 20 years. All of the therapists believed that they played an important role in the lives of their clients. They reported that their clients thought having chronic pain meant the loss of valued life roles; for these clients, who were more often male, life did not appear to be worth living. Large numbers of their clients were depressed. The situation was even more complicated when the clients received compensation because of their chronic pain. They knew that if they improved, they would probably lose their compensation. "It was difficult for people to move forward in the pain management process while they had a chance of being financially compensated by remaining in high levels of pain." Some clients who did not improve had a lack of acceptance of their situation and little readiness for change. Likewise, some avoided activities, afraid that they would exacerbate the pain. It was not uncommon for clients to fixate on the need for a cure, rather than willfully participate in an exercise program. Faced with such challenging clients, the occupational therapists commented that they used a number of strategies such as goal setting, pacing, relaxation techniques, and cognitive behavior therapy. The therapists also needed to teach the clients to accept the fact that they are dealing with chronic pain that was not going away. Still, the results, especially in clients who were depressed, were not always notable or meaningful. Yet, clients with good family support tended to better manage their pain. The researchers concluded that "examining the narratives of therapist-participants adds to knowledge about chronic pain management."[9]

Some Occupational Therapists Need to Learn More about Pain

In a study published in 2016 in the journal *Disability and Rehabilitation*, researchers from Alberta, Canada wanted to learn if Canadian occupational therapists have sufficient levels of knowledge about pain or if the gaps that were found in earlier studies were still evident. The researchers electronically disseminated a self-report survey, which was open from May to July 2014, to all members of the Canadian Association of Occupational Therapists. Only practicing clinicians, who worked in a variety of settings, were included in the study. Three hundred twenty-four therapists completed the entire survey. Over 45 percent of the therapists had 10 years of experience or less. The researchers determined that the therapists selected the correct answers for two-thirds of the test items; in one-third of the test, only 85 percent or fewer therapists selected the correct responses. Interestingly, while 99.4 percent of the therapists indicated that the patient was the best judge of his or her pain, 17.7 percent of the therapists thought they could help determine if the patient was lying about pain. Among a sizable number of therapists there was a prevailing belief that patients tend to overstate their pain. "Respondents seem to fluctuate between placing a high premium on patient self-reported pain and issues of veracity." In addition, the researchers observed deficits in the areas of acute and chronic pain, pediatric pain, pain assessment, and medications. The researchers noted that it is "concerning that this study identified similar knowledge gaps as those identified in previous studies."[10]

NOTES

1. Lagueux, Émilie, Andréa Dépelteau, and Julie Masse. "Occupational Therapy's Unique Contribution to Chronic Pain Management: A Scoping Review." *Pain Research and Management* 2018 (2018): Article ID 5378451.

2. Uyeshuri Simon, Ashley, and Chantelle E. R. Collins. "Lifestyle Redesign® for Chronic Pain Management: A Retrospective Clinical Efficacy Study." *American Journal of Occupational Therapy* 71, no. 4 (2017): 7104190040p1–7104190040p7.

3. Siegel, Patricia, Melissa Tencza, Beverly Apodaca, and Janet L. Poole. "Effectiveness of Occupational Therapy Interventions for Adults with Rheumatoid Arthritis: A Systematic Review." *Journal of Occupational Therapy* 71, no. 1 (2017): 7101180050p1–7101180050p11.

4. Hesselstrand, Malin, Kersti Samuelsson, and Gunilla Liedberg. "Occupational Therapy Interventions in Chronic Pain—A Systematic Review." *Occupational Therapy International* 22 (2015): 183–194.

5. Dorsey, Julie, and Michelle Bradshaw. "Effectiveness of Occupational Therapy Interventions for Lower-Extremity Musculoskeletal Disorders: A Systematic Review." *Journal of Occupational Therapy* 71, no. 1 (2017): 7101180030p1–7101180030p11.

6. Kipping, Belinda, and Kate Miller. "Occupational Therapists' Role in Facilitating Pain Management in Children with Burn Injuries." *Australian Occupational Therapy Journal* 64, Supplement 1 (2017): 35–38.

7. Mohammadi, Ahmad, Afsoon Hassani Mehraban, and Shahla A. Damavandi. "Effect of Play-Based Occupational Therapy on Symptoms of Hospitalized Children with Cancer: A Single-Subject Study." *Asia-Pacific Journal of Oncology Nursing* 4, no. 2 (April–June 2017): 168–172.

8. Swift, Catherine, Clare Hocking, Annette Dickinson, and Margaret Jones. "Facilitating Open Family Communication When a Parent Has Chronic Pain: A Scoping Review." *Scandinavian Journal of Occupational Therapy* 26, no. 2(2019): 103–120.

9. van Huet, Helen, Ev Innes, and Roger Stancliffe. "Occupational Therapists Perspectives of Factors Influencing Chronic Pain Management." *Australian Occupational Therapy Journal* 60, no. 1 (2013): 56–65.

10. Reyes, Angelica N., and Cary A. Brown. "Occupational Therapists' Pain Knowledge: A National Survey." *Disability and Rehabilitation* 38, no. 13 (2016): 1309–1317.

REFERENCES AND FURTHER READINGS

Dorsey, Julie, and Michelle Bradshaw. "Effectiveness of Occupational Therapy Intervention for Lower-Extremity Musculoskeletal Disorders: A Systematic Review." *American Journal of Occupational Therapy* 71, no. 1 (2017): 7101180030p1–7101180030p11.

Hesselstrand, Malin, Kersti Samuelsson, and Gunilla Liedberg. "Occupational Therapy Interventions in Chronic Pain—A Systematic Review." *Occupational Therapy International* 22 (2015): 183–194.

Kipping, Belinda, and Kate Miller. "Occupational Therapists' Role in Facilitating Pain Management in Children with Burn Injuries." *Australian Occupational Therapy Journal* 64, Supplement 1 (2017): 35–38.

Lagueux, Émilie, Andréa Dépelteau, and Julie Masse. "Occupational Therapy's Unique Contribution to Chronic Pain Management: A

Scoping Review." *Pain Research and Management* 2018 (2018): Article ID 5378451.

Mohammadi, Ahmad, Afsoon Hassani Mehraban, and Shahla A. Damavandi. "Effect of Play-Based Occupational Therapy in Symptoms of Hospitalized Children with Cancer: A Single-Subject Study." *Asia-Pacific Journal of Oncology Nursing* 4, no. 2 (April–June 2017): 168–172.

Reyes, Angelica N., and Cary A. Brown. "Occupational Therapists' Pain Knowledge: A National Survey." *Disability and Rehabilitation* 38, no. 13 (2016): 1309–1317.

Siegel, Patricia, Melissa Tencza, Beverly Apodaca, and Janet L. Poole. "Effectiveness of Occupational Therapy Intervention for Adults with Rheumatoid Arthritis: A Systematic Review." *American Journal of Occupational Therapy* 71, no. 1 (2017): 7101180050p1–7101180050p.11.

Swift, Catherine, Clare Hocking, Annette Dickinson, and Margaret Jones. "Facilitating Open Family Communication When a Parent Has Chronic Pain: A Scoping Review." *Scandinavian Journal of Occupational Therapy* 26, no. 2 (2019): 103–120.

Uyeshiro Simon, Ashley, and Chantelle E. R. Collins. "Lifestyle Redesign® for Chronic Pain Management: A Retrospective Clinical Efficacy Study." *American Journal of Occupational Therapy* 71, no. 4 (2017): 7104190040p1–7104190040p7.

van Huet, Helen, Ev Innes, and Roger Stancliffe. "Occupational Therapists Perspectives of Factors Influencing Chronic Pain Management." *Australian Occupational Therapy Journal* 60, no. 1 (2013): 56–65.

Opioids and Opiates

INTRODUCTION

An opiate is a drug naturally derived from the flowering opium poppy plant. Examples are codeine, morphine, and heroin. Opioid is a broader term that includes any substance, natural or synthetic, that binds to the brain's opioid receptors—to the parts of the brain that are responsible for controlling pain, rewards, and addictive behavior. Some examples of synthetic opioids are hydrocodone, oxycodone, fentanyl, and methadone. Though these terms have often been used interchangeably, the term "opiate" is becoming obsolete. "Opioids" is now the term used to describe opioids and opiates.

Also known as narcotics, opioids are common medications that have been repeatedly demonstrated to relieve pain and relax the body. They are frequently prescribed to help people dealing with moderate to severe pain associated with surgery, accidents, falls, and chronic illnesses and medical problems, such as cancer pain, chronic back pain, and osteoarthritis.

Opioids bind to and activate opioid receptors on cells in many areas of the brain, as well as the spinal cord and other organs of the body, especially organs involved in feeling pain and pleasure. After the opioids attach to these receptors, they block pain signals from the brain to the body, and they release dopamine into the body.

Not everyone uses opioids for medically approved reasons. In fact, opioids are often misused. For example, opioids may be used in a way not approved by the medical provider. People sometimes take someone else's opioid medication, and it is not at all uncommon for people to take opioids simply for a "high." People who misuse opioids may swallow them as usual, or they may crush pills, open capsules, dissolve the power into water, snort the powder, or inject the liquid into a vein. Countless numbers of people misuse opioid medications every day. People who overdose on opioids, and may be at risk for death, may be treated with a medication known as naloxone, which is sold as a nasal spray or handheld auto-injector. It works by binding to opioid receptors and blocking the effects of the opioids. Opioid misuse, addiction, and overdoses are huge public health problems in the United States. Opioid misuse may lead to heroin use; this occurs when people have problems obtaining prescriptions for opioids or are unable to pay for their opioid prescriptions and turn to heroin.

Though the annual prescribing rates of opioids have been going down, according to the Centers for Disease Control and Prevention, in 2017, there were almost 58 opioid prescriptions written for every 100 Americans. More than 17 percent of Americans had at least one opioid prescription filled, with an average of 3.4 opioid prescriptions per person. The average number of days per prescription continues to increase, with an average of 18 days in 2017.[1]

ADMINISTRATION AND REGULATION

Legal opioids are prescribed by medical providers. Generally, they are prescribed for a relatively short period of time. However, in some instances, they are needed for longer time periods. While the oral administration is the easiest, opioids may be administered in several other ways including intravenous, intramuscular, subcutaneous, rectal, inhaled, topical, and sublingual.

Opioids are schedule II controlled medications that are legally issued only by a physician, dentist, podiatrist, veterinarian, midlevel practitioner, or other registered practitioner. Practitioners who prescribe opioids must be registered with the Drug Enforcement Administration (DEA). It is the responsibility of the practitioner to prescribe a controlled substance properly; similarly, it is the responsibility of the pharmacist to dispense the prescription correctly. Opioids require a written prescription signed by the practitioner; an oral order may only be used in an emergency situation for a 72-hour supply. A prescription for opioids must be dated and signed. It must include the patient's full name and address and the practitioner's full name, address, and DEA registration number. The prescription must also include the drug name, strength, dosage for the quantity prescribed, directions for use, and number of refills, if allowed. The preference is for opioid prescriptions to be electronically signed and faxed to the pharmacy.

Although some states and many insurance companies limit the amount of opioids that may be dispensed during a 30-day period of time, there are no federal limits. In 2016, Massachusetts became the first state to pass a law limiting first-time opioid prescriptions to seven days. Since then, many more states have passed laws that restrict the prescribing and dispensing of opioids for acute pain.

While opioids tend to be expensive, often several dollars per pill, they are usually covered by insurance, at least for a specific period of time. People who take opioids for noncancer-related problems may find that their medical provider is reluctant to continue to prescribe such medication and their insurer no longer wants to pay for the potentially addictive drugs.

BENEFITS AND RISKS

It is well known that opioids provide excellent relief for short-term pain. People who have undergone surgery or have broken a bone will be spared untold pain by taking opioids for a few days. In addition, taking an opioid medication will enable them to rest more comfortably and begin rehabilitation in a more timely manner.

However, not all pain is short-term pain. It has been estimated that about 40 percent of Americans suffer from some type of chronic pain; about 10 percent suffer from debilitating pain. Also, standard treatments do not provide relief to everyone. Without a doubt, medical providers feel an obligation to address their patients' pain. Furthermore, people who have been suffering from nonstop pain are desperate for a lifeline.

On the other hand, it is well known that opioids have a number of problematic side effects. These include drowsiness, confusion, nausea, constipation, dry mouth, euphoria, increased sensitivity to pain, itching, sweating, and slowed breathing. When breathing is slowed, too little oxygen may reach the brain, a condition called hypoxia. Hypoxia appears to have short- and long-term psychological and neurological effects including brain damage, coma, and death.

It is not uncommon for people taking opioids to develop a tolerance. Over time, they may require higher doses to achieve the same pain relief.

Women who are pregnant should realize that the growing fetus may develop a dependence on opioids and may need to go through withdrawal after birth. In addition, women who use opioids have an increased risk of miscarriage and having a baby with lower birth weight. (Pregnant women who seek treatment for their addiction from providers who offer methadone and buprenorphine tend to have better outcomes than those who attempt to quit suddenly by themselves.)

Pharmaceutical fentanyl is a synthetic opioid pain reliever that is approved for severe pain. It is 50 to 100 times more potent than morphine. Most cases of fentanyl-related problems are associated with products that have been made illegally. To enhance the euphoric effects, illegal drug marketers may mix fentanyl with heroin or cocaine.

Heroin is an illegal, highly addictive opioid drug. Though it is usually injected, heroin may be smoked and snorted. Injecting heroin increases the risk of acquiring viral infections such as HIV, hepatitis B, and hepatitis C and bacterial infections involving the skin, bloodstream, and heart. People tend to use heroin together with other drugs or alcohol, which increases the risk of an overdose. A heroin overdose may cause slow breathing, coma, and death.

The repeated misuse of opioids may lead to substance use disorder; people with a substance use disorder tend to be unable to meet their work, school, or home responsibilities. Yet, withdrawal from opioids is associated with a host of different medical concerns including muscle and bone pain, sleep problems, diarrhea and vomiting, cold flashes and goose bumps, uncontrollable leg movements, and severe cravings. There are medications, such as lofexidine, that may help reduce opioid withdrawal symptoms.

It is not an exaggeration to say that the misuse of opioids in the United States is a serious national health crisis. Information listed on the website of the National Institute on Drug Abuse noted that roughly 21 to 29 percent of people prescribed opioids for chronic pain misuse them. Between 8 and 12 percent develop an opioid use disorder. About 4 to 6 percent who misuse prescription opioids transition to heroin, and about 80 percent of people who use heroin first misused prescription opioids. Data obtained in 2018 found that everyday on average 128 people in the United States die from overdosing on opioids. It has been estimated that the total economic burden of the misuse of prescription opioids is U.S. $78.5 billion per year.[2]

RESEARCH FINDINGS

Oral Oxycodone Is a Safe and Effective Postoperative Pain Medication

In a review published in 2017 in the journal *Pain Physician*, researchers from Hong Kong evaluated 26 clinical studies that examined the use of oral oxycodone to relieve postoperative pain. Thirteen of the studies had a randomized double-blind trial design, and 10 had a placebo control arm. Seventeen studies were randomized trials with an active comparator. Three studies compared a prospective cohort with a retrospective historical cohort. One open-label study compared results from two prospective cohorts. The types of surgery varied widely and included abdominal surgery, joint arthroplasty, foot surgery, spine surgery, and breast surgery. There were even studies on caesarean sections, retinal surgery, and dental surgery. The researchers learned that when compared to placebos, the oral oxycodone provided superior pain relief and the use of less rescue medication. When compared to intravenous opioids, oral oxycodone provided comparable or better pain control and, in some instances, a reduced need for rescue medication. However, oral oxycodone was inferior to rofecoxib in treating pain from dental surgery. The researchers concluded that "more randomized, double-blind, controlled trials comparing oral oxycodone with other standard analgesics in different postsurgical pain models are needed to determine the most effective approach in each scenario."[3]

Yet, Many People Do Not Take Their Prescribed Opioids after Surgery

In a systematic review published in 2017 in *JAMA Surgery*, researchers from Baltimore, Maryland (USA), examined why people failed to take all of the opioids they are prescribed after a surgical procedure. The researchers located six eligible intermediate quality studies that had a total of 810 subjects; all of the subjects lived in the United States. The number of subjects in each study ranged from 30 to 250, and the studies involved seven different types of surgical procedures including obstetrical, thoracic, orthopedic, and urologic. There were cross-sectional and cohort studies, as well as randomized, controlled studies of adult patients who were prescribed at least one oral opioid medication after inpatient or outpatient discharge. The researchers noted that between two-thirds and nine-tenths of the subjects reported unused opioids. Why did they take such small amounts of their medications? Between 71 and 83 percent noted that they had adequate pain control; between 16 percent and 29 percent indicated a concern for side effects. Only one study addressed the risk of addiction, and about 8 percent of thoracic surgery patients avoided opioids for that reason. The majority of subjects stored opioids in the medicine cabinet or other box. That was followed by a cupboard or wardrobe. It is important to note that 73 to 77 percent of the opioids were in unlocked locations. Only between 4 and 30 percent of the subjects planned to dispose or actually disposed of their opioids. The researchers commented that "the combination of unused opioids, poor-storage practices, and lack of disposal sets the stage for the diversion of opioids for nonmedical use."[4]

Opioids Appear to Be Useful in the Treatment of Noncancer Pain for Up to Three Months

In a systematic review and meta-analysis published in 2018 in the *Journal of Pain Research*, researchers from Massachusetts and Rhode Island (USA) evaluated the efficacy of any type of opioid medication (administered via the oral, transdermal nasal, sublingual, or transmucosal routes) to treat chronic noncancer pain. Fifteen randomized, double-blind, placebo-controlled trials met the researchers' criteria; they included trials on various types of chronic nonmalignant pain, such as chronic low back pain and osteoarthritis. Studies of acute or postsurgical pain were excluded. Fourteen trials were considered to be high quality; the most often used opioid was hydrocodone. The researchers learned that when compared to placebos, opioid medication was found to be statistically significant for measurements of pain, such as pain intensity, improvements in pain, patient's global impression of change, and patient's global assessment of study medication. The researchers concluded that "there is an ample evidence base supporting the efficacy of opioid analgesics for at least 3 months duration, a standard period for the evaluation of treatments for chronic pain and other chronic disorders."[5]

Sublingual Fentanyl Tablets Appear Useful for Breakthrough Cancer Pain

In a multicenter, prospective, observational, open-label study published in 2018 in the journal *Drugs in R & D*, researchers from Spain assessed the ability of sublingual fentanyl tablets to help cancer patients with breakthrough pain, or a sudden increase in pain in people who already have chronic pain. The initial cohort consisted of 81 subjects with either locally advanced cancer or metastatic cancer; all of the subjects were regularly experiencing breakthrough cancer pain. Thirty-nine subjects were already taking oxycodone/naloxone, and 29 were taking fentanyl. All of the subjects were provided sublingual fentanyl tablets to take when they experienced this pain. All pain relief and quality of life outcomes were reviewed at 3 days, 7 days, 15 days, and 30 days, when the trial ended. Sixty-nine subjects completed the trial. The mean age was 69.7 years, and 58 percent were female. The researchers learned that pain relief was achieved within minutes, and pain intensity values decreased. Interestingly, the subjects who were already taking fentanyl had better relief than those who were already taking oxycodone/naloxone. When the subjects were grouped according to cancer stage, pain intensity outcomes were better for those with metastatic cancer than for locally advanced cancer. The researchers concluded that the use of sublingual fentanyl tablets for treating breakthrough cancer pain was effective and safe, "regardless of their cancer stage and background opioid medication."[6]

There Appears to Be No Evidence that Morphine, Fentanyl, Oxycodone, or Codeine Affect Patient Consciousness, Appetite, and Thirst When Used to Treat Cancer Pain

In a systematic review published in 2014 in the *Cochrane Database of Systematic Reviews*, researchers from the United Kingdom wanted to learn more about the impact of opioids on consciousness, appetite, and thirst in end-stage cancer patients. They were concerned that morphine, fentanyl, oxycodone, and codeine may impair patient consciousness and lead to earlier death. In addition, they worried that the effect of these opioids on appetite and thirst may result in unnecessary suffering. The researchers located 77 relevant studies with 5,619 subjects. Most of the studies were small and had the potential risk of bias. In 60 of the studies, the individual treatment groups had fewer than 50 subjects. The mean age of the subjects tended to be between 50 and 70 years. Several problems in the reporting of adverse events were observed, such as the failure to report adverse events in all of the subjects who received medication and the failure to note how adverse events were tallied. Still, the researchers found no direct evidence that opioids affected the subjects' consciousness, appetite, or thirst. However, the researchers learned that people with cancer pain who were treated with these opioids often had somnolence (drowsiness), dry mouth, and anorexia. The researchers concluded that adverse events "cannot always be attributed unequivocally to the use of opioids."[7]

The Use of Hydrocodone May Not Significantly Impair Driving

In a double-blind, placebo-controlled crossover study published in 2018 in the journal *Traffic Injury Prevention*, researchers from Iowa and Missouri (USA) evaluated the influence of hydrocodone/acetaminophen (Norco, 10mg/325mg) and the antianxiety medication alprazolam (Xanax, 1mg) on driving. The cohort consisted of eight adults who had valid driver licenses and drove at least 5,000 miles per year. All passed a general physical and psychological examination and were found to have no evidence of a chronic disease that would affect driving. The subjects were evenly split by gender and had a mean age of 30 years. At baseline, the subjects were given a 10-panel urine drug screen. During four study visits, which were at least five days apart, the researchers administered a placebo, alprazolam alone, hydrocodone/acetaminophen, and the combination of the drugs during a standardized simulated driving protocol. Using the Stanford Sleepiness Scale, the researchers assessed levels of drowsiness before and after the approximately 35-minute simulator drive. The drive involved driving from an urban environment to an interstate and then a rural road. During the final 10 minutes, they drove on a straight two-lane rural road at night. Though alprazolam clearly impaired driving, the changes associated with the hydrocodone preparation ranged from very small to medium. Still, the researchers cautioned that the sample was small. With such a small sample, it is "more difficult to draw conclusions on the narcotic effects." Nevertheless, the effects of the hydrocodone medication were "much less pronounced" than the effects of the antianxiety medication.[8]

In the Emergency Department, a Single Dose of Oral Opioid Worked about as Well as Nonopioid Analgesics for Acute Moderate to Severe Extremity Pain

In a randomized, single-center, double-blind, clinical trial published in 2017 in *JAMA*, researchers from New York compared the effectiveness of different single doses of opioid or nonopioid oral medications for acute moderate to severe extremity pain in an emergency department in Bronx, New York. The cohort consisted of 411 emergency department patients with acute extremity pain; slightly less than half were women. Sixty percent were Latino, and 31 percent were Black. While awaiting further care, the subjects received either 400 mg of ibuprofen and 1,000 mg of acetaminophen, 5 mg of oxycodone and 325 mg of acetaminophen, 5 mg of hydrocodone and 300 mg of acetaminophen, or 30 mg of codeine and 300 mg of acetaminophen. Patients were asked to give numeric pain ratings after one hour and again after two hours. The researchers learned that, over time, the pain intensity declined in all forms of treatment. None of the differences between the analgesics was statistically significant or minimally clinically important. The researchers observed that their "findings support the inference that there are no clinically meaningful differences between the analgesic effects of these 4 analgesics and suggest that a combination of ibuprofen and acetaminophen represents an alternative to oral opioid analgesics for the treatment of acute extremity pain in the ED [emergency department]."[9]

There Are Many Adverse Effects Associated with the Medium- to Long-Term Use of Opioids for Chronic Noncancer Pain

In an overview published in 2017 in the *Cochrane Database of Systematic Reviews*, researchers from Canada examined past *Cochrane* reviews of the adverse effects associated with the use of opioids for chronic noncancer pain for medium to longer periods of time. The researchers included 16 reviews in their analysis; of these, 14 presented with unique quantitative data. The 14 reviews investigated 14 different opioids that were administered for at least two weeks. Although most of the studies continued for 6 to 16 weeks, the longest study was 13 months in duration. The quality of the studies tended to be high. The 14 reviews included a total of 61 studies with 18,679 randomized subjects. When compared to placebos, the review found that taking opioids significantly increased the risk of experiencing adverse events and a serious adverse event. When compared to nonopioid pain medications, people who took opioids also had a greater risk of adverse events. Many adverse events were associated more with opioids than placebos. These included constipation, dizziness, drowsiness, fatigue, hot flashes, increased sweating, nausea, pruritus (severe itching of the skin), and vomiting. When placebos were used as a comparison, the "absolute event rate" for any adverse events with opioids was 78 percent, with an absolute rate of 7.5 percent for any serious event. "Based on the adverse events identified, clinically relevant benefit would need to be clearly demonstrated before long-term use could be considered in people with CNCP [chronic non-cancer pain] in clinical practice."[10]

While It Is Not Always Easy for Practitioners to Identify Who Is More Likely to Become Addicted to Opioids, There Are a Few Indicators

In a systematic review published in 2019 in *JAMA Network*, researchers from Ireland, Canada, Italy, and New York City and North Carolina (USA) wanted to learn how physicians could differentiate between patients at higher or lower risk for addiction to opioids. Six high-quality studies were included in the qualitative synthesis, and four high-quality studies were included in the quantitative synthesis. From these studies, the researchers learned that a history of any pain disorder, a personality disorder, a somatoform disorder, a psychotic disorder, and nonopioid substance use disorder were associated with an increased risk of prescription opioid addiction. On the other hand, only the absence of a mood disorder seemed to reduce the likelihood of opioid addiction. Meanwhile, the researchers observed that people who obtained a new prescription for any opioid for 30 days or more (as opposed to fewer than 30 days) as well as those who had prescriptions for doses greater than 120 morphine milligram equivalents or more had an increased risk of developing opioid use disorder. The researchers realized that determining which patients could safely take opioids was quite difficult. "While a history of substance use disorder, certain mental health diagnoses, and concomitant prescription of certain psychiatric medications appeared useful for identifying patients at higher risk, few quality studies were available and no symptoms, signs, or screening tools were particularly useful for identifying those at lower risk."[11]

Opioids Are About as Useful as Nonopioid Analgesics for Chronic Back Pain, Chronic Hip Pain, and Knee Osteoarthritis

In a 12-month, randomized, clinical trial published in 2018 in *JAMA*, researchers from Minnesota and Indiana compared the use of opioids to nonopioid medications for the pain associated with chronic back pain, chronic hip pain, or knee osteoarthritis. The initial cohort consisted of 240 subjects who had moderate to severe chronic back pain, chronic hip pain, or knee osteoarthritis pain, despite analgesic use. Sixty-five percent had chronic back pain, and 35 percent had either chronic hip pain or knee osteoarthritis pain. They were recruited from 62 Minneapolis Veterans Affairs primary care clinicians between June 2013 to December 2015.

They had a mean age of 58.3 years, and 32 subjects were women. Subjects on long-term opioids were excluded. The subjects were placed on opioids or nonopioid medications. In the opioid group, the first step was immediate-release morphine, oxycodone, or hydrocodone/acetaminophen; for the nonopioid group, the first step was acetaminophen (paracetamol) or a nonsteroidal anti-inflammatory drug. According to the needs of each subject, medications were changed, added, adjusted within the assigned treatment group. Follow-up rates were 92 percent at 3 months, 97 percent at 6 months, 90 percent at 9 months, and 98 percent at 12 months. The findings are truly notable. When compared to the treatment with nonopioids over a 12-month period of time, the treatment with opioids did not offer superior pain relief. At the same time, the opioid medications caused significantly more medication-related adverse symptoms. The researchers commented that "opioids did not demonstrate any advantage over nonopioid medications that could potentially outweigh their greater risk of harms." Their findings "do not support initiation of opioid therapy for moderate to severe chronic back pain or hip or knee osteoarthritis pain."[12]

NOTES

1. Centers for Disease Control and Prevention. www.cdc.gov.

2. National Institute on Drug Abuse. https://www.drugabuse.gov.

3. Cheung, Chi Wai, Stanley Sau Ching Wong, Qiu Qiu, and Xianyu Wang. "Oral Oxycodone for Acute Postoperative Pain: A Review of Clinical Trials." *Pain Physician* 20 (2017): SE33–SE52.

4. Bicket, Mark C., Jae J. Long, Peter J. Pronovost, et al. "Prescription Opioids Commonly Unused after Surgery: A Systematic Review." *JAMA Surgery* 152, no. 11 (November 1, 2017): 1066–1071.

5. Meske, Diana S., Oluwadolapo D. Lawal, Harrison Elder, et al. "Efficacy of Opioids versus Placebo in Chronic Pain: A Systematic Review and Meta-Analysis of Enriched Enrollment Randomized Withdrawal Trials." *Journal of Pain Research* 11 (2018): 923–934.

6. Guitart, Jordi, María Isabel Vargas, Vicente De Sanctis, et al. "Efficacy and Safety of Sublingual Fentanyl Tablets in Breakthrough Cancer Pain Management According to Cancer Stage and Background Opioid Medication." *Drugs in R & D* 18 (2018): 119–128.

7. Wiffen, Philip J., Sheena Derry, and R. Andrew Moore. "Impact of Morphine, Fentanyl, Oxycodone or Codeine on Patient Consciousness,

Appetite and Thirst When Used to Treat Cancer Pain." *Cochrane Database of Systematic Reviews* 5 (May 29, 2014): CD011056.

8. Brown, Timothy L., Gary Milavetz, Gary Gaffney, and Andrew Spurgin. "Evaluating Drugged Driving: Effects of Exemplar Pain and Anxiety Medications." *Traffic Injury Prevention* 19, Supplement 1 (February 28, 2018): S97–S103.

9. Chang, Andrew K., Polly E. Bijur, David Esses, et al. "Effect of a Single Dose of Oral Opioid and Nonopioid Analgesics on Acute Extremity Pain in the Emergency Department." *JAMA* 38, no. 17 (November 7, 2017): 1661–1667.

10. Els, C., T. D. Jackson, D. Kunyk, et al. "Adverse Events Associated with Medium- and Long-Term Use of Opioids for Chronic Non-Cancer Pain: An Overview of Cochrane Reviews." *Cochrane Database of Systematic Reviews* 10 (2017): CD012509.

11. Klimas, Jan, Lauren Gorfinkel, Nadia Fairbairn, et al. "Strategies to Identify Patient Risk of Prescription Opioid Addiction When Initiating Opioids for Pain." *JAMA Network Open* 2, no. 5 (May 2019): e193365.

12. Krebs, Erin E., Amy Gravely, Sean Nugent, et al. "Effect of Opioid vs Nonopioid Knee Osteoarthritis Pain: The SPACE Randomized Clinical Trial." *JAMA* 319, no. 9 (March 6, 2018): 872–882.

REFERENCES AND FURTHER READINGS

Bicket, Mark C., Jane J. Long, Peter J. Pronovost, et al. "Prescription Opioids Commonly Unused after Surgery: A Systematic Review." *JAMA Surgery* 152, no. 11 (November 1, 2017): 1066–1071.

Brown, Timothy L., Gary Milaveta, Gary Gaffney, and Andrew Spurgin. "Evaluating Drugged Driving: Effects of Exemplar Pain and Anxiety Medications." *Traffic Injury Prevention* 19, Supplement 1 (February 28, 2018): S97–S103.

Centers for Disease Control and Prevention. www.cdc.gov.

Chang, Andrew K., Polly E. Bijur, David Esses, et al. "Effect of a Single Dose of Oral Opioid and Nonopioid Analgesics on Acute Extremity Pain in the Emergency Department: A Randomized Clinical Trial." *JAMA* 318, no. 17 (November 7, 2017): 1661–1667.

Cheung, Chi Wai, Stanley Sau Ching Wong, Qiu Qiu, and Xianyu Wang. "Oral Oxycodone for Adults Postoperative Pain: A Review of Clinical Trials." *Pain Physician* 20 (2017): SE33–SE52.

Els, C., T. D. Jackson, D. Kunyk, et al. "Adverse Effects Associated with Medium- and Long-Term Use of Opioids for Chronic Non-Cancer Pain: An Overview of Cochrane Reviews." *Cochrane Database of Systematic Reviews* 10 (2017): CD012509.

Guitart, Jordi, María Isabel Vargas, Vicente De Sanctis, et al. "Efficacy and Efficacy of Sublingual Fentanyl Tablets in Breakthrough Cancer Pain Management According to Cancer Stage and Background Opioid Medication." *Drugs in R & D* 18 (2018): 119–128.

Klimas, Jan, Lauren Gorfinkel, Nadia Fairbairn, et al. "Strategies to Identify Patient Risks of Prescription Opioid Addiction When Initiating Opioids for Pain." *JAMA Network Open* 2, no. 5 (May 2019): e193365.

Krebs, Erin E., Amy Gravely, Sean Nugent, et al. "Effect of Opioid vs. Nonopioid Medications on Pain-Related Function in Patients with Chronic Back Pain in Hip or Knee Osteoarthritis Pain: The SPACE Randomized Clinical Trial." *JAMA* 319, no. 9 (March 6, 2018): 872–882.

Meske, Diana S., Oluwadolapo D. Lawal, Harrison Elder, et al. "Efficacy of Opioids versus Placebo in Chronic Pain: A Systematic Review and Meta-Analysis of Enriched Enrollment Randomized Withdrawal Trials." *Journal of Pain Research* 11 (2018): 923–934.

National Institute on Drug Abuse. https://www.drugabuse.gov.

Wiffen, Phillip, Sheena Derry, and R. Andrew Moore. "Impact of Morphine, Fentanyl, Oxycodone or Codeine on Patients Consciousness, Appetite and Thirst When Used to Treat Cancer Pain." *Cochrane Database of Systematic Reviews* 5 (May 29, 2014): CD011056.

Pain-Relieving Foods and Beverages

INTRODUCTION

It is well known that some foods are healthier than others. Obviously, it is better to eat a grilled, skinless chicken breast with steamed broccoli and rice than a three-cheese, pepperoni pizza; and fresh fruit is a healthier choice for dessert than three scoops of whole-fat ice cream.

One of the many reasons that some foods and beverages are better alternatives is that they appear to support good health. In some instances, they have properties or components that enable them to reduce inflammation. For example, berries have lots of vitamins and antioxidants called flavonoids; flavonoids fight inflammation. And green tea contains epigallocatechin gallate (EGCG), the most powerful type of catechin, which has similar anti-inflammation properties. Salmon is an excellent source of omega-3 fatty acids, a type of nutrient that reduces inflammation and eases joint pain.

Why is this important? A good deal of chronic pain is a result of chronic inflammation. The list of illnesses associated with inflammation is too long to note, but it includes rheumatoid arthritis and other types of joint diseases, back pain, allergies, psoriasis, chronic peptic ulcer, active and chronic hepatitis, diabetes, Crohn's disease, ulcerative colitis, chronic obstructive pulmonary disease, vasculitis, some cancers, sinusitis, and chronic periodontitis.

When people include more anti-inflammatory foods and beverages in their diets, they have the potential to decrease the levels of pain that they are experiencing. Though foods and beverages alone may be sufficient to relieve mild pain, they will probably not eliminate moderate to severe pain. Still, anti-inflammatory foods and beverages will help people to better deal with and manage their pain. Some foods are even useful as a poultice, as will become evident later in this entry.

There are many examples of anti-inflammatory foods. These include fatty fish, broccoli, avocados, mushrooms, grapes, extra virgin olive oil, dark chocolate, tomatoes, and cherries. The foods and beverages included in this entry are cinnamon, flaxseed, garlic, and green tea.

ADMINISTRATION AND REGULATION

The best way to support pain reduction is to incorporate many different anti-inflammatory foods in the diet. When this is not possible, some may be available as a supplement or a poultice. At the same time, it is important to reduce the intake of foods that increase inflammation, such as fatty foods, red meat and processed meats, French fries, white bread, white pasta, high fructose corn syrup, soda and other sugar-sweetened beverages, margarine, shortening, lard, and foods with simple sugars. These changes must be ongoing. If not, the inflammation will return, as will the pain.

While there are many governmental regulations concerning food, there are no specific regulations associated with anti-inflammatory foods. There are far fewer regulations of supplements. It should be noted that healthier anti-inflammatory foods tend to be more expensive than foods that foster inflammation. That is why many people, especially people with lower incomes, all too often eat the less desirable food choices that support inflammation and pain.

BENEFITS AND RISKS

Of course, the goal is to find lots of enjoyable foods and beverages that reduce pain and inflammation. But, not everyone can consume even smaller amounts of these foods. Millions of people have food allergies; they may react to even tiny amounts of a certain foods, such as milk, eggs, wheat, peanuts, and soybeans. Reactions may vary from hives and rashes to severe breathing problems and death. Fortunately, most anti-inflammatory foods are not common allergens. Still, any food has the potential to be an allergen.

Far more common than food allergies are food intolerances. Food intolerances occur when people develop uncomfortable responses, especially uncomfortable gastrointestinal problems, when they ingest certain foods. Though people may develop intolerance to almost any food, common food intolerances include dairy, gluten, and foods with caffeine, such as caffeinated coffee and tea. Still, healthy foods may be problematic for some. For example, when some people consume garlic, they experience side effects such as bad breath, a burning sensation in the mouth or stomach, heartburn, gas, nausea, vomiting, body odor, and diarrhea. These side effects may be even worse with raw garlic. And, there have been reports of excessive bleeding after surgery in people who consume garlic.

RESEARCH FINDINGS

Cinnamon

Cinnamon May Help Primary Dysmenorrhea or Menstrual Pain

In a randomized, double-blind clinical trial published in 2018 in the journal *Complementary Therapies in Clinical Practice*, researchers from Iran examined the use of cinnamon for menstrual pain. The cohort consisted of 80 single female college students who lived in the dormitories of a medical sciences university. All of the women had regular menstrual cycles but suffered from menstrual pain. For two menstrual cycles, the 40 women in the intervention group, who had a mean age of 22.2 years, took 1,000 mg cinnamon three times per day during the first 72 hours of menstruation; the 40 women in the control group, who had a mean age of 22.3 years, followed the same protocol but took 1,000 mg of starch. Subjects were assessed after each cycle, and changes in pain levels were noted. Both groups experienced reductions in pain, but the researchers found that pain reduction was significantly higher in the cinnamon group. The researchers concluded, "that using Cinnamon 3 g daily can significantly reduce the severity of menstrual pain and is safe."[1]

In a randomized, double-blind clinical trial published in 2015 in the *Journal of Clinical & Diagnostic Research*, different researchers from Iran compared the effect of cinnamon and ibuprofen for menstrual pain. The cohort consisted of 114 women with "moderate" menstrual pain; all of the subjects were college students who lived in dormitories. Thirty-eight subjects were assigned to take 420 mg cinnamon capsules 3 times each day; 38 subjects were placed on 400 mg ibuprofen three times each day; and 38 subjects took placebo capsules containing starch. The women in all three groups had similar characteristics. Pain intensity and duration were monitored at baseline and nine additional times during the first 72 hours of the menstrual cycle of each subject. The mean pain severity and the mean duration of pain were less for the women in the cinnamon and ibuprofen groups than for the women in the control group. However, cinnamon was less effective than ibuprofen. The researchers concluded that "due to the lack of adverse events in this study, cinnamon can be used as a safe and non-pharmacological treatment for primary dysmenorrheal pain."[2]

Cinnamon May Help the Pain Associated with Rheumatoid Arthritis

In a randomized, double-blind clinical trial published in 2018 in the *Journal of the American College of Nutrition*, researchers also from Iran investigated the use of cinnamon for women with rheumatoid arthritis. For eight weeks, 36 women with rheumatoid arthritis took four capsules per day of 500 mg cinnamon powder (n=18) or a starch placebo (n=18). They took two capsules after breakfast and two after dinner. No adverse effects were reported; only one subject in the cinnamon group reported mild gastric discomfort. The researchers determined that by the end of the trial, the mean score for pain decreased significantly in the cinnamon group. Furthermore, the differences remained after adjustments were made for menopausal status. The researchers concluded that "the regular intake of cinnamon supplement may be used as a pharmacological agent in the treatment of RA."[3]

Flaxseed

Flaxseed May Be Useful for Breast Pain

In a "quasi"-randomized clinical trial published in 2017 in the *Journal of Education and Health Promotion*, researchers from Iran investigated the use of flaxseed, evening primrose oil, and vitamin E for periodic breast pain. All of the 90 subjects, who had a mean age of 30 years, had cyclical breast pain for at least five consecutive days in two previous menstrual cycles. The women were divided into three groups. At baseline, the women in all three groups had about the same levels of breast pain. The women in the first group took 30 g of powdered flaxseed everyday; the women in the second group took two 1,000 mg capsules of evening primrose oil everyday; and the women in the third group took one capsule of 400 IU vitamin E each day. The trial continued for two menstrual cycles. During this time, five women in the flaxseed group reported side effects, such as diarrhea and nausea. The researchers learned that while all three options reduced breast pain, only the flaxseed results were statistically significant. The researchers commented that the reductions for flaxseed were "impressive."[4]

In a randomized, triple-blind, two-month, placebo-controlled trial published in 2016 in the journal *Complementary Therapies in Medicine*, researchers again from Iran compared the use of flaxseed and chasteberry (*Vitex agnus*) for cyclic breast pain. The cohort consisted of 159 women with cyclic breast pain who were referred to health centers in Tabriz, Iran; they were placed in one of three groups of 53 women. The women had a mean age of 32.6 years, and almost half of the women were overweight. The first group of women took 25 g of flaxseed powder per day and placebo chasteberry tablets; the second group of women took one 3.2 to 4.8 mg chasteberry tablet per day and placebo flaxseed; the third group of women took two placebo tablets. The subjects were personally visited at the end of each menstrual cycle. Only one woman, who was in the double placebo group, failed to complete the trial. During the trial, two gastrointestinal adverse events were reported in the flaxseed group. At the same time, although the women in both the flaxseed and chasteberry groups reported significant reductions in the severity and duration of breast pain, the reduction was greater in the women taking flaxseed. The researchers underscored the need for additional, longer-term studies on the use of flaxseed and chasteberry for cyclic breast pain.[5]

A Flaxseed Compress May Help People with Hand Osteoarthritis

In a randomized, controlled intervention trial published in 2019 in the journal *Clinical Rheumatology*, researchers from Turkey examined the usefulness of a flaxseed compress for people with hand osteoarthritis who have had pain for at least one month. The cohort consisted of subjects who were seen at a rheumatology outpatient clinic between January 15, 2017, and May 15, 2018. The subjects, with a mean age of 63.84 years, were all diagnosed with primary hand osteoarthritis; the mean duration of disease was 81.95 months. The subjects, who were almost all female and had similar demographic characteristics, were placed in one of three groups. The 33 subjects in the first group were treated with flaxseed poultice compresses; the 29 subjects in the second group were treated with hot compresses; and the 20 subjects in the third group were controls who received no treatment. The interventions were applied once a day for seven consecutive days. The researchers learned that when compared to the hot compress group or the controls, the subjects in the flaxseed poultice compress group had significant reductions in pain. "The use of flaxseed poultice compresses was beneficial for reducing pain and increasing hand functions in patients with hand OA [osteoarthritis]."[6]

Garlic

Garlic Appears to Have Limited Use for the Pain Associated with Peripheral Arterial Occlusive Disease

In a systematic review published in 2013 in the *Cochrane Database of Systematic Reviews*, researchers from the United Kingdom evaluated the use of garlic for the pain associated with peripheral arterial occlusive disease or the blockage or narrowing of an artery in the legs (rarely arms), usually due to atherosclerosis. After a search of the medical literature for lower limb studies, the researchers located only one relevant trial with 78 male and female subjects. For 12 weeks, the subjects consumed either two coated tablets of 200 mg standardized garlic powder twice daily or a placebo. By the end of the trial, the level of pain free walking increased in the subjects in the garlic group from 161 to 207 meters; in the placebo group that increase went from 172 to 203 meters. The difference was not statistically significant. As a result, the researchers concluded that, "at this stage, garlic as a therapy for the treatment of peripheral arterial occlusive disease cannot be recommended."[7]

Garlic May Not Help People with Knee Osteoarthritis

In a randomized, double-blind, placebo-controlled, single-center, parallel-design trial published in 2018 in the *International Journal of Clinical Practice*, researchers from Iran assessed the ability of garlic to help overweight or obese women who suffer from mild to moderate knee osteoarthritis. The initial cohort consisted of 80 women, between the ages of 50 and 75 years, with medically diagnosed knee ostcoarthritis. For 12 weeks, the women took either odorless garlic tablets that were the equivalent of 2,500 mg of fresh garlic or identical placebo/lactose tablets. Thirty-nine subjects in the garlic group and 37 subjects in the placebo group completed the trial; the mean age of the women in the garlic group was 58.9 years, and the mean age of the women in the placebo group was 58.5 years. Pain assessments were administered. By the end of the trial, the researchers learned that while the garlic group had significantly lower levels of stiffness, there was no significant difference between the groups in terms of pain. The women in the garlic group did not have significantly less pain than the women in the placebo group. The researchers underscored the need for more clinical trials on the use of garlic for osteoarthritis.[8]

Fresh Raw Garlic May Burn the Oral Mucosa

In a report published in 2017 in the *Journal of the American Dental Association*, dentists from Pittsburgh, Pennsylvania (USA) described a 49-year-old man who used crushed raw garlic to relieve tooth pain. When he appeared at the emergency dental clinic, his primary symptom was maxillary right tooth pain. During the examination, the dentist observed a chemical burn. Upon questioning, the man revealed that, in an attempt to self-treat, he placed crushed raw garlic near the area of his dental pain. Apparently, members of the man's family told him about the "supposed analgesic effects of raw garlic." The dentist commented that garlic is "a rarely reported cause of unintentional therapeutic chemical burns."[9]

Green Tea

Green Tea May Help People with Knee Osteoarthritis

In a randomized, double-arm, parallel group, open-label active-controlled clinical trial published in 2018 in the journal *Clinical Nutrition*, researchers from Iran evaluated the use of green tea for people with mild to moderate knee osteoarthritis. The initial cohort consisted of 50 subjects. For four weeks, 25 subjects were assigned to take daily doses of green tea extract and diclofenac (a nonsterioidal anti-inflammatory medication), and the other 25 took only diclofenac. The mean age of the subjects in the combination group was 56.65 years, and the mean age of the subjects in the diclofenac group was 53.05 years. At baseline, there were no significant differences between the subjects in the two groups. Forty subjects were included in the analyses. The researchers learned that the subjects in the combination group had significant reductions in the symptoms associated with knee osteoarthritis, including pain. However, the combination therapy had no effect on stiffness. The researchers concluded that there is a need for more studies that have more subjects and continue for a longer period of time.[10]

Green Tea Appears to Help People with Rheumatoid Arthritis

In a trial published in 2016 in the *Journal of Physical Therapy Science*, researchers from Saudi Arabia and Egypt evaluated the ability of green tea and supervised exercise to help people dealing with rheumatoid arthritis. The cohort consisted of 120 Saudi subjects with a mean age of 60.7 years; all of the subjects had their rheumatoid arthritis diagnosis for at least 10 years. For six months, the subjects were treated with green tea alone or in combination with infliximab, a medication used to treat several autoimmune illnesses, or a supervised aerobic exercise program. Green tea was supplemented at a dose of four to six cups per day; infliximab was administered by intravenous infusions. The subjects in the supervised aerobic exercise program used a treadmill for 45 to 60 minutes three times per week. Various assessments were conducted on all of the subjects. The researchers learned that all three treatments resulted in significant improvement in "clinical and biochemical parameters." When the subjects drank green tea combined with infliximab or exercise, there were additional benefits, such as significant improvements in disease activity parameters including C-reactive protein and swollen and tender joints. For those hoping to have a nondrug option, the combination of green tea and exercise proved to be particularly useful. "Scores revealed more clinical improvement in the disease activity of rheumatoid arthritis patients treated with green tea along with exercise."[11]

Green Tea May or May Not Be Useful for Exercise-Induced Muscle Soreness

In a randomized, triple-blind, placebo-controlled trial published in 2018 in the journal *Physiology & Behavior*, researchers from Brazil wanted to determine if green tea would reduce exercise-induced muscle soreness. The cohort consisted of 20 untrained men who do not perform regular exercise. Ten men with a mean age of 25 years were assigned to an intervention group, and 10 men with a mean age of 23 years were assigned to a placebo group. All of the men performed exercises to induce delayed-onset muscle soreness (DOMS) at baseline and after 15 days. During that time, the men in the intervention group took 500 mg per day of green tea supplementation, and the men in the placebo group took a placebo. Both groups had similar exercise routines. The researchers learned that green tea reduced muscle damage but not muscle soreness. The green tea had "positive effects on muscle recovery after strenuous exercise." However, did it help relieve pain? It was not clear.[12]

NOTES

1. Jahangirifar, Maryam, Mahboubeh Taebi, and Mahrokh Dolatian. "The Effect of Cinnamon on Primary Dysmenorrhea: A Randomized, Double-Blind Clinical Trial." *Complementary Therapies in Clinical Practice* 33 (November 2018): 56–60.

2. Jaafarpour, Molouk, Masoud Hatefi, Ali Khani, and Javaher Khajavikhan. "Comparative Effect of Cinnamon and Ibuprofen for Treatment of Primary Dysmenorrhea: A Randomized Double-Blind Clinical Trial." *Journal of Clinical & Diagnostic Research* 9, no. 4 (April 2015): QC04–QC07.

3. Shishehbor, Farideh, Mahnaz Rezaeyan Safar, Elham Rejaei, and Mohammad Hosein Haghighizadeh. "Cinnamon Consumption Improves Clinical Symptoms and Inflammatory Markers in Women with Rheumatoid Arthritis." *Journal of the American College of Nutrition* 37, no. 8 (2018): 685–690.

4. Jaafarnejad, Farzaneh, Elham Adibmoghaddam, Seyyed Ahmad Emami, and Azadeh Saki. "Compare the Effect of Flaxseed, Evening Primrose Oil and Vitamin E on Duration of Periodic Breast Pain." *Journal of Education and Health Promotion* 6 (2017): 85.

5. Mirghafourvand, Mojgan, Sakineh Mohammad-Alizadeh-Charandabi, Parivash Ahmadpour, and Yousef Javadzadeh. "Effects of *Vitex agnus* and Flaxseed on Cyclic Mastalgia: A Randomized Controlled Trial." *Complementary Therapies in Medicine* 24 (February 2016): 90–95.

6. Sava, B. B., G. B. Alparslan, and C. Korkmaz. "Effect of Flaxseed Poultice Compress Application on Pain and Hand Functions of Patients with Hand Osteoarthritis." *Clinical Rheumatology* 38, no. 7 (July 2019): 1961–1969.

7. Jepson, R. G., J. Kleijnen, and G. C. Leng. "Garlic for Peripheral Arterial Occlusive Disease." *Cochrane Database of Systematic Reviews* 4 (2013): CD000095.

8. Salimzadeh, Ahmed, Elham Alipoor, Sahar Dehghani, et al. "The Effect of 12-Week Garlic Supplementation on Symptom Relief in Overweight or Obese Women with Knee Osteoarthritis." *International Journal of Clinical Practice* 72, no. 6 (June 2018): e13208.

9. Vargo, Richard J., Blake M. Warner, Anitha Potluri, and Joanne L. Prasad. "Garlic Burn of the Oral Mucosa: A Case Report and Review of Self-Treatment Chemical Burns." *Journal of the American Dental Association* 148, no. 10 (October 2017): 767–771.

10. Hashempur, M. H., S. Sadrneshin, S. H. Mosavat, and A. Ashraf. "Green Tea (*Camellia sinensis*) for Patients with Knee Osteoarthritis: A Randomized Open-Label Active-Controlled Clinical Trial." *Clinical Nutrition* 37, no. 1 (February 2018): 85–90.

11. Alghadir, Ahmad, Sami A. Gabr, and Einas S. Al-Eisa. "Green Tea and Exercise Interventions as Nondrug Remedies in Geriatric Patients with Rheumatoid Arthritis." *Journal of Physical Therapy Science* 28 (2016): 2820–2829.

12. da Silva, Willian, Álvaro S. Machado, Mauren A. Souza, et al. "Effect of Green Tea Extract Supplementation on Exercise-Induced Delayed Onset Muscle Soreness and Muscular Damage." *Physiology & Behavior* 194 (October 1, 2018): 77–82.

REFERENCES AND FURTHER READINGS

Alghadir, Ahmad, Sami A. Gabr, and Einas A. Al-Eisa. "Green Tea and Exercise Interventions as Nondrug Remedies in Geriatric Patients with Rheumatoid Arthritis." *Journal of Physical Therapy Science* 28 (2016): 2820–2829.

da Silva, Willian, Álvaro S. Machado, Mauren A. Souza, et al. "Effect of Green Tea Extract Supplementation on Exercise-Induced Delayed Onset Muscle Soreness and Muscular Damage." *Physiology & Behavior* 194 (October 1, 2018): 77–82.

Hashempur, M. H., S. Sadrneshin, S. H. Mosavat, and A. Ashraf. "Green Tea (*Camellia sinensis*) for Patients with Knee Osteoarthritis: A Randomized Open-Label Active-Controlled Clinical Trial." *Clinical Nutrition* 37, no. 1 (February 2018): 85–90.

Jaafarnejad, Farzaneh, Elham Adibmoghaddam, Seyyed Ahmad Emami, and Azadeh Saki. "Compare the Effect of Flaxseed, Evening Primrose Oil and Vitamin E on Duration of Periodic Breast Pain." *Journal of Education and Health Promotion* 6 (2017): 85.

Jaafarpour, Molouk, Masoud Hatefi, Ali Khani, and Javaher Khajavikhan. "Comparative Effect of Cinnamon and Ibuprofen for Treatment of Primary Dysmenorrhea: A Randomized Double-Blind Clinical Trial." *Journal of Clinical & Diagnostic Research* 9, no. 4 (April 2015): QC04–QC07.

Jahangirifar, Maryam, Mahboubeh Taebi, and Mahrokh Dolatian. "The Effect of Cinnamon on Primary Dysmenorrhea: A Randomized, Double-Blind Clinical Trial." *Complementary Therapies in Clinical Practice* 33 (November 2018): 56–60.

Jepson, R. G., J. Kleijnen, and G. C. Leng. "Garlic for Peripheral Arterial Occlusive Disease." *Cochrane Database of Systematic Reviews* 4 (April 2013): CD000095.

Mirghafourvand, Mojgan, Sakinen Mohammed-Alizadeh-Charandabi, Parivash Ahmadpor, and Yousef Javadzadeh. "Effects of *Vitex agnus* and Flaxseed on Cyclic Mastalgia: A Randomized Controlled Trial." *Complementary Therapies in Medicine* 24 (February 2016): 90–95.

Salimzadeh, Ahmed, Elham Alipoor, Sahar Dehghani, et al. "The Effect of 12-Week Garlic Supplementation on Symptom Relief in Overweight or Obese Women with Knee Osteoarthritis." *International Journal of Clinical Practice* 72, no. 6 (June 2018): e13208.

Savaş, B. B., G. B. Alparslan, and C. Korkmaz. "Effect of Flaxseed Poultice Compress Application on Pain and Hand Functions of Patients with Hand Osteoarthritis." *Clinical Rheumatology* 38 (2019): 1961–1969.

Shishehbor, Farideh, Mahnaz Rezaeyan Safar, Elham Rajaei, and Mohammad Hosein Haghighizadeh. "Cinnamon Consumption Improves Clinical Symptoms and Inflammatory Markers in Women with Rheumatoid Arthritis." *Journal of the American College of Nutrition* 37, no. 8 (2018): 685–690.

Vargo, Richard J., Blake M. Warner, Anitha Potluri, and Joanne L. Prasad. "Garlic Burn of the Oral Mucosa: A Case Report and Review of Self-Treatment Chemical Burns." *Journal of the American Dental Association* 148, no. 10 (October 2017): 767–771.

Physical Therapy

INTRODUCTION

Physical therapy is a healthcare specialty that primarily addresses the needs of people with functional mobility problems. A physical therapist, who is licensed in the state in which she or he works, evaluates, assesses, and treats these problems.

Physical therapists treat people of all ages who have an injury or illness that causes pain, physical impairment, and the limitation or loss of function. Some of the problems treated by physical therapists include after fracture rehabilitation, sports injuries, carpal tunnel syndrome, stroke, amputations, cystic fibrosis, chronic obstructive pulmonary disease, post-myocardial infarction, back pain, multiple sclerosis, traumatic brain injuries, concussion, temporomandibular (TMJ), rotator cuff tears, lymphedema, urinary incontinence, burns, and arthritis. The goal is to reduce pain, return the patient to maximal functioning, and prevent any additional injury. Physical therapy may be a stand-alone treatment, or it may be combined with other treatments, such as massage therapy or acupuncture.

In the United States, modern physical therapy emerged at the end of the 19th century. However, it really grew in numbers and importance when the polio epidemic became widespread in 1916. At the time, there was a tremendous need for people to carry out muscle testing and muscle re-education, in order to restore function to those affected by the disease. The need grew even greater when the country entered World War I and injured soldiers returned home.

ADMINISTRATION AND REGULATION

A first visit to a physical therapist will begin with history of the functional mobility problem(s), a description of other medical problems, and a review of any tests that have already been taken. The physical therapist will conduct an examination and evaluate the injury or illness for concerns, such as pain, flexibility, posture, muscle and joint motion and performance, and mobility. Then, she or he will discuss short-term and long-term treatment goals and develop in-office and at-home treatment and exercise plans.

Physical therapists use a wide variety of techniques to help patients decrease their levels of pain and stiffness, improve motion, strength, and mobility. The treatments may include therapeutic exercises, patient education, ice, heat, ultrasound, and electrical stimulation (E-stim). (Electrical stimulation uses topical electrodes on the skin to reduce pain and increase functional capabilities. One type of E-stim is transcutaneous electrical nerve stimulation or TENS.)

Physical therapists work in a variety of different settings. These include hospitals, sports training facilities and teams, outpatient clinics or offices, skilled nursing facilities, athletic and fitness centers, schools, hospices, occupational settings, government agencies, research centers, and in inpatient rehabilitation settings. Some physical therapists treat patients in the patients' homes.

It has been estimated that about nine million adults in the United States use physical therapy services each year. Costs vary, but most insurance plans cover physical therapy. Still, there may well be a copayment required. People without insurance pay an average of $125 per session. The average length of care is 7 to 10 sessions.

Physical therapists are licensed by the state in which they work. They have earned a master's degree or a clinical doctorate from an accredited university, and they must pass the state-administered national licensing examination to practice. Though physical therapists who have already earned a master's degree may continue to practice, new students must now complete the clinical doctorate. They may also be certified specialists in specific areas of physical therapy, such as neurological, cardiovascular, pulmonary, or orthopedics.

BENEFITS AND RISKS

Physical therapy has a number of potential benefits for people dealing with pain. First and foremost, physical therapy may relieve pain and reduce the need for medication, especially opioid medication. It may help avoid surgery and improve mobility and movement, while also facilitating recovery from injury, surgery, trauma, stroke, or paralysis. Physical therapists may teach patients how to prevent falls, improve balance, and manage

age-related medical problems. Most likely, a physical therapist will assign at home exercises. In order to be effective and beneficial, these exercises must be completed as assigned.

Still, there are a few risks with physical therapy. These are more likely to occur if the physical therapist fails to properly supervise the patient or uses poor or improper techniques. Patients may experience injury from manipulations or burns from heating sources. In addition, there may be injury from stretching or exercises.

RESEARCH FINDINGS

Physical Therapy Exercises Are an Excellent Means to Treat Subacromial or Shoulder Blade (Scapula) Pain

In a systematic review published in 2016 in *British Journal of Sports Medicine*, researchers from Brazil and Spain reviewed 64 high-quality randomly controlled trials and "quasi"-randomly controlled trials on the use of physical therapy for shoulder blade pain, functioning, and range of motion. Diagnoses were made based on clinical symptoms or imaging tests. The researchers included studies with all types of active or passive physical therapy interventions. Three of the trials were follow-ups of initial studies. The researchers learned that physical therapy, which focused on stretching and strengthening exercises, appeared to be as effective as arthroscopic surgery and better than no treatment or placebo treatment to improve pain, function, and range of motion in short-, mid-, and long-term time periods. Among the five groups of physical therapy treatments employed, exercises and manual therapy were the most effective. (The other types were physical resources, taping, and acupuncture.) The researchers commented that patients should participate in a physical therapy program before having surgery for scapula pain. These physical therapy exercises should be viewed as the first treatments. "Rehabilitation with exercises is easy to apply, low cost and presents low risk to the patient since it consists of a non-invasive treatment."[1]

Earlier Referrals to Physical Therapy for Low Back Pain Appear to Be Associated with Reduced Use of Opioid Medication

In a retrospective study published in 2017 in the *Journal of the American Board of Family Medicine*, researchers based in Salt Lake City, Utah

(USA), wanted to learn more about the benefits of early referrals to physical therapists for low back pain. The cohort consisted of 454 Medicaid enrollees, with a mean age of 40.4 years; all of the mostly female subjects had new-onset low back pain. A primary care provider referred 215 (47%) for physical therapy. Eighty-one of these subjects (37%) had at least one low back pain-related physical therapy visit within 90 days of referral. While the researchers did not find an association between prior opioid use and receiving a physical therapy consult, a physical therapy consult was associated with a reduced chance of an opioid prescription after the physical therapy visit. According to the researchers, "this is a potentially important finding in light of the current opioid epidemic."[2]

Early Physical Therapy for Recent-Onset Low Back Pain May Have Only Modest Results

In a randomized clinical trial published in 2015 in *JAMA*, researchers from Salt Lake City, Utah, and Peoria, Illinois (USA), evaluated the early use of physical therapy for patients with low back pain. Two hundred twenty subjects were recruited between March 2011 and November 2013. All of the subjects received education in low back care. One hundred eight subjects had four physical therapy sessions, and 112 subjects had the usual care. Thirteen of the subjects who received physical therapy reported a total of 20 adverse effects, such as increased pain and stiffness. While the early intervention of physical therapy resulted in statistically significant improvement in disability, the improvement was "modest" and "did not achieve the minimum differences considered clinically important at the individual patient level."[3]

Adding Trigger Point Treatment to Regular Physical Therapy Does Not Improve Pain Outcomes in Rotator Cuff Pathology

In a randomized, controlled, double-blind, prospective clinical trial published in 2019 in the *Journal of Back and Musculoskeletal Rehabilitation*, researchers from Turkey evaluated if the addition of myofascial trigger point treatment to regular physical therapy would improve the management of pain and other problems associated with rotator cuff pathology. Forty-six patients with rotator cuff tears satisfied all of the inclusion requirements; they were placed in one of two groups. All of the patients, who were recruited from May 2016 through September 2017, received the same conservative physical therapy, twice each week for six weeks. But, the patients in the first group also received myofascial trigger point treatment. Forty-one patients were included in the final analysis. The mean age of the subjects in the first group was 50 years; the mean age of the subjects in the second group was 54.10 years. The researchers found that, after the treatments, the subjects in both groups experienced improvements in pain, range of motion, and functioning. However, there were no significant differences between the groups in these improvements; the myofascial trigger point treatment did not have a significant impact on the clinical outcomes. Nevertheless, the researchers concluded "the inclusion of trigger point treatment in patients with rotator cuff pathologies may lead to results that are more positive in terms of pain management."[34]

Physical Therapy May Be Useful for People with Tension Headaches

In a randomized, controlled trial published in 2018 in the journal *Neurología*, researchers from Spain investigated the ability of two programs to ease tension headaches. The first program combined physical therapy (cervical spine kinesiotherapy and posture correction) with relaxation techniques (Schultz's Autogenic Training); the second program consisted only of relaxation training. The cohort consisted of 152 university students, with a mean age of 20.42 years, who had a diagnosis of tension-type headache. There were 84 women and 68 men. The students were divided into two groups of 76 students. Each group had 59 students who took medication to manage their headaches and 17 who did not. In a single session, the therapists provided oral and written instructions for the subjects to do the exercises in their own homes. The students in the combined treatment group were told to perform one session of relaxation exercises and another of physiotherapy daily for four weeks; the students in the relaxation only group were told to perform their exercises once daily for four weeks. Weekly follow-up sessions were held, and during the three months following the post-treatment evaluation, the frequency of home sessions was reduced to three times per week. The subjects were provided a headache diary in which to note periodic recordings of their headaches. The researchers learned that both groups obtained good short- and medium-term results. However, the combination group had more significant improvements in headache frequency and intensity. The researchers commented that, "it would be interesting to assess to what extent the benefits are maintained over a longer period of time, such as six months or one year after therapy."[5]

Physical Therapy May Have Some Benefit for Low Back Pain and Pelvic Pain in Pregnant Women

In a systematic review published in 2012 in the journal *Acta Obstetricia et Gynecologica Scandinavica*, researchers from Australia wanted to determine if physical therapy would help pregnant women with low back pain or pelvic pain. The researchers located four randomly controlled trials with 566 subjects that met their inclusion criteria. They were all of moderate quality and published in either obstetric or physical therapy scientific journals, with a physical therapist as the primary provider. Sample sizes varied, and the duration of interventions ranged from one to 12 weeks. The subjects ranged in gestational ages across the three trimesters. The results demonstrated the usefulness of physical therapy. For example, the researchers learned that women who participated in group exercises for 60 minutes once a week for 12 weeks, including twice-daily home pelvic floor muscle contractions and education, had better self-reported outcomes than the members of a control group, who received only information. And, individual home exercises three times per day for one week improved functional outcomes for pregnant subjects with pubic symphysis pain. The researchers noted that although there is good evidence that physical therapy is useful, there is a need for further research on "other treatment modalities used by physical therapists and establish an appropriate, reliable and valid functional outcome measure to assess low back and pelvic pain in pregnancy."[6]

Physical Therapy May or May Not Be Useful for Pregnancy-Related Low Back and/or Pelvic Pain after Delivery

In a systematic review published in 2013 in the journal *Physiotherapy Theory and Practice*, researchers from Brazil and Spain hoped to determine if physical therapy would help women with pregnancy-related low back or pelvic girdle pain after delivery. The researchers found only four trials, with 341 subjects, that met their criteria. Though they included different interventions, all of the trials employed exercise for motor control and to increase stability in the lumbopelvic region. And, they all had at least one control group and a low risk of bias. Two were conducted in the

Netherlands, one in Norway, and one in Sweden. All of the studies involved women in the postpartum period who were suffering from low back pain or pelvic girdle pain during pregnancy or just after delivery. The researchers learned that "individual guidance and adjusted exercises" may help people with pelvic girdle pain. Yet, with so few studies, it is near impossible to draw clear conclusions. "More randomized clinical trials on this topic, with high quality, are in need."[7]

Early Use of Physical Therapy for the Onset of Musculoskeletal Painful Conditions May Decrease Costs and Improve Outcomes

In a systematic review published in 2016 in the *Journal of Orthopaedic & Sports Physical Therapy*, researchers from Philadelphia, Pennsylvania, Stockton, California, and New York City (USA) wanted to learn if the early initiation of physical therapy for painful musculoskeletal conditions would decrease costs and improve outcomes. As a result, they compared the early and delayed initiation of physical therapy for these conditions. The cohort consisted of 14 studies; of these, 12 addressed low back pain, one focused on low back pain and neck pain, and one examined neck pain. Four of the studies were randomized, controlled trials, and 10 were nonrandomized or cohort studies. Sample sizes varied widely, as did the populations and the definitions of timing. The researchers observed that earlier physical therapy was associated with decreased costs and reduced medical utilization, including imaging, opioid medications, injections, and surgery. In fact, all of the studies consistently demonstrated that the early use of physical therapy was not associated with unfavorable outcomes, increased medical utilization, more physical therapy visits, or increased costs. The researchers concluded that their findings "suggest that there is no risk and potential cost savings associated with patients receiving physical therapy consultation within the acute time frame."[8]

When Compared to TENS, Diadynamic Current Did Not Help People with Nonspecific Low Back Pain

In a double-blind, randomized, controlled trial published in 2018 in the *Journal of Bodywork & Movement Therapies*, researchers from Iran compared the immediate nonspecific low back pain relieving effects of Diadynamic current to TENS. The cohort consisted of 30 subjects who suffered from nonspecific low back pain for more than three months. Subjects who used pain medication during the previous 24 hours were excluded. Fifteen subjects received a Diadynamic current treatment for 10 minutes, and 15 received a TENS treatment for 15 minutes. The subjects were unaware of the kinds of electrical stimulation they received. Pain levels were assessed before and after the treatments. Additional pain assessments were made 20 minutes after the electrical stimulation and again after 48 hours. The researchers found that pain was significantly decreased only in the TENS group after 20 minutes from the termination of the current. "Within the framework of this study we could conclude that the Diadynamic current had no positive effect on prompt relief of pain in patients suffering from NSLBP [nonspecific low back pain]."[9]

The Use of Electrotherapies Does Not Appear to Increase the Effectiveness of Neck Stabilization Exercise for Chronic Neck Pain

In a prospective, randomized, controlled, single-blind, multicenter clinical trial published in 2018 in the journal *Spine*, researchers from Turkey wanted to learn if people with at least three months of chronic neck pain would benefit from electrotherapies added to their neck stabilization exercises. The cohort consisted of 81 subjects with chronic neck pain; they were assigned to one of three groups. The members of the first group had neck stabilization exercises; the members of the second group had TENS and neck stabilization exercises; and the members of the third group had interferential current (IFC) and neck stabilization exercises. Physical therapy modalities were applied for 15 sessions in all groups. Assessments were made of pain levels, limits of cervical range of motion, quality of life, mood, levels of disability, and the need for analgesics. The researchers found that the subjects in all three treatment groups improved in the issues assessed. No statistically significant differences were found between the groups. Although TENS and IFC are effective treatments for people with chronic neck pain, "they have no advantage over NSE [neck stabilization exercises]."[10]

Manual Therapy and Stabilizing Exercises, Two Types of Physical Therapy, Are Useful for Head and Rounded Shoulder Postures

In a randomized, controlled trial published in 2019 in the journal *BMC Musculoskeletal Disorders*, researchers from Iran wanted to learn if manual therapy and stabilizing exercises would help people with forward head and rounded shoulder postures, which are sources of pain and dysfunction. The cohort consisted of 60 married women, between the ages of 32 and 42 years, with neck pain and forward head and rounded shoulder postures. Having been recruited through physicians, orthopedic surgeons, and physical therapists, the women were placed in one of three groups. For six weeks, the 20 women in the first group performed stabilizing exercises and received manual therapy; the 20 women in the second group performed stabilizing exercises; and the 20 women in the third group performed home exercises. One month after the programs ended, there was a follow-up. All of the subjects completed the trial. The researchers learned that the subjects in the first two groups had significant within-group improvements in pain, function, and head and shoulder posture. However, the improvements in pain and function were more effective in the first group than the second group. So, the combination of stabilizing exercises and manual therapy was more useful than the stabilizing exercises alone. The researchers concluded that additional research is needed on the effectiveness of these treatments for chronic neck pain. Still, it does appear that manual therapy is beneficial "as a supplementary method to the stabilizing intervention in the treatment of neck pain."[11]

Focused Low-Intensity Pulsed Ultrasound Therapy May Benefit Those with Knee Osteoarthritis

In a randomized, placebo-controlled clinical trial published in 2016 in the journal *Scientific Reports*, researchers from China investigated the use of low-intensity pulsed ultrasound therapy for people with knee osteoarthritis. The initial cohort consisted of 106 subjects with bilateral knee osteoarthritis. Fifty-three subjects were assigned to received diclofenac sodium sustained-release (a nonsteroidal anti-inflammatory medication) and low-intensity pulsed ultrasound treatments, and 53 received the same medication and sham ultrasound treatments. Forty-nine subjects completed the intervention group, and 48 finished the control group. Both the actual and sham 20-minute ultrasound treatments were held daily for 10 days, and assessments were conducted at the end of the 10 days and during 4- and 12-week follow-ups. Whereas at baseline, the subjects had similar levels of pain, at the end of the 10 days and at follow-ups, the actual intervention group had significant improvements in levels of pain. There were no ultrasound-related adverse effects. The researchers concluded that low-intensity pulsed ultrasound therapy "is a safe and effective treatment modality for relieving pain and improving the functions and quality of life of patients with KOA [knee osteoarthritis]."[12]

Ultrasound May or May Not Be Useful for Joint Pain

In a systematic review published in 2020 in the journal *Pain Medicine*, researchers from New York City, Cleveland, Ohio, Palo Alto, California, (USA), and Taiwan examined studies on the use of low-intensity ultrasound for chronic knee, shoulder, and hip pain. The researchers identified eight randomized controlled trials for knee pain and seven randomized controlled trials for shoulder pain. They were unable to locate a hip trial that met their criteria. All of the included trials were written in English and had subjects who were at least 18 years old; the trials all compared ultrasound to another treatment or placebo. The eight knee pain trials had mixed results. Ultrasound therapy had better pain relief than placebos, but other modalities were sometimes more useful. All seven of the trials on shoulder pain found good evidence that ultrasound therapy offered pain relief. However, in four of the trials, ultrasound therapies were not as effective as other modalities. The veracity of these results is further complicated by the fact that ultrasound therapy is often combined with other therapies. Still, the researchers concluded that "low-intensity ultrasound is a safe modality to consider when treating osteoarthritis of the knee, hip, and shoulder."[13]

Ultrasound Therapy May or May Not Help Myofascial Pain Syndrome

In a systematic review and meta-analysis published in 2017 in the *Journal of Pain Research*, researchers from China assessed the ability of ultrasound therapy to ease the pain associated with myofascial pain syndrome. (Myofascial pain is the pain associated with the strong membranes that wrap, connect, and support the body's muscles. The most common complaint with this disorder is neck and upper back pain.) The cohort consisted of 10 randomized controlled trials with 428 subjects; only 8 of these could be included in the meta-analysis. The mean age of the subjects ranged from 21 to 49 years. Nine trials compared ultrasound to sham ultrasound, and one trial compared ultrasound to a blank control. The trials were published between 1997 and 2015. The risk of bias was low for three trials, high for three trials, and unclear for four trials. While the trials supported the usefulness of ultrasound for pain relief, the researchers noted that as a result of the high risk of bias and the heterogeneity of the studies, "the current evidence is not clear enough to support US [ultrasound] as an effective method to treat MPS [myofascial pain syndrome]."[14]

NOTES

1. Haik, M. N., F. Alburquerque-Sendin, R. F. Moreira, et al. "Effectiveness of Physical Therapy Treatment of Clearly Defined Subacromial Pain: A Systematic Review of Randomised Controlled Trials." *British Journal of Sports Medicine* 50, no. 18 (September 2016): 1124–1134.

2. Thackeray, Anne, Rachel Hess, Josette Dorius, et al. "Relationship of Opioid Prescriptions to Physical Therapy Referral and Participation for Medicaid Patients with New-Onset Low Back Pain." *Journal of the American Board of Family Medicine* 30, no. 6 (November–December 2017): 784–794.

3. Fritz, Julie M., John S. Magel, Molly McFadden, et al. "Early Physical Therapy vs Usual Care in Patients with Recent-Onset Low Back Pain: A Randomized Clinical Trial." *JAMA* 314, no. 14 (2015): 1459–1467.

4. Akbaba, Y. A., E. K. Mutlu, S. Altun, et al. "The Effectiveness of Trigger Point Treatment in Rotator Cuff Pathology: A Randomized Controlled Double-Blind Study." *Journal of Back and Musculoskeletal Rehabilitation* 32, no. 3 (2019): 519–527.

5. Álvarez-Melcón, A. C., R. Valero-Alcaide, M. A. Atin-Arratibel, et al. "Effects of Physical Therapy and Relaxation Techniques on the Parameters of Pain in University Students with Tension-type Headache: A Randomised Controlled Clinical Trial." *Neurología* 33, no. 4 (May 2018): 233–243.

6. Richards, E., G. van Kessel, R. Virgara, and P. Harris. "Does Antenatal Physical Therapy for Pregnant Women with Low Back Pain or Pelvic Pain Improve Functional Outcomes? A Systematic Review." *Acta Obstetricia et Gynecologica Scandinavica* 91, no. 9 (September 2012): 1038–1045.

7. Ferreira, Caroline Wanderley Souto, and Francisco Alburquerque-Sendin. "Effectiveness of Physical Therapy for Pregnancy-Related Low Back and/or Pelvic Pain After Delivery: A Systematic Review." *Physiotherapy Theory and Practice* 29, no. 6 (2013): 419–431.

8. Ojha, H. A., N. J. Wyrsta, T. E. Davenport, et al. "Timing of Physical Therapy Initiation for Nonsurgical Management of Musculoskeletal Disorders and Effects on Patient Outcomes: A Systematic Review."

Journal of Orthopaedic & Sports Physical Therapy 46, no. 2 (February 2016): 56–70.

9. Ebadi, S., N. N. Ansari, T. Ahadi, et al. "No Immediate Analgesic Effect of Diadynamic Current in Patients with Nonspecific Low Back Pain in Comparison to TENS." *Journal of Bodywork & Movement Therapies* 22, no. 3 (July 2018): 693–699.

10. Yesil, H., S. Hepquler, U. Dundar, et al. "Does the Use of Electrotherapies Increase the Effectiveness of Neck Stabilization Exercises for Improving Pain, Disability, Mood, and Quality of Life in Chronic Neck Pain? A Randomized, Controlled, Single-Blind Study." *Spine* 43, no. 20 (October 15, 2018): E1174–E1183.

11. Fathollahnejad, Kiana, Amir Letafatkar, and Malihe Hadadnezhad. "The Effect of Manual Therapy and Stabilizing Exercises on Forward Head and Rounded Shoulder Postures: A Six-Week Intervention with a One-Month Follow-Up Study." *BMC Musculoskeletal Disorders* 20(2019): 86–93.

12. Jia, Lang, Yan Wang, Jinyun Chen, and Wenzhi Chen. "Efficacy of Focused Low-Intensity Pulsed Ultrasound Therapy for the Management of Knee Osteoarthritis: A Randomized, Double Blind, Placebo-Controlled Trial." *Scientific Reports* 6 (2016): 35453.

13. Aiyer, Rohit, Selaiman A. Noori, Ke-Vin Chang, et al. "Therapeutic Ultrasound for Chronic Pain Management in Joints: A Systematic Review." *Pain Medicine* 21, no. 7 (2020): 1437–1448.

14. Xia, Peng, Xiaoju Wang, Qiang Lin, et al. "Effectiveness of Ultrasound Therapy for Myofascial Pain Syndrome: A Systematic Review and Meta-Analysis." *Journal of Pain Research* 10 (2017): 545–555.

REFERENCES AND FURTHER READINGS

Aiyer, Rohit, Selaiman A. Noori, Ke-Vin Chang, et al. "Therapeutic Ultrasound for Chronic Pain Management in Joints: A Systematic Review." *Pain Medicine* 21, no. 7 (2020): 1437–1448.

Akbaba, Y. A., E. K. Mutlu, S. Altun, et al. "The Effectiveness of Trigger Point Treatment in Rotator Cuff Pathology: A Randomized Controlled Double-Blind Study." *Journal of Back and Musculoskeletal Rehabilitation* 32, no. 3 (2019): 519–527.

Álvarez-Melcón, A. C., R. Valero-Alcaide, M. A. Atin-Arratibel, et al. "Effects of Physical Therapy and Relaxation Techniques on the Parameters of Pain in University Students with Tension-Type

Headache: A Randomised Controlled Clinical Trial." *Neurologia* 33, no. 4 (May 2018): 233–243.

Ebadi, S., N. N. Ansari, T. Ahadi, et al. "No Immediate Analgesic Effect of Diadynamic Current in Patients with Nonspecific Low Back Pain in Comparison to TENS." *Journal of Bodywork & Movement Therapies* 22, no. 3 (July 2018): 693–699.

Fathollahnejad, Kiana, Amir Letafatkar, and Malihe Hadadnezhad. "The Effect of Manual Therapy and Stabilizing Exercises on Forward Head and Rounded Shoulder Postures: A Six-Week Intervention with a One-Month Follow-Up Study." *BMC Musculoskeletal Disorders* 20 (2019): 86–93.

Ferreira, Caroline Wanderley Souto, and Francisco Alburquerque-Sendin. "Effectiveness of Physical Therapy for Pregnancy-Related Low Back and/or Pelvic Pain After Delivery: A Systematic Review." *Physiotherapy Theory and Practice* 29, no. 6 (2013): 419–431.

Fritz, Julie M., John S. Magel, Molly McFadden, et al. "Early Physical Therapy vs Usual Care in Patients with Recent-Onset Low Back Pain: A Randomized Clinical Trial." *JAMA* 314, no. 14 (2015): 1459–1467.

Hai, M. N., F. Alburquerque-Sendin, R. F. Moreira, et al. "Effectiveness of Physical Therapy Treatment of Clearly Defined Subacromial Pain: A Systematic Review of Randomised Controlled Trials." *British Journal of Sports Medicine* 50, no. 18 (September 2016): 1124–1134.

Jia, Lang, Yan Wang, Jinyun Chen, and Wenzhi Chen. "Efficacy of Focused Low-Intensity Pulsed Ultrasound Therapy for the Management of Knee Osteoarthritis: A Randomized, Double Blind, Placebo-Controlled Trial." *Scientific Reports* 6 (2016): 35453.

Ojha, H. A., N. J. Wyrsta, T. E. Davenport, et al. "Timing of Physical Therapy Initiation for Nonsurgical Management of Musculoskeletal Disorders and Effects on Patient Outcomes: A Systematic Review." *Journal of Orthopaedic & Sports Physical Therapy* 46, no. 2 (February 2016): 56–70.

Richards, E., G. van Kessel, R. Virgara, and P. Harris. "Does Antenatal Physical Therapy for Pregnant Women with Low Back Pain or Pelvic Pain Improve Functional Outcomes? A Systematic Review." *Acta Obstetricia et Gynecologica Scandinavica* 91, no. 9 (September 2012): 1038–1045.

Thackeray, Anne, Rachel Hess, Josette Dorius, et al. "Relationship of Opioid Prescriptions to Physical Therapy Referral and Participation for Medicaid Patients with New-Onset Low Back Pain." *Journal of the American Board of Family Medicine* 30, no. 6 (November–December 2017): 784–794.

Xia, Peng, Xiaoju Wang, Qiang Lin, et al. "Effectiveness of Ultrasound Therapy for Myofascial Pain Syndrome: A Systematic Review and Meta-Analysis." *Journal of Pain Research* 10 (2017): 545–555.

Yesil, H., S. Hepguler, U. Dundar, et al. "Does the Use of Electrotherapies Increases the effectiveness of Neck Stabilization Exercises for Improving Pain, Disability, Mood, and Quality of Life in Chronic Neck Pain? A Randomized, Controlled, Single-Blind Study." *Spine* 43, no. 20 (October 2018): E1174–E1183.

Reiki

INTRODUCTION

Reiki, which is also known as palm healing or hands-on healing, is a type of energy healing. It involves the transfer of universal energy from the practitioner's palms to the patient. (Universal energy is known as qi and pronounced as "chi.") Energy healing supposedly targets the energy field around the body.

With Reiki, which means universal life energy in Japanese, the practitioner moves energy by placing his or her hands on or over the patient. If the patient feels uncomfortable being touched, the entire process may be completed with hands placed three or four inches from the body. In some cases, distant Reiki is performed, and the practitioner may be physically quite far from the patient.

According to Reiki practitioners, following a physical injury, energy can stagnate in the body. These energy blocks may result in medical problems, such as pain. Energy medicine is believed to increase and improve the flow of energy throughout the body, thereby removing energy blocks. In this way, it is similar to other forms of energy medicine, such as acupuncture and acupressure. Unfortunately, this energy is unable to be measured by modern scientific techniques. So, at least some practitioners of Western medicine may not find it credible.

Though it has been used for thousands of years, the current form of Reiki was designed in 1922 by a Japanese Buddhist monk named Mikao Usui. During his lifetime, Usui taught the method to about two thousand people. The practice entered the United States via Hawaii (which was not yet a state) in the 1940s and then to Europe in the 1980s.

ADMINISTRATION AND REGULATION

During a Reiki session, the patient/client sits in a comfortable chair or lies on a table, fully clothed. Background music may or may not be played.

Practitioners then place their hands over specific areas of the body, including the head, limbs, and torso; the hands usually remain at each location for two to five minutes. Practitioners contend that while they hold their hands over the different areas of the body, a transfer of energy occurs. The practitioner's hands may become warm, and they may tingle. Each position is held until the practitioner believes that the energy has stopped flowing. Then, the practitioner moves on to the next area of the body. Some practitioners use crystals and chakra healing wands. Sessions may last between 15 and 90 minutes, and the number of sessions may be limited or continue for an indefinite period of time.

Entering a Reiki program does not require any specific prior training, education, or experience. Instead, Reiki training, which is also known as the "attunement process," consists of a master transferring attunement energy and healing techniques to the student. Many private Reiki education companies offer Reiki certification. Still, in most states, no license or certification is required. No single organization sets national standards for education, training, credentials, and certification. People without a background in health care may become Reiki practitioners.

People who already practice some form of traditional or integrative health care, such as physical therapists, massage therapists, nurses, and acupuncturists, tend to be the practitioners who pursue training in Reiki. Training is available at the beginning, intermediate, and master levels. Costs associated with Reiki visits will be a function of the background and training of the practitioner as well as the location of the practice. Though insurers may provide some coverage for Reiki when it is combined with another type of treatment, do not assume that insurers will pay for treatments that include only Reiki. Before beginning Reiki treatments, it is best to check with the insurer.

While there are no current reliable statistics on how often Reiki is used, it is known that hundreds of hospitals and health-care facilities offer this treatment. And, countless others include it as part of traditional, complementary, or integrative care.

BENEFITS AND RISKS

Reiki is thought to aid in relaxation, assist the body's natural healing processes, and support and improve both physical and psychological well-being. As a result, it is useful for chronic pain, but it is also supposedly helpful for people dealing with cancer, heart disease, anxiety, depression, infertility, autism, Crohn's disease, and fatigue syndromes.

There do not appear to be any risks associated with the actual practice of Reiki. However, a few negative side effects have been reported. While music may be played during a session, there tends to be little, limited, or no talking. Some people may find the silence uncomfortable, even awkward. And though most people feel profoundly relaxed from Reiki, some may feel excessive fatigue and headache, stomachache, or weakness. It is important to remember that Reiki is not an alternative to medical treatment. People who have a specific medical concern should receive appropriate treatment while pursing Reiki.

RESEARCH FINDINGS

Reiki May Help People with the Pain Associated with Knee Replacement Surgery

In a randomized, blinded, sham-controlled, pilot trial published in 2017 in the journal *Holistic Nursing Practice*, researchers from several locations in the United States but based in Arizona wanted to learn if Reiki would be useful for the pain associated with knee replacement surgery. The cohort consisted of 45 male and female patients who ranged in age from 50 to 85 years; they were admitted to an acute care hospital for scheduled single knee replacement surgery, "a procedure that is quite painful and that usually involves powerful pain management protocols." Fifteen subjects received three or four 30-minute Reiki treatments plus standard care; a second group of 15 subjects received three or four 30-minute sham Reiki sessions plus standard care; and a third group received three or four sessions of "quiet time" plus standard care. For all of the subjects, the first treatment was one hour before surgery, with subsequent treatments at 24, 48, and 72 hours (if not already discharged) after surgery. A variety of assessments were conducted before and after all treatments. The researchers observed a "trend of pain reduction" in the Reiki subjects that was not seen in the other subjects, and the subjects in the Reiki group used the least amount of pain medication. Likewise, the subjects in the Reiki group had the highest percentage of discharges at 48 hours rather than 72 hours, indicating they had fewer problems requiring longer hospitalizations. The researchers commented that "the reduction of patients' pain in the hospital environment is an important dimension of a caring-healing environment and can enhance the patient experience and satisfaction with care and pain management."[1]

In another trial published in 2016 in the journal *Nursing*, researchers from Pennsylvania and Delaware (USA) examined the same pain issue in knee replacement surgeries at a 311-bed acute care hospital located outside of Philadelphia. Apparently, Reiki, which was promoted as a complementary therapy, was already well-received at this hospital. The 43 patients who were hospitalized for total knee replacements were randomly placed in a Reiki treatment group ($n = 23$) or a nontreatment group ($n = 20$). The researchers used a 10-point pain sensitivity rating to measure levels of pain. The subjects in the Reiki treatment group received Reiki treatments before and after their surgeries as well as the usual care; the subjects in the nontreatment group received the usual care. Subjects in both groups had the same access to pain medication. On the day of discharge, a questionnaire was distributed to measure the satisfaction with Reiki and the hospital experience. The researchers learned that almost all the Reiki sessions resulted in statistically significant reductions in pain. No statistically significant differences were found in the use of pain medications. The researchers concluded that "Reiki may be an effective component in the management of surgical patients' postoperative pain."[2]

Reiki Seems to Support Physical and Psychological Health, Including Pain Relief

In a study published in 2019 in the *Journal of Alternative and Complementary Medicine*, researchers from Massachusetts, Arizona, and Michigan (USA) assessed the ability of a single session of Reiki to improve physical and psychological health. Pain was among the physical health factors that were reviewed. The cohort consisted of 99 Reiki practitioners throughout the United States. They gave Reiki sessions to their clients that lasted between 45 and 90 minutes; a total of 1,411 Reiki sessions were included in the final analyses. The mean age of the clients was 49.0 years; 1,143 were female, and 246 were male. Eighty-three percent identified as Caucasian, and 49 percent reported that they were Christian, and 33 percent said that they were spiritual but not religious. In order to evaluate the effectiveness of the sessions, assessments were conducted immediately before the sessions began and immediately after the sessions ended. The researchers learned that statistically significant improvements were obtained for all outcomes measured, including pain. The researchers concluded that Reiki "can provide immediate relief for many health conditions."[3]

Reiki Therapy Seems to Help People Deal with Pain

In a systematic review published in 2014 in the journal *Pain Management Nursing*, researchers from Pittsburgh, Pennsylvania (USA) investigated the use of Reiki for pain. The cohort consisted of seven studies that met their criteria. The sample sizes for these studies ranged from 16 to 160 subjects (median = 24) for a total of 328 subjects. Forty-three percent of the subjects were women, and the mean age for the overall sample was 63 years. Three studies included people with cancer, two studies were in a surgical setting, and two studies examined adults in a community setting. Reiki treatments ranged from 25 to 90 minutes; the average treatment length was 48 minutes. While the researchers acknowledged that the studies included in the review had design flaws "common to research involving complementary therapies," there was still good evidence that Reiki therapy may reduce pain. "Continued research using Reiki therapy with larger sample sizes, consistently randomized groups, and standardized treatment protocols is recommended."[4]

In a meta-analysis published in 2018 in the journal *Complementary Therapies in Clinical Practice*, a researcher from Turkey located four clinical trials that met her criteria for using Reiki to deal with pain. All of the trials had experimental and control groups. There were 104 subjects in the Reiki groups and 108 subjects in the control groups. Researchers collected the data in two of the four studies, which were double-blind, randomized, and controlled. Three studies used a visual analogue scale (VAS), and one used a 10-point face pain scale. Although the number of studies was small, the researcher determined that Reiki was an effective complementary therapy to reduce pain. However, she was unable to be more specific on the types of pain that best respond to Reiki. The researcher concluded that "this meta-analysis revealed that Reiki was an effective approach in relieving the pain."[5]

Cancer Patients Who Experience a Variety of Concerns, Including Pain, May Benefit from Reiki

In a study published in 2016 in the *Clinical Journal of Oncology Nursing*, researchers from Illinois (USA) investigated the benefits of Reiki, yoga, and massage at a cancer resource center (LivingWell Cancer Resource Center in Geneva, Illinois). The cohort consisted of 150 subjects with cancer who participated in Reiki, yoga, or massage. Relief from pain was one of the benefits measured on a 10-point scale. Ninety-one percent of the subjects were women, and 9 percent were men. Initially, there were 50 subjects in the Reiki group, 50 in the yoga group, and 50 in the massage group. The subjects were told to complete a questionnaire before and after participating in one of the three services. At the time of the data collection, 75 percent of the subjects were either newly diagnosed with cancer or had completed their prescribed medical treatment; 21 percent were undergoing chemotherapy, and 4 percent were having radiation treatment. The subjects in all three groups improved, but the subjects in the Reiki group had the best improvements in pain. The researchers commented that "patients with cancer who experience pain should be encouraged to partake in Reiki."[6]

Reiki May Help People with Low Back Pain from a Herniated Disc

In a study published in 2018 in the *Journal of Evidence-Based Integrative Medicine*, researchers from Iran compared the usefulness of Reiki and physical therapy for people who have low back pain from an orthopedic surgeon diagnosed herniated disc. The initial cohort consisted of 60 subjects with hernia disc low back pain; they had an average age of 45 years. The subjects were randomly assigned to receive Reiki therapy and drug therapy, physical therapy and drug therapy, or drug therapy alone; there were 20 subjects in each group. The drug therapy consisted of a 75 mg nonsteriodal anti-inflammatory drug (indomethacin) and a 500 mg muscle relaxant (methocarbamol) every eight hours for a week. The subjects in the Reiki group received three 15-minute distance energy-healing sessions on consecutive days; the subjects in the physical therapy group had 7 to 10 sessions of physical therapy. The researchers found no significant difference in managing pain between Reiki and physical therapy. However, Reiki combined with medication managed pain better than medication alone. The researchers concluded that "Reiki is more cost-effective and faster treatment" than physical therapy.[7]

Reiki Seems to Help Hospitalized Patients Deal with Symptoms, Such as Pain

In a retrospective study published in 2018 in the *Journal of Alternative and Complementary Medicine*, researchers from New Hampshire

(USA) examined the use of single sessions of Reiki or massage therapy for patients hospitalized in a 396-bed rural academic and tertiary medical center. Patients were classified as having a cancer or noncancer diagnosis. Patients received 20-minute sessions of either Reiki or massage between June 1, 2010, and December 8, 2015. Sessions were tailored to meet the individual needs of each patient. Patients were asked to complete a questionnaire that included questions on pain, nausea, fatigue, and other medical problems. The final analyses included 1,585 patient encounters. Though the patients ranged widely in ages, the average age was 53 years. About 62 percent were male, and 59 percent had a primary diagnosis of cancer. Reiki encounters tended to have older patients than massage encounters and more noncancer diagnoses. The researchers learned that all of the studied symptoms, including pain, improved after Reiki or massage. Thus, the researchers found that Reiki improved pain by 49.2 percent. Oncology patients reported a 41.3 percent improvement, and cardiology patients reported a 41.8 percent improvement. The researchers concluded that "hospitals interested in trying to improve patients' experiences and symptom control nonpharmacologically should consider adding either a Reiki or massage therapy program."[8]

Reiki May or May Not Be Useful for Pain from a Cesarean Section

In a systematic review and meta-analysis published in 2017 in the journal *Sao Paulo Medical Journal*, researchers from Brazil tested the ability of Reiki and prayer to help women who are experiencing pain following a cesarean section (the surgical delivery of babies). The researchers included three randomized, controlled trials and quasi-randomized, controlled trials in English or Portuguese. They had 343 subjects and were conducted in Canada, Turkey, and Iran. Sample sizes ranged from 40 to 80, and the women were in their 20s or 30s. All three of the studies found that Reiki and prayer were significantly better than the standard care for treating the pain of caesarean section. Regular and distant Reiki appeared to work equally well. The researchers cautioned that their findings were based only a very small number of studies, and they underscored the need for more high-quality randomized, controlled trials. "Low-certainty evidence suggested that use of Reiki and prayer meditation might be associated with pain reduction."[9]

Reiki Does Not Appear to Help Children with Postoperative Pain from Dental Procedures

In a double-blind, single-site, randomized, controlled pilot trial published in 2014 in the journal *Complementary Therapies in Clinical Practice*, researchers from Seattle, Washington (USA), wanted to learn if Reiki would help children better cope with the pain associated with dental procedures. The cohort consisted of 38 children, who ranged in age from 9 to 48 months. Forty-two percent were males. Before their dental procedures, they received either 20 to 30 minutes of Reiki therapy or sham Reiki therapy. Sixty-five percent of the procedures corrected or reconstructed the palate in a child with a cleft palate (palatoplasty). All of the children received the standard surgery and postsurgery pain care. Age-appropriate pain scores were collected. The researchers found no statistically significant differences between the groups. They concluded that "young patients undergoing palatoplasty and elective dental procedures found no evidence of benefit from a single session of preoperative Reiki in terms of reducing pain intensity, analgesic requirements, incidence of side effects, and perioperative family satisfaction."[10]

Reiki Does Not Appear to Be Useful for Fibromyalgia

In a factorial designed, randomized, sham-controlled trial published in 2008 in *the Journal of Alternative and Complementary Medicine*, researchers from Seattle, Washington (USA), examined the use of Reiki for people with fibromyalgia. One hundred initial subjects with fibromyalgia were recruited from the Seattle area; they were primarily Caucasian women with college degrees. The subjects were placed in one of four groups. The subjects in the first group received a 30-minute direct contact Reiki treatment; the subjects in the second group received a distant Reiki treatment by a master practitioner who sat about two feet away. The subjects in the third group received a sham direct contact Reiki, and the subjects in the fourth group received a sham two-feet treatment by actors who mimicked what the practitioners did. The subjects received two weekly treatments for eight weeks, or a total of 16 treatments. All of the people who collected, monitored, and analyzed the data were blinded to treatment groups. Seventy-six percent of the subjects completed the full course of treatment. Subjective pain was measured by visual analog scale at weeks 4, 8, and 20 (after the treatment ended). Although almost half of the subjects reported that they were certain that Reiki could relieve the symptoms of fibromyalgia, Reiki did not appear to have any effect on pain. "Baseline demographic characteristics, clinical features, and treatment expectations did not differ across the 4 treatments."[11]

NOTES

1. Baldwin, Ann Linda, Anne Vitale, Elise Brownell, et al. "Effects of Reiki on Pain, Anxiety, and Blood Pressure in Patients Undergoing Knee Replacement: A Pilot Study." *Holistic Nursing Practice* 31, no. 2 (March-April, 2017): 80–89.

2. Notte, Barbara Byrna, Carol Fazzini, and Ruth A. Mooney. "Reiki's Effect on Patients with total Knee Anthroplasty: A Pilot Study." *Nursing* 46, no. 2 (February 2016): 17–23.

3. Dyer, Natalie, Ann L. Baldwin, and William L. Rand. "A Large-Scale Effectiveness Trial of Reiki for Physical and Psychological Health." *Journal of Alternative and Complementary Medicine* 25, no. 12 (December 2019): 1156–1162.

4. Thrane, Susan, and Susan M. Cohen. "Effect of Reiki Therapy on Pain and Anxiety in Adults: An In-Depth Literature Review of Randomized Trials with Effect Size Calculations." *Pain Management Nursing* 15, no. 4 (December 2014): 897–908.

5. Demir Doğan, Melike. "The Effect of Reiki on Pain: A Meta-Analysis." *Complementary Therapies in Clinical Practice* 31 (May 2018): 384–387.

6. Rosenbaum, Mark S., and Jane Van de Velde. "The Effects of Yoga, Massage, and Reiki on Patient Well-Being at a Cancer Resource Center." *Clinical Journal of Oncology Nursing* 20, no. 3 (June 1, 2016): E77–E81.

7. Jahantiqh, Farnaz, Abdolghani Abdollahimohammad, Mohammadreza Firoouzkouhi, and Vahid Ebrahiminejad. "Effects of Reiki Versus Physiotherapy on Relieving Lower Back Pain and Improving Activities Daily Living of Patients with Intervertebral Dis Hernia." *Journal of Evidence-Based Integrative Medicine* 23 (2018): NA.

8. Vergo, Maxwell T., Briane M. Pinkson, Kathleen Broglio, et al. "Immediate Symptoms Relief after a First Session of Massage Therapy or Reiki in Hospitalized Patients: A 5-Year Clinical Experience from a Rural Academic Medical Center." *Journal of Alternative and Complementary Medicine* 24, no. 8 (2018): 801–808.

9. Ferraz, G. A. R., M. R. K. Rodrigues, S. A. M. Lima, et al. "Is Reiki or Payer Effective in Relieving Pain During Hospitalization for Cesarean? A Systematic Review and Meta-Analysis of Randomized Controlled Trials." *Sao Paulo Medical Journal* 135, no. 2 (2017): 123–132.

10. Kundu, Anjana, Yuting Lin, Assaf P. Oron, and Ardith Z. Doorenbos. "Reiki Therapy for Postoperative Oral Pain in Pediatric Patients: Pilot Data from a Double-Blind, Randomized, Clinical Trail." *Complementary Therapies in Clinical Practice* 20, no. 1 (February 2014): 21–25.

11. Assefi, Nassim, Andy Bogart, Jack Goldberg, and Dedra Buchwald. "Reiki for the Treatment of Fibromyalgia: A Randomized Controlled Trial." *The Journal of Alternative and Complementary Medicine* 14, no. 9 (2008): 1115–1122.

REFERENCES AND FURTHER READINGS

Assefi, Nassin, Andy Bogart, Jack Goldberg, and Dedra Buchwald. "Reiki for the Treatment of Fibromyalgia: A randomized Controlled Trial." *The Journal of Alternative and Complementary Medicine* 14, no. 9 (2008): 1115–1122.

Baldwin, Ann Linda, Anne Vitale, Elise Brownell, et al. "Effects of Reiki on Pain, Anxiety, and Blood Pressure in Patients Undergoing Knee Replacement: A Pilot Study." *Holistic Nursing Practice* 31, no. 2 (March-April, 2017): 80–89.

Demir Doğan, Melike. "The Effect of Reiki on Pain: A Meta-Analysis." *Contemporary Therapies in Clinical Practice* 31 (2018): 384–387.

Dyer, Natalie, Ann L. Baldwin, and William L. Rand. "A Large-Scale Effectiveness Trial of Reiki for Physical and Psychological Health." *Journal of Alternative and Complementary Medicine* 25, no. 12 (December 2019): 1156–1162.

Ferraz, G. A. R., M. R. K. Rodrigues, S. A. M. Lima, et al. "Is Reiki or Prayer Effective in Relieving Pain During Hospitalization for Cesarean? A Systematic Review and Meta-Analysis of Randomized Controlled Trials." *Sao Paulo Medical Journal* 135, no. 2 (2017): 123–132.

Jahantiqh, Farnaz, Abdolghani Abdollahimohammad, Mohammadreza Firouzkouhi, and Vahid Ebrahiminejad. "Effects of Reiki versus Physiotherapy on Relieving Lower Back Pain and Improving Activities Daily Living of Patients with Intervertebral Disc Hernia." *Journal of Evidence-Based Integrative Medicine* 23 (2018): NA.

Kundu, Anjana, Yuting Lin, Assaf P. Oron, and Ardith Z. Doorenbos. "Reiki therapy for Postoperative Oral Pain in Pediatric Patients: Pilot Data from a Double-Blind, Randomized Clinical Trial." *Complementary Therapies in Clinical Practice* 20, no. 1 (February 2014): 21–25.

Notte, Barbara Byrne, Carol Fazzini, and Ruth A. Mooney. "Reiki's Affect on Patients with Total Knee Arthroplasty: A Pilot Study." *Nursing* 46, no. 2 (February 2016): 17–23.

Rosenbaum, Mark S., and Jane Van de Velde. "The Effects of Yoga, Massage, and Reiki on Patient Well-Being at a Cancer Resource Center." *Clinical Journal of Oncology Nursing* 20, no. 3 (June 1, 2016): E77–E81.

Thrane, Susan, and Susan M. Cohen. "Effect of Reiki therapy on Pain and Anxiety in Adults: An In-Depth Literature Review of Randomized Trials with Effect Size Calculations." *Pain Management Nursing* 15, no. 4 (December 2014): 897–908.

Vergo, Maxwell T., Briane M. Pinkson, Kathleen Broglio, et al. "Immediate Symptom Relief after a First Session of Massage Therapy or Reiki inn Hospitalized Patients: A 5-Year Clinical Experience from a Rural Academic Medical Center." *Journal of Alternative and Complementary Medicine* 24, no. 8 (218): 801–808.

Relaxation Techniques

INTRODUCTION

Though relaxation techniques are probably best known for helping people cope with stress, they may play a role in dealing with a host of different health concerns, including the management of chronic pain, such as chronic headaches in adults, teens, and children, which may be debilitating. Scientists believe that the human brain can only focus on a certain amount of input. When some of the input is redirected, as takes place during relaxation techniques, pain may drop from the foreground into the background.

Learning the basics of relaxation techniques is actually fairly easy, generally low cost or free, and these techniques may be practiced in almost any setting. Once the basics are learned, they may be employed at the first signs of pain and may help prevent the pain from worsening.

Generally, relaxation techniques involve refocusing attention on something that is calming and increasing awareness of the body. There are several types of relaxation techniques. These include autogenic training, biofeedback, deep breathing, guided imagery, progressive relaxation, and self-hypnosis. Relaxation techniques are never intended to replace medical treatments. However, they may well be an important addition to such care.

A wide variety of practitioners may incorporate relaxation techniques into their practices. These include physicians, psychologists, social workers, nurses, physical therapists, massage therapists, and complementary health providers. Not all types of relaxation techniques work equally well for all people. It is a good idea to experiment with different techniques to find the ones that work best.

ADMINISTRATION AND REGULATION

Like other skills, relaxation techniques must be learned and practiced. People who practice relaxation techniques often are more likely to obtain benefits, especially if they are dealing with an ongoing health problem, such as chronic pain. While in-person relaxation techniques classes are sometimes available at hospitals, wellness centers, health-care clinics, community centers, and other places where people gather, thanks to the many offerings online, these techniques may be easily practiced at home.

As has been noted, there are several types of relaxation techniques. Autogenic means something that comes from within you. With autogenic training, people use both visual imagery and body awareness to move themselves into a deep state of relaxation. People imagine a peaceful place and then focus on different physical sensations, such as warmth and heaviness in the limbs or natural breathing or a calm heartbeat. Using electronic devices, biofeedback measures body functions, such as muscle tension and heart rate, and focuses on learning to control them. During deep breathing, people may close their eyes and take slow, deep, even breaths, inhaling as much air and oxygen-as they can and then slowly exhaling. For guided imagery, people are taught to direct their attention to pleasant images, rather than stressful or unpleasant thoughts. Progressive relaxation or progressive muscle relaxation, which involves 5 seconds of tightening followed by 30 seconds of relaxing various muscle groups starting with the toes or head and progressing to the head or toes. This type of relaxation technique may be combined with guided imagery or breathing exercises. And in self-hypnosis, people are taught to have a relaxation response to a phrase or a nonverbal cue. It may distract people from their pain or alter the perception of pain.

Although there are many online educational programs on relaxation techniques, there do not appear to be any state or federal regulations. The relaxation techniques programs seem to be entirely unregulated. There is no way to know how often relaxation techniques are used.

BENEFITS AND RISKS

Researchers have determined that relaxation techniques reduce the perception of pain, such as the pain associated with surgical procedures and chronic migraines. As a result, people who are dealing with chronic pain who regularly practice relaxation techniques may well experience a reduction in pain.

Relaxation techniques are generally considered safe for most healthy people. Still, there have been reports of negative reactions, such as increases in anxiety, intrusive thoughts, or the fear of losing control. Other potential negative side effects include heart palpitations, muscle twitching, and uncontrolled crying spells. In rare instances, people with epilepsy, a history of abuse or trauma, or certain psychiatric problems, such as schizophrenia, may experience a worsening of their symptoms. People with serious physical or psychiatric problems should probably consult with their health-care provider before beginning a relaxation program.

RESEARCH FINDINGS

Relaxation Techniques Combined with Physical Therapy May Help People with Tension Headaches

In a randomized, controlled trial published in 2018 in the journal *Neurología*, researchers from Spain tested the ability of relaxation techniques alone and in combination with physical therapy to help university students with tension-type headaches, a somewhat common medical problem. The cohort consisted of 152 university students, with 84 women (55.3%) and 68 men (44.7%). They ranged in age from 18 to 25 years and had a mean age of 20.42 years. The students were placed in a group that completed daily relaxation techniques or in a group that completed daily relaxation techniques and had neck physical therapy and posture training. Each group had 59 subjects who were taking medication to control headaches and 17 who were not. All of the students completed the four-week study; no one was lost to follow-up. They kept diaries in which they made end of day notations of their headaches and analgesic use. The students in both groups had a statistically significant reduction in headaches; the reduction was more pronounced in the combination therapy group. Both groups had decreases in the amounts of analgesic medication. The frequency of headaches was reduced by 45 percent in the combination group and by 32 percent in the relaxation techniques group. The duration of pain was reduced by 25 percent in the combination group and by 22 percent in the relaxation techniques group. Also, the amount of pain medication was reduced by 44 percent in the combination group and by 29 percent in the relaxations techniques group. The researchers commented that "it would be interesting to assess to what extent the benefits are maintained over a longer period such as 6 months or one year after therapy."[1]

People with Arthritis and Other Rheumatic Diseases May Benefit from Guided Imagery

In a systematic review published in 2015 in the journal *Pain Management Nursing*, researchers from Morgantown, West Virginia (USA), wanted to learn if guided imagery would be useful for the millions of people who suffer from arthritis and other rheumatoid diseases. They assembled a cohort of seven randomized, controlled trials that included 306 enrolled subjects and 287 subjects who completed the interventions. The trials ranged in size from 28 to 58 participants; the average age of the subjects was 62.9 years. Only two of the studies included men. The guided imagery was delivered via audio technology that differed in nature and content in the various studies. All of the trials used self-report surveys to measure the primary and secondary outcomes. And, all of the trials found statistically significant results for guided imagery; they all supported the use of guided imagery as a therapeutic tool for pain. In addition, guided imagery was found to have other benefits, such as improving psychological well-being and mobility. The researchers noted that "time permitting, nursing or other health personnel could co-develop guided imagery scripts with patients in order to maximize the impact of imagery on patient outcomes."[2]

Women with Multiple Sclerosis May Benefit from Relaxation Techniques

In a single-blind, randomized, clinical trial published in 2016 in the *Journal of Complementary and Integrative Medicine*, researchers from Iran compared the ability of relaxation techniques and foot reflexology to help women with multiple sclerosis deal with pain. (Reflexology is a system of massage that is used to relieve tension and treat illness. It is based on the theory that there are reflex points in the feet, hands, and head that are linked to every part of the body.) The initial cohort consisted of 75 subjects with neurologist diagnosed multiple sclerosis. Twenty-five subjects were placed in each group—relaxation, foot reflexology, and control. The interventions were performed twice each week for four weeks; each intervention continued for 40 minutes. The subjects in the control group received routine care. Data were collected before and after the interventions and two months after the interventions ended. The researchers found significant differences between the pain intensity scores between the intervention groups and the control group immediately after the study. However, after two months, the improvement was no longer evident. And, reflexology offered more pain relief than relaxation techniques. Nevertheless, "these two methods can be recommended as effective techniques."[3]

Imagery Training May Benefit Athletes Who Have First-Time Anterior Cruciate Ligament (ACL) Reconstruction

In an article published in 2019 in the *Journal of Sport Rehabilitation*, researchers from San Diego, California (USA), reviewed four studies that investigated the use of imagery training for athletes with first-time anterior cruciate ligament reconstructions. The researchers explained that the ACL is a major stabilizing ligament of the knee joint. Would imagery help them reduce the fear of reinjury and the perception of pain? The researchers located four randomized, controlled trials that met their criteria. The largest sample size was 30; they were all small studies. The researchers learned that fear of reinjury may play a strong role in preventing athletes from working to return to their previous skill level. Yet, from these trials, the researchers determined that imagery combined with physical therapy may help promote greater activation of the quadriceps muscles and reduce the laxity of the ligaments. This, in turn, may promote greater knee function. The researchers observed that it is important to address the psychological elements during the early stages of recovery. It may well "be effective in reducing pain and increasing the range of motion." Furthermore, "guided imagery has been shown to be associated with reduction of reinjury anxiety, lowered stress levels, increased muscle activation, and decreased pain perception."[4]

Guided Imagery May Help People with Pain from Hip or Knee Joint Replacement Surgery

In a randomized, controlled trial published in 2015 in *The Permanente Journal*, researchers from New Jersey and Nebraska (USA) examined the combination of a specific type of structured touch and guided imagery to help people recovering from joint replacement surgery. (The structured touch, known as the "M" Technique, uses a set sequence and number of strokes and a consistent level of pressure on the hands and feet.) The cohort consisted of 225 male and female patients, between the ages of 38 and 90 years, who had elective hip or knee replacement surgery at a New Jersey community hospital. The patients were assigned to one of three groups, with 75 patients in each group—the M group, guided imagery group, and the usual care group. The study sample was 33.9 percent men and 66.1 percent women; 31.3 percent had hip replacement and 68.7 percent had knee replacement. Patients in the M group received the therapy for 18 to 20 minutes before surgery; patients in the guided imagery group received instructions on the protocol and were provided with headphones and a

MP3 player using two tracts for presurgery guided imagery. Immediately after the surgery ended and during the next two days, the interventions were repeated. All but one of the patients was included in the analyses. From the assessments that they conducted, the researchers learned that M and guided imagery provided pain relief, but M was better than guided imagery. The patients in the M group had higher satisfaction scores than those in the guided imagery group; still, the patients in the guided imagery group were more satisfied than the usual care group. The researchers commented that "a major strength of this study is the success of applying integrative interventions under routine conditions."[5]

Children May Benefit from Relaxation Techniques before Surgery

In a trial published in 2019 in the *European Journal of Pediatrics*, researchers from Italy investigated the use of relaxation-guided imagery before children have surgery. They wanted to learn if it would reduce preoperative anxiety and postoperative pain. The cohort consisted of 60 children between the ages of 6 and 12 years who were having minor surgery under general anesthesia. They were recruited between March 2017 and May 2018 at Meyer Children's Hospital in Florence, Italy. Thirty children were randomly assigned to the experimental group and received 15 minutes of relaxation-guided imagery before their surgery, and 30 were in the control group where they received the usual care. The researchers noted that the psychologist who performed the relaxation techniques had "significant clinical experience in delivering non-pharmacological techniques." From assessments that were conducted of preoperative anxiety and postoperative pain, the researchers learned that the relaxation techniques reduced the anxiety and pain, but the association was not statistically significant. The researchers wondered if the lack of statistical significance was at least partially a result of the small sample size. The researchers underscored the need "to investigate the feasibility of this non-pharmacological intervention in a surgical context, with the aim of developing specific protocols."[6]

Relaxation Techniques May Offer Some Assistance to Women during Labor

In a systematic review published in 2018 in the *Cochrane Database of Systematic Review*, researchers based in Australia investigated the use of relaxation techniques, yoga, music, and mindfulness for women dealing with the pain associated with childbirth (labor). The researchers included 19 studies with 2,519 women. Fifteen of these studies (with 1,731 women) contributed data. All of the studies were randomized, controlled trials or quasi-randomized, controlled trials or cluster trials. Unfortunately, the evidence from these trials ranged from low to very low quality. Hence, the results need to be interpreted with caution. Still, the researchers found that during the latent phase of labor, relaxation techniques reduced the intensity of pain. Four trials reported on the efficacy of relaxation techniques during active labor. There was high heterogeneity between the trials and very low-quality results, suggesting "that there was no strong evidence that the effects were any different between groups for this outcome." In addition, there were very low-quality findings that women receiving relaxation reported greater satisfaction with pain relief during labor. The researchers noted that relaxation techniques may play a role in pain reduction, "although the quality of evidence varies between very low and low."[7]

Relaxation Techniques May Help People with the Pain from Sickle-Cell Disease

In a randomized pilot trial published in 2016 in the *Journal of Advanced Nursing*, researchers from Illinois and Pennsylvania (USA) tested the feasibility of using a guided audio-visual relaxation intervention for reducing pain and stress in adults with sickle-cell disease. The researchers explained that medications alone may be unable to control the ongoing pain associated with sickle-cell disease. The initial cohort consisted of 28 patients; there were 15 in the experimental group and 13 in the control group. For two weeks, subjects in the experimental group were told to use the intervention at least once daily and to track pain and stress before and after use. Subjects in the control group were told to track pain and stress daily. The researchers were able to analyze data from 27 subjects—15 in the experimental group and 12 in the control group. The mean age of the subjects was 31.7 years, and 85 percent were African American. Seventy percent were female. The researchers learned that the subjects used the tablets on 71 percent of the study days, not as often as they had hoped the subjects would. Still, "although the dose of the intervention varied substantially," by the end of the trial, the subjects in the experimental group had significantly lower composite pain scores. The researchers concluded that the relaxation intervention "shows promise for reducing sickle-cell pain and warrants a larger randomized clinical trial to determine its efficacy."[8]

Relaxation Techniques May or May Not Be Useful for People Having Abdominal Surgery

In a systematic review and meta-analysis published in 2019 in the journal *Experimental and Therapeutic Medicine*, researchers from China assessed the usefulness of relaxation techniques for people having painful abdominal surgery. No restrictions were placed on the types of relaxation techniques and the types of abdominal surgery. Twelve studies were included in the qualitative review, and seven had sufficient data to be included in the meta-analysis. The researchers determined that the patients in the relaxation techniques groups had significantly greater pain relief than those who did not participate in relaxation techniques (controls). Only minor variations were observed between the different types of relaxation techniques. Unfortunately, only one of the studies was high quality. The methodology of the remaining studies "was questionable with absence of proper randomization and the blinding of outcome assessment." Further, only one study included more than 100 subjects per group. So, the studies tended to have fewer participants; a few had less than 20 participants in each group. And, there were differences in the pain scales used, and the lengths of the relaxation techniques varied. The researchers commented that despite the studies demonstrating significant pain relief from relation techniques, there is a notable "lack of high-quality scientific evidence substantiating its routine use."[9]

NOTES

1. Álvarez-Melcón, A. C., R. Valero-Alcaide, M. A. Atín-Arratibel, et al. "Effects of Physical Therapy and Relaxation Techniques on the Parameters of Pain in University Students with Tension-Type Headache: A Randomized Controlled Clinical Trial." *Neurología* 33, no. 4 (May 2018): 233–243.

2. Giacobbi, P. R., Jr., M. Stabler, J. Stewart, et al. "Guided Imagery for Arthritis and Other Rheumatoid Diseases: A Systematic Review of Randomized Controlled Trials." *Pain Management Nursing* 16, no. 5 (October 2015): 792–803.

3 Nazari, Fatemeh, Mozhgan Soheili, Sayed Mohsen Hosseini, and Vahid Shaygannejad. "A Comparison of the Effects of reflexology and Relaxation on Pain in Women with Multiple Sclerosis." *Journal of Complementary and Integrative Medicine* 13, no. 1 (2016): 65–71.

4. Rodriguez, Rosa M., Ashley Marroquin, and Nicole Cosby. "Reducing Fear of Reinjury and Pain Perception in Athletes with First-Time Anterior Cruciate Ligament Reconstructions by Implementing Imagery Training." *Journal of Sport Rehabilitation* 28 (2019): 385–389.

5. Forward, John Brent, Nancy Elizabeth Greuter, Santa J. Crisall, and Houston F. Lester. "Effect of Structured Touch and Guided Imagery for Pain and Anxiety in Elective Joint Replacement Patients—A Randomized Controlled Trial: M-TIJRP." *The Permanente Journal* 19, no. 4 (Fall 2015): 18–28.

6. Vagnoli, Laura, Alessandra Bettini, Bena Amore, et al. "Relaxation-Guided Imagery Reduces Perioperative Anxiety and Pain in Children: A Randomized Study." *European Journal of Pediatrics* 178 (2019): 913–921.

7. Smith, Caroline A., Kate M. Levett, Carmel T. Collins, et al. "Relaxation Techniques for Pain Management in Labour." *Cochrane Database of Systematic Reviews* 3, no. 3 (March 2018): CD009514.

8. Ezenwa, Miriam O., Yingwei Yao, Christopher G. Engeland, et al. "A Randomized Controlled Pilot Study Feasibility of Tablet-Based Guided Audio-Visual Relaxation Intervention for Reducing Stress and Pain in Adults with Sickle Cell Disease." *Journal of Advanced Nursing* 72, no. 6 (June 2016): 1452–1463.

9. Ju, Wanxia, Lili Ren, Jun Chen, and Yuman Du. "Efficacy of Relaxation Therapy as an Effective Nursing Intervention for Post-Operative Pain Relief in Patients Undergoing Abdominal Surgery: A Systematic Review and Meta-Analysis." *Experimental and Therapeutic Medicine* 18 (2019): 2909–2916.

REFERENCES AND FURTHER READINGS

Álvarez-Melcón, A. C., R. Valcro-Alcaide, M. A. Atín-Arratibel, et al. "Effects of Physical Therapy and Relaxation Techniques on the Parameters of Pain in University Students with Tension-Type Headache: A Randomised Controlled Clinical Trial." *Neurología* 33, no. 4 (May 2018): 233–243.

Ezenwa, Miriam O., Yingwei Yao, Christopher G. Engeland, et al. "A Randomized Controlled Pilot Study Feasibility of Tablet-Based Guided Audio-Visual Relaxation Intervention for Reducing Stress and Pain in Adults with Sickle Cell Disease." *Journal of Advanced Nursing* 72, no. 6 (June 2016): 1452–1463.

Forward, John Brent, Nancy Elizabeth Greuter, Santa J. Crisall, and Houston F. Lester. "Effect of Structured Touch and Guided Imagery for Pain and Anxiety in Elective Joint Replacement Patients—A Randomized Controlled Trial: M-TIJRP." *The Permanente Journal* 19, no. 4 (Fall 2015): 18–28.

Giacobbi, P. R., Jr., M. Stabler, J. Stewart, et al. "Guided Imagery for Arthritis and Other Rheumatic Diseases: A Systematic Review of Randomized Controlled Trials." *Pain Management Nursing* 16, no. 5 (October 2015): 792–803.

Ju, Wanxia, Lili Ren, Jun Chen, and Yuman Du. "Efficacy of Relaxation Therapy as an Effective Nursing Intervention for Post-Operative Pain Relief in Patients Undergoing Abdominal Surgery: A Systematic Review and Meta-Analysis." *Experimental and Therapeutic Medicine* 18 (2019): 2909–2916.

Nazari, Fatemeh, Mozhgan Soheili, Sayed Mohsen Hosseini, and Vahid Shaygannejad. "A Comparison of the Effects of Reflexology and Relaxation on Pain in Women with Multiple Sclerosis." *Journal of Complementary and Integrative Medicine* 13, no. 1 (March 2016): 65–71.

Rodriguez, Rosa M., Ashley Marroquin, and Nicole Cosby. "Reducing Fear of Reinjury and Pain Perception in Athletes with First-Time Anterior Cruciate Ligament Reconstructions by Implementing Imagery Training." *Journal of Sport Rehabilitation* 28 (2019): 385–389.

Smith, Caroline A., Kate M. Levett, Carmel T. Collins, et al. "Relaxation Techniques for Pain Management in Labour." *Cochrane Database of Systematic Reviews* 3, no. 3 (March 2018): CD009514.

Vagnoli, Laura, Alessandra Bettini, Bena Amore, et al. "Relaxation-Guided Imagery Reduces Perioperative Anxiety and Pain in Children." *European Journal of Pediatrics* 178 (2019): 913–921.

Yoga

INTRODUCTION

Rooted in Indian philosophy, yoga is an ancient physical and spiritual discipline that originated in India more than 5,000 years ago. The word "yoga" comes from the Sanskrit "yuj," which means to yoke, join, or unite. Yoga is believed to promote physical and mental well-being. As practiced in the United States, yoga combines physical, mental, and spiritual elements. It emphasizes postures (asanas), breathing techniques (pranayama), and meditation (dyana). Yoga experts tend to stress that it is best to concentrate initially on the physical aspects of postures and breathing; in time, they say, the mediation component becomes easier.

There are many different types of yoga. In the United States, the most common is Hatha yoga. With its gentle, slow, and smooth movements, it focuses on holding the poses and breathing. Considered an excellent type of yoga for beginners, Hatha yoga includes stretching and working with muscles. Although similar to Hatha yoga, Iyengar yoga directs attention to body alignment and balance. Poses are held longer, and extra materials, such as straps, blankets and blocks, may be used. With Kundalini yoga, there is a rapid movement through the poses and an emphasis on breathing, chanting, and meditation. It may well be too challenging for beginners. Bikram yoga or hot yoga is practiced in a room that is heated to about 105 degrees Fahrenheit. The goal of this type of yoga is to loosen muscles and sweat, which practitioners believe cleanses the body of toxins. And Ashtanga yoga, or power yoga, is an aggressive workout in which participants quickly move from pose to pose. More like a traditional workout, it is physically demanding.

It has been estimated that there are between 250,000 and 650,000 certified yoga teachers in the United States. Many of these people completed the training to improve their yoga skills, not to actually teach. There are about 3,000 yoga schools in the country.

In the United States, yoga is very popular. During the past 12 months, about one in seven adults practiced yoga. About one in 12 children between the ages of 4 and 17 years practiced this discipline.

ADMINISTRATION AND REGULATION

Yoga classes are taught in many locations, such as fitness clubs, churches and other houses of worship, public community and recreation centers, public schools, and yoga studios. Of course, for those who wish to practice at home, many different types of classes, workout routines, and instructional videos for particular poses are available online. There is also the option of in home or office private instruction.

Yoga instructors train at a registered yoga school at the 200-hour or 500-hour level. Two hundred hours of training is the minimum to earn certification. It is generally recommended that people pursue the 500 hours of training, especially if they wish to rise in the field or own their own facility. On average, individual yoga classes cost about $90–$100 for 60 minutes. But that will vary based on location. To reduce costs, people who enjoy yoga classes and attend frequently should enroll in an ongoing program, fitness center, or studio, which may average about $100 to $200 per month. However, there may be less expensive options at local churches and community centers. The yoga industry appears to be largely self-regulated. There are no laws that prevent someone from teaching without certification.

BENEFITS AND RISKS

People who practice yoga tend to extoll its many benefits. These include supporting good health habits, overall physical and emotional health, sleep, and balance. Yoga may also relieve low back pain and neck pain and reduce pain from carpal tunnel syndrome, headaches, arthritis and fibromyalgia. Some contend that yoga is beneficial for menopausal symptoms, anxiety, depression, smoking cessation, weight loss, and to manage chronic conditions, such as cancer, diabetes, high blood pressure, multiple sclerosis, chronic obstructive pulmonary disease, and asthma. People who practice yoga often maintain that they better manage their stress and eat, or try to eat, a healthier diet.

For most people, yoga is considered a safe form of activity, especially under the guidance of a qualified certified instructor. Yet, it is important to note that injuries, such as sprains and strains, may occur. The risk of injury with yoga is far less than that with higher impact activities. Still, people 65 years and older are more likely than younger people to be injured. To reduce the injury risk, yoga beginners should avoid extreme postures, such as headstands and forceful breathing. Hot yoga or yoga purposely practiced in a hot environment increases the risk of overheating and dehydration. Before beginning yoga, women who are pregnant, older people, and people with special health concerns should discuss yoga with their medical providers. In many cases, they will be able to practice yoga, but some modifications may be advised. Also, it is always best to start slowly, with the easiest postures.

RESEARCH FINDINGS

Yoga Appears to Benefit People with Rheumatoid Arthritis

In a study published in 2017 in the *Journal of Alternative and Complementary Medicine*, researchers from Philadelphia, Pennsylvania, and San Francisco, California (USA), wanted to learn more about the effects yoga has on people with rheumatoid arthritis, a chronic inflammatory autoimmune disease that is characterized by pain, stiffness, loss of physical function, fatigue, depression, and reduced quality of life. The cohort consisted of 17 adults; most of the subjects were white females with an average age of 56 years. In general, the subjects have been dealing with rheumatoid arthritis for 21 years, with the range spanning from 5 to 44 years. The telephone interviews used a structured guide and open-ended questions. The interviews were conducted by a single researcher, and they lasted for about 30 minutes. The subjects reported that their yoga sessions, which usually took place three times per week for 56 minutes, included stretching, strengthening, aerobic physical exertion, breathing exercises, meditation, positive verbal statements from the instructor, spirituality, and chanting. The sessions were held in a gym, a yoga studio, or at home. The average number of years practiced was 12.6. According to the subjects, who preferred the physical components of yoga over the spirituality or chanting, there were a number of benefits associated with their yoga practice. These included improvements in pain, flexibility, strength, energy, pain, and sleep disturbances. The subjects reported using yoga as a tool to manage their physical, mental, and emotional symptoms; they experienced improvement from both gentle and vigorous yoga. The researchers concluded that their study "adds strength to the growing body of research suggesting that yoga is an acceptable complementary therapy that may be able to affect physical and psychosocial symptoms in adults with RA [rheumatoid arthritis]."[1]

Yoga May or May Not Be Useful for Neck Pain

In a systematic review and meta-analysis published in 2019 in the journal *Medicine*, researchers based in China wanted to learn if yoga is useful for chronic nonspecific neck pain, a very common medical problem. A total of 10 randomized controlled trials and quasi-randomized controlled trials with 686 subjects met the researchers' criteria. The trials, which were published between 2010 and 2018 and were from researchers in Turkey, India, Korea, Sweden, United States, Germany, and China, included different types of yoga. The researchers learned that yoga seemed to have a positive effect on several neck and neck-related issues, such as neck pain intensity, pain-related functional disability, and cervical range of motion. Still, the researchers commented that the quality of the trials was not high and the sample size "was limited." The average sample size was only 68.8. In addition, "the characteristics, the intervention program, and the outcome measurements instruments of the studies were different." As a result, the researchers concluded that they may only cautiously recommend yoga for chronic neck pain.[2]

Yoga May Have Some Benefits for People with Chronic Low Back Pain

In a 12-week, single-blind, three-group, randomized trial published in 2017 in the journal *Annals of Internal Medicine*, researchers from Boston, Massachusetts, Pittsburgh, Pennsylvania, Seattle, Washington, and Santa Monica, California (USA), compared the use of yoga, physical therapy, and education for moderate to severe chronic low back pain. The 320 predominantly low-income, racially diverse adults with nonspecific chronic low back pain received either 12 weekly yoga classes, 15 physical therapy visits, or an educational book and newsletter. After the 12 weeks ended, the subjects participated in a 40-week maintenance phase in which the yoga participants were randomly assigned to a weekly drop-in yoga class or home practice, and the physical therapy participants were randomly assigned to attend five booster sessions or home practice. The researchers learned that at 12 weeks the yoga and physical therapy subjects were 21 and 22 percentage points less likely, respectively, than the education participants to use pain medication. These were clinically significant improvements. Also, the yoga and physical therapy improvements were maintained at one year, "regardless of whether patients were assigned to ongoing yoga classes, PT [physical therapy] booster sessions, or home practice only. The researchers concluded that a structured yoga program for patients with cLBP [chronic low back pain] may be a reasonable alternative to PT depending on patient preferences, availability, and cost."[3]

In a prospective randomized, comparative trial published in 2019 in the *Journal of Alternative and Complementary Medicine*, researchers from India compared the effectiveness of Hatha yoga to conventional therapeutic exercises (CTE) for reducing back pain intensity and back-related dysfunction in people with chronic nonspecific low back pain. The cohort consisted of 70 subjects, between the ages of 18 and 55 years, who had chronic nonspecific low back pain with a pain rating of 4 or more (on a scale of 0 to 10) for at least 12 weeks. They were placed in groups who participated in six standardized 35-minute weekly Hatha yoga sessions or six 35-minute weekly sessions of CTE. All of the subjects were asked to practice at home for 30 minutes on their nonclass days and during the six weeks before follow-up. Assessments were conducted at baseline, after 6 weeks, and at the 12-week follow-up. Thirty-five subjects completed the entire trial and follow-up. The researchers learned that the subjects in both groups had significant improvements in back pain intensity and back-related dysfunction. There were no statistically significant differences between the groups. So, both interventions were equally effective. "Yoga provided comparable improvement in terms of pain intensity and back-related dysfunction."[4]

In an analysis published in 2017 in the *Cochrane Database of Systematic Reviews*, researchers from several locations but based in Baltimore, Maryland (USA), noted that nonspecific low back pain is a common, "potentially disabling" condition that is generally treated with self-care and nonprescription medication. The researchers wanted to learn if yoga would also be useful. The cohort consisted of 12 randomized, controlled trials with 1080 subjects that compared yoga to any other intervention or no intervention. Seven trials compared yoga to a nonexercise intervention, three trials compared yoga to an exercise intervention, and two trials compared yoga to both exercise and nonexercise interventions. Seven trials were conducted in the United States, three in India, and two in the United Kingdom. Because participants and providers were not blinded, all the trials were at a high risk of performance and detection bias. When yoga was compared to nonexercise controls (nine trials with 810 subjects), the researchers found low-certainty evidence that yoga produced small to moderate improvements in back-related function at three and six months. However, yoga was only "slightly more effective" for pain at three and six months, and the results did not reach clinical importance. The researchers could not determine if there was any difference between yoga and other exercises for back-related function or pain or whether yoga and exercise was more effective than exercise alone. As might be expected, yoga was associated with more adverse events than the nonexercise controls, but it was not associated with serious adverse events. The researchers concluded that "there is a need for additional high-quality research to improve confidence in estimates of effects, to evaluate long-term outcomes, and to provide additional information on comparisons between yoga and other exercise for chronic non-specific low back pain."[5]

Though They Tend to Be Minor, Yoga Injuries Are Somewhat Common

In a cross-sectional national online survey published in 2019 in the journal *BMC Complementary and Alternative Medicine*, researchers from Germany and Australia wanted to learn more about the injuries sustained by German yoga practitioners. (The survey was conducted from January to June 2016.) The cohort consisted of 1702 yoga practitioners; of these, 88.9 percent were female. The practitioners were asked details about their yoga practice and about any acute or chronic injuries they have sustained. The researchers learned that 364 yoga practitioners reported 702 acute adverse effects, occurring after a mean of 7.6 years of yoga practice. On average, 0.60 injuries were reported for every 1,000 hours of yoga practice. Almost all of the reported acute adverse effects occurred with the musculoskeletal system; the most commonly reported yoga practices that were associated with acute adverse effects were hand, shoulder, and headstands. Other positions linked to adverse effects were forward and backward bends and sitting. It is not surprising that the researchers found that injuries were more common in the yoga practices that emphasized postures, especially rigorous postures, over meditation and breathing. Perhaps, the researchers theorized, "emphasizing the importance of non-physical aspects of yoga to align with traditional practice may be one way to reduce the risk of adverse effects." And, the researchers underscored the fact that when yoga is compared to other sports and exercises "the overall injury rate per 100 practice hours appears to be relatively low."[6]

Yoga May Help Shoulder and Arm Pain in Patients with Breast Cancer

In a prospective, randomized, controlled, single-blind trial published in 2018 in the journal *Complementary Therapies in Clinical Practice*, researchers from Turkey investigated the ability of yoga to reduce shoulder arm pain that is sometimes experienced by women receiving treatment for breast cancer. The cohort consisted of 42 patients between the ages of 18 and 65 years who completed a demographic data questionnaire. The 22 patients in Group 1 participated in a 10-week Hatha yoga exercise program; the women attended a program supervised by a certified trainer two days per week, each class lasting for one hour. The 20 patients in Group 2 had no yoga intervention. The rate of adherence to the yoga treatment was very high, about 95 percent. The researchers learned that the subjects in Group 1 had a significant improvement in the pain intensity of their arms and shoulders. That improvement was maintained 2.5 months after the yoga sessions ended. The subjects in the control group did not have this improvement. The researchers concluded that yoga "was an effective and safe exercise for alleviating pain (both shoulder and arm)."[7]

Yoga Seems to Be Useful for Primary Dysmenorrhea

In a randomized, controlled trial published in 2017 in the *Journal of Bodywork & Movement Therapies*, researchers based in Thailand examined the use of yoga for dysmenorrhea, the pain and discomfort that may be associated with the menstrual cycle. The cohort consisted of 34 volunteers between the ages of 18 and 22 years who had dysmenorrhea. For 12 weeks, 17 women practiced yoga poses, and 17 women served as controls. The women in the yoga group practiced their selected poses sequentially for one 30-minute session before breakfast/dinner or at least two hours after breakfast/dinner, twice each week. The yoga group used long sitting, standing, prone, plank, and supine poses. Each subject was given a booklet entitled, "Yoga for Primary Dysmenorrhea." The researchers noted that, although yoga is better learned from yoga teachers, the booklet provided the information needed to complete the poses at home. The yoga participants kept an exercise diary and were offered weekly 10 minute telephone calls to provide support. All of the participants completed the trial. The researchers determined that yoga reduced the severity of the primary dysmenorrhea symptoms. And, they concluded that "yoga may be a suitable complementary treatment for PD [primary dysmenorrhea]."[8]

Practicing Yoga May Help Pregnant Women Have Less Pain During Labor and Delivery

In a randomized, controlled, single-blind trial published in 2017 in *Complementary Therapies in Clinical Practice*, researchers from Iran evaluated the ability of yoga to help pregnant women deal with the pain associated with labor and delivery. The initial cohort consisted of 60 women between the ages of 18 and 35 who were pregnant for the first time; they were placed in a yoga group or a control group. The women in the yoga group were asked to perform one hour of supervised yoga exercise classes three times per week starting at the 26th week of gestation and continuing until the end of their 37th week of gestation. The women in the control group received the usual prenatal care. The researchers learned that analgesic use during the first stage of labor was the same in both groups. However, as the labor progressed, the women in the yoga group had significantly less pain and significantly shorter second and third stages of labor than the women in the control group. The researchers concluded that "yoga during pregnancy may contribute to a reduction [in the] pain of labor and improved adequacy of childbirth."[9]

In a single-blind, parallel, randomized, controlled trial published in 2018 in the *Journal of Alternative and Complementary Medicine*, researchers from India also tested the hypothesis that prenatal yoga alleviates labor pain and improves birth outcomes. The cohort consisted of 200 women who were pregnant with their first child; all of the women had been pregnant for at least 30 weeks. One hundred women were placed in the yoga group and 100 were controls. The women in the yoga group participated in a series of 30-minute practice sessions at the 30th, 32nd, 34th, 36th, 37th, 38th, and 39th weeks of gestation. In addition, each subject received a self-study yoga booklet and was asked to practice at home at least twice weekly. The yoga teacher was a well-trained yoga therapist. The women in the control group did not practice any yoga. Analyses were conducted on 75 women in each group. The researchers commented that the subjects "were meticulously monitored." The researchers found that the yoga subjects had reduced labor pain, a shorter labor, fewer caesarian births, and a better tolerance of pain during active labor. The researchers concluded that "yoga is a noninvasive, easy to learn mind-body medicine and complementary health practice, effective in alleviation of labor pain and possibly improving birth outcome."[10]

Yoga May Help the Symptoms Associated with Knee Osteoarthritis

In a systematic review published in 2016 in the journal *Evidence-Based Complementary and Alternative Medicine*, researchers based in China assessed the effects of yoga on pain, mobility, and quality of life in people with knee osteoarthritis. Their cohort consisted of a total of nine articles, with six studies, that included 372 subjects with knee osteoarthritis. The number of participants in the intervention and control groups ranged from 11 to 125; the mean age of the subjects varied from 51 to 71 years. One study was deemed to be of good quality, seven were of medium quality, and one was of poor quality. The researchers learned that in all of the studies yoga relieved pain, and they noted that yoga appears to be a "safe and tolerable exercise" for people with knee osteoarthritis.[11]

NOTES

1. Greysen, Heather M., S. Ryan Greysen, Kathryn A. Lee, et al. "A Qualitative Study Exploring Yoga Practice in Adults with Rheumatoid Arthritis." *Journal of Alternative and Complementary Medicine* 23, no. 6 (2017): 487–493.

2. Li, Yunxia, Siyuan Li, Jieqiong, and Sue Yuan. "Effects of Yoga on Patients with Chronic Nonspecific Neck Pain: A PRISMA Systematic Review and Meta-Analysis." *Medicine* 98, no. 8 (2019): e14649.

3. Saper, Robert B., Chelsey Lemaster, Anthony Delitto, et al. "Yoga, Physical Therapy, or Education for Chronic Low Back Pain: A Randomized Noninferiority Trial." *Annals of Internal Medicine* 167 (2017): 85–94.

4. Neyaz, O., L. Sumila, S. Nanda, and S. Wadhwa. "Effectiveness of Hatha Yoga versus Conventional Therapeutic Exercises for Chronic

Nonspecific Low-Back Pain." *Journal of Alternative and Complementary Medicine* 25, no. 9 (September 2019): 938–945.

5. Wieland, L. Susan, Nicole Skoetz, Karen Pilkington, et al. "Yoga Treatment for Chronic Non-Specific Low Back Pain." *Cochrane Database for Systematic Reviews* 1 (January 2017): CD010671.

6. Cramer, Holger, Daniela Quinker, Dania Schumann, et al. "Adverse Effects of Yoga: A National Cross-Sectional Survey." *BMC Complementary and Alternative Medicine* 19 (2019): Article 190.

7. Eyigor, S., R. Uslu, S. Apaydin, et al. "Can Yoga Have Any Effect on Shoulder and Arm Pain and Quality of Life in Patients with Breast Cancer? A Randomized, Controlled, Single-Blind Trial." *Complementary Therapies in Clinical Practice* 32 (2018): 40–45.

8. Yonglitthipagon, Ponlapat, Somruthai Muansiangsai, Wilanee Wongkhumngern, et al. "Effect of Yoga on the Menstrual Pain, Physical Fitness, and Quality of Life of Young Women with Primary Dysmenorrhea." *Journal of Bodywork & Movement Therapies* 21, no. 4 (2017): 840–846.

9. Jahdi, Fereshteh, Fatemeh Sheikhan, Hamid Haghani, et al. "Yoga During Pregnancy: The Effects in Labor Pain and Delivery Outcomes (A Randomized Controlled Trial)." *Complementary Therapies in Clinical Practice* 27 (2017): 1–4.

10. Bolanthakodi, Chethana, Chitra Raghunandan, Arvind Saili, et al. "Prenatal Yoga: Effects on Alleviation of Labor Pain and Birth Outcomes." *Journal of Alternative and Complementary Medicine* 24, no. 12 (2018): 1181–1188.

11. Kan, Laidi, Jiaqi Zhang, Yonghong Yang, and Pu Wang. "The Effects of Yoga on Pain, Mobility, and Quality of Life in Patients with Knee Osteoarthritis: A Systematic Review." *Evidence-Based Complementary and Alternative Medicine* 2016 (2016): Article ID 6016532.

REFERENCES AND FURTHER READINGS

Bolanthakodi, Chethana, Chitra Raghunandan, Arvind Saili, et al. "Prenatal Yoga: Effects of Alleviation of Labor Pain and Birth Outcomes." *Journal of Alternative and Complementary Medicine* 24, no. 12 (2018): 1181–1188.

Cramer, Holger, Daniela Quinker, Dania Schumann, et al. "Adverse Effects of Yoga: A National Cross-Sectional Survey." *BMC Complementary and Alternative Medicine* 19 (2019): Article 190.

Eyigor, S., R. Uslu, S. Apaydin, et al. "Can Yoga Have Any Effect on Shoulder and Arm Pain and Quality of Life in Patients with Breast

Cancer? A Randomized, Controlled, Single-Blind Trial." *Complementary Therapies in Clinical Practice* 32 (August 2018): 40–45.

Greysen, Heather M., S. Ryan Greysen, Kathryn A. Lee, et al. "A Qualitative Study Exploring Community Yoga Practice in Adults with Rheumatoid Arthritis." *Journal of Alternative and Complementary Medicine* 23, no. 6 (2017): 487–493.

Jahdi, Fereshteh, Fatemeh Sheikhan, Hamid Haghani, et al. "Yoga during Pregnancy: The Effects on Labor Pain and Delivery Outcomes (A Randomized Controlled Trial)." *Complementary Therapies in Clinical Practice* 27 (2017): 1–4.

Kan, Laidi, Jianqi Zhang, Yonghong Yang, and Pu Wang. "The Effects of Yoga on Pain, Mobility, and Quality of Life in Patients with Knee Osteoarthritis: A Systematic Review." *Evidence-Based Complementary and Alternative Medicine* 2016 (2016): Article ID 6016532.

Neyez, O., L. Sumila, S. Nanda, and S. Wadhwa. "Effectiveness of Hatha Yoga versus Conventional Therapeutic Exercises for Chronic Nonspecific Low-Back Pain." *Journal of Alternative and Complementary Medicine* 25, no. 9 (September 2019): 938–945.

Saper, Robert B., Chelsey Lemaster, Anthony Delitto, et al. "Yoga, Physical Therapy, or Education for Chronic Low Back Pain: Randomized Noninferiority Trial." *Annals of Internal Medicine* 167, no. 2 (2017): 85–94.

Wieland, L. Susan, Nicole Skoetz, Karen Pilkington, et al. "Yoga Treatment for Chronic Non-Specific Low Back Pain." *Cochrane Database of Systematic Reviews* 1 (January 2017): CD010671.

Yonglitthipagon, Ponlapat, Somruthai Muansiangsai, Wilanee Wongkhumngern, et al. "Effect of Yoga on the Menstrual Pain, Physical Fitness, and Quality of Life of Young Women with Primary Dysmenorrhea." *Journal of Bodywork & Movement Therapies* 21, no. 4 (2017): 840–846.

Yunxia, Li, Siyuan Li, Jieqiong Jiang, and Sue Yuan. "Effects of Yoga on Patients with Chronic Nonspecific Neck Pain: A PRISMA Systematic Review and Meta-Analysis." *Medicine* 98, no. 8 (2019): e14649.

Glossary

Acute myocardial infarction
Heart attack, which usually occurs when a blood clot blocks the flow of blood in one of the coronary arteries supplying oxygen to the heart.

Acute renal colic
Acute severe pain that occurs when urinary stones block part of the urinary tract, generally a ureter (kidneys, ureters, bladder, and urethra).

Ai Chi
A water-based total body strengthening and relaxation program

Analgesic
Medication for reducing pain.

Ankylosing spondylitis
A chronic inflammatory disease characterized by low back pain, enthesitis, and asymmetrical peripheral arthritis.

Antipyretic
Medication for reducing fever.

Apgar score
Newborn evaluation test that has five components—color, heart rate, reflexes, muscle tone, and respiration. It is given one minute after birth and five minutes after birth.

Arthroplasty
Reconstruction or replacement of a joint.

Benign essential blepharospasm
The painful abnormal contraction of eye muscles.

Breakthrough pain
Sudden increase in pain in patients who already have chronic pain.

Cannabinoid receptors
Located throughout the body, these are part of the endocannabinoid system, which is involved in a variety of physiological processes including pain-sensation.

Cannabinoids
Any group of closely related compounds which include cannabinol and the active constituents of cannabis.

Cannula
Thin tube inserted into a blood vessel or body cavity in order to administer medicine.

Cervicogenic headache
Pain that develops in the neck but is felt in the head.

Cold pressor task
Placing a hand or forearm in cold water, a stimulus that produces a slowly mounting pain of mild to moderate intensity.

Cord avulsion
The tearing of the umbilical cord from its insertion site on the placenta, making the delivery of the placenta more difficult.

Dysmenorrhea
Pain and discomfort associated with menstrual cycles.

Dyspareunia
Difficult or painful sexual intercourse.

Dyspepsia
Indigestion.

Effleurage massage
A type of massage in which there are circular strokes with the palm of the hand.

Electrical stimulation
Uses topical electrodes on the skin to reduce pain and increase functional capabilities. One type is transcutaneous electrical nerve stimulation or TENS.

Endodontic pain
Is mainly caused by the inflammation of the pulp tissue from dental caries deep in the tooth.

Endometriosis
An illness characterized by the presence of endometrial tissue outside the cavity of the uterus.

Epicondylitis
Also known as tennis elbow, the inflammation of the tissue connecting the forearm muscle to the elbow.

Erythema
Superficial reddening of the skin.

Fibromyalgia
A multi-symptomatic disorder characterized by chronic widespread pain, fatigue, sleep and balance issues, cognitive impairment, depression, and anxiety.

Idiopathic
Any disease or condition that arises spontaneously for which the cause is unknown.

Kinesiophobia
A term used in rehabilitation, it is the fear of pain during movement.

Motor control exercise
Used to manage nonspecific low back pain, this type of exercise focuses on the activation of the deep spine muscles. Patients are taught how to isolate the deep spinal muscles while maintaining normal respiration.

Nulliparous
A woman who has never given birth or has given birth to a child who was unable to survive outside the womb.

Palatoplasty
A surgical procedure to correct or reconstruct the palate in a person with cleft palate.

Patellofemoral pain syndrome
This occurs when the nerves sense pain in the soft tissues and bone around the kneecap.

Photophobia
Extreme sensitivity to light.

Primiparous
Pregnant for the first time.

Reflexology
A system of massage that is used to relieve tension and treat illness that is based on the theory that there are reflex points in the feet, hands, and head linked to every part of the body.

Refractory headaches
Incapacitating headaches that are resistant to medical treatment.

Regional analgesia
Analgesia that numbs part of the body.

Retro walking
Walking backward on the ground or a treadmill.

Rheumatoid arthritis
A chronic inflammatory autoimmune disease of the joints that is characterized by pain, stiffness, reduced quality of life, fatigue, depression, and loss of physical function.

Rotator cuff
Group of muscles that surround the shoulder joint.

Somnolence
Drowsiness.

ST-elevation myocardial infarction
Classic heart attack with changes noted on the electrocardiogram.

TENS (transcutaneous electrical nerve stimulation)
The electrical stimulation of the skin to relieve pain by interfering with the neural transmission of signals from underlying pain receptors.

Trigemial nerve
The largest of 12 cranial nerves, the main function of this nerve is to transmit sensory information to the skin, sinus, and mucus membranes. It also stimulates movement of jaw muscles.

Index

*Note: Page numbers in **bold** indicate main entries.*

About the Authors

Myrna Chandler Goldstein, MA, has been a freelance writer and independent scholar for over 30 years. She is the author of several Greenwood books, including *Dietary Supplements: Fact versus Fiction* and *Vitamins and Minerals: Fact versus Fiction*.

Mark A. Goldstein, MD, is the Chief Emeritus of the Division of Adolescent and Young Adult Medicine at Massachusetts General Hospital and associate professor of pediatrics at Harvard Medical School. Dr. Goldstein is currently editor-in-chief of *Current Pediatrics Reports*, and he is researching and writing a book on technology, COVID-19, and adolescents with Myrna Chandler Goldstein.